RESPIRATORY PHYSIOLOGY

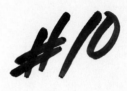

RESPIRATORY PHYSIOLOGY

N. BALFOUR SLONIM, M.D., Ph.D.

Director, Cardiopulmonary Diagnostic Laboratory,
Denver, Colorado

LYLE H. HAMILTON, Ph.D.

Principal Scientist, Wood VA Center; Professor of Physiology and Director,
Clinical Physiology Section, The Medical College of Wisconsin,
Milwaukee, Wisconsin

FOURTH EDITION

With **111** illustrations and **17** tables

The C. V. Mosby Company

ST. LOUIS · TORONTO · LONDON   1981

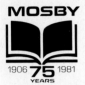

MOSBY

1906 **75** 1981
YEARS

A TRADITION OF PUBLISHING EXCELLENCE

Editor: John E. Lotz
Design: Susan Trail
Production: Debbie Wedemeier

FOURTH EDITION

Copyright © 1981 by The C.V. Mosby Company

Previous editions copyrighted 1967, 1971, 1976

Printed in the United States of America

The C.V. Mosby Company
11830 Westline Industrial Drive, St. Louis, Missouri 63141

Library of Congress Cataloging in Publication Data

Slonim, N. Balfour, 1923-
     Respiratory physiology

     Bibliography: p.
     Includes index.
     1. Respiration. I. Hamilton, Lyle H., 1924-
II. Title. [DNLM: 1. Respiration. WF 102 S634r]
QP121.S6   1981   612′.2   81-11055
ISBN 0-8016-4668-5   AACR2

C/VH/VH 9 8 7 6 5 4   01/B/048

To the breath of life
and every thing that hath breath

PREFACE

The major objective of this text is to present clearly and concisely the physiology of respiration. We have stressed fundamental principles and also indicated the applications of the basic science to the clinical practice of medicine. We have further attempted to identify and to propound the pressing problems of the field and to distinguish established fact from unproved speculation. We hope that the reader will share our fascination with this vital subject. We aim to pique his or her curiosity about the unanswered questions of respiratory physiology.

The traditional rigid boundaries that scientists have drawn between adjacent disciplines in the biomedical field now appear arbitrary, unnatural, and restrictive. Although originally necessary as a scaffold to delineate practical areas of work, these boundaries persist as a tribute to the instinct of territoriality. They cut through the complex structure of the biomedical field, blocking communication, interrupting continuities, obscuring patterns, impeding progress, and hindering recognition of interrelationships. We have expanded and extended this fourth edition in the direction of the new organ system biology. To accomplish this, examples of applied clinical physiology, as well as material from the basic biosciences, are woven into the text where they fit into the development of the central physiologic theme.

The present material is the product of experience gained in both teaching physiology and practicing medicine. This book is designed primarily for medical students, but it should also prove useful to physicians, physiologists, environmental scientists, and bioengineers. Paramedical personnel, such as nurses, anesthetists, respiratory therapists, and physical therapists, will find some sections of particular interest.

Almost all the illustrations have been drawn especially for this book. The illustrative material includes electron micrographs of healthy human lung. In addition to the standard material, the text contains material on the respiratory aspects of hydrogen ion regulation (Chapter 11), the respiratory physiology of the newborn (Chapter 15), respiratory physiology in unusual atmospheres and environments (Chapter 16), and the clinical evaluation of pulmonary function (Chapter 17). The Appendix includes a table of symbols and abbreviations for respiratory physiology and a set of equations for use in respiratory calculations. A glossary of key terms and concepts follows the Appendix.

We are keenly aware that mathematics is the language of science and thus of physiology, lending itself to objective, precisely quantitative, and unambiguous expression. In this regard we have aimed for a realistic balance, to avoid the delusion of mathematical precision on the one hand and the misfortune of unnecessary complication on the other.

We use torr instead of mm Hg and °C instead of °F. To eliminate ambiguity, units that measure different dimensions and imply sequential arithmetic operations including more than one division are given in the form A $\times$ $B^{-1} \times C^{-2} \times D^{-3}$. For example, the units of respiratory resistance are given as cm $H_2O \times$ liter^{-1} $\times$ sec^{-1} instead of cm H_2O/liter/sec or cm H_2O/(L $\times$ sec), and the units of cardiac index are given as liters $\times$ min^{-1} $\times$ M^{-2} instead of liters/min/M^2 or liters/(min $\times$ M^2).

Our main objective is to present the current state of the science of respiratory physiology. It is beyond the scope of this book to offer rigorous evidence for our statements and conclusions or to give details of the evolutionary development of the facts, principles, and concepts of respiratory physiology. However, "Historic Review," a section in the Introduction, discusses some of the major contributors to respiratory physiology and their work.

We are sorry to have had to omit, for the sake of brevity, the names of many contributors to the field of respiratory physiology, as well as the specific references to their published works. However, we believe that the inclusion of such a large and constantly increasing volume of detail would defeat the objective of this book. We have attempted to reach a compromise by listing selected references for further study in a section at the end of the book.

We acknowledge with pleasure the capable and dedicated assistance of Luba Ilczyszyn-Horodyskyj and Sylvia Welytok in the preparation of our manuscript and of Carole R. Hilmer for many of the illustrations in this fourth edition. Our sincere appreciation also goes to numerous reviewers whose frank criticism has been invaluable in the revision, and the improvement, of our text.

N. Balfour Slonim
Lyle H. Hamilton

CONTENTS

LIST OF TABLES

RESPIRATORY PHYSIOLOGY

INTRODUCTION

ON PHYSIOLOGY

We define physiology broadly as the science of processes and functions of living biologic systems. Its roots are in anatomy, biochemistry, and biophysics, and its spreading branches bear the blossoms and fruit of clinical medicine. The physiologist studies sensors, intercommunicating neurohumoral pathways, effectors, feedback control systems, and the differentiating and integrating intermediation of the central nervous system. All physiologic explanations involve the elements of cell function and biologic control mechanisms that, in turn, reduce to sequences of physicochemical events. The application of feedback control theory to physiology is a step toward thinking in terms of dynamic processes.

There are two stages of conceptualization in the evolution of a science—early static description and entity thinking and a later stage of thinking in terms of dynamic process and function. As knowledge accumulates and the unity of science is discovered, the classic artificial boundaries between the departmentalized disciplines basic to physiology blur and then disappear. Having served their original purpose, these carefully defended borders now appear less and less meaningful. On analysis today, physiologic processes resolve inevitably into the more basic biologic sciences of biochemistry, biophysics, and anatomy—the science of structure. In this resolution process pharmacologic tools are often used as molecular dissecting needles with which to unravel physiologic processes. At molecular level the apparent dichotomy disappears as structure and function fuse into a single identity. Synthetically, physiologic processes are the manifestation of highly organized molecular processes; analytically, physiologic processes resolve inevitably into biochemical and biophysical events.

Of basic importance to physiology are the concepts of internal environment, homeostasis, and steady state. Many different feedback control systems operate to assure the fitness of the internal environment, or *milieu interieur,* and the constancy of its regulated quantities throughout a wide range of environmental conditions. When an environmental influence perturbs a biologic system, appropriate counterreactions begin. Homeostasis is a consequence of successful counterreactions, both physiologic and behavioral, to environmental influences; it is thus the tendency to maintain a condition of relative constancy, or stability, of the internal environment of the organism through a series of interacting physiologic processes. It is this mean physiologic state that maintains the organism as a viable entity distinct from its external environment. The essence of physiology is regulation.

Thermodynamically, a living biologic system is an open system in a steady state. Such a system is to a large extent self-regulatory. If a stimulus is applied to it, it reacts to reestablish the steady state or, if the stimulus continues to act, it assumes a different steady state. The whole organism, its organs, its cells, and the

1

reaction systems within the cell are all open systems.

Physiologically, a steady state is a balanced condition of responsive adjustment to any particular environmental condition, influence, or stress. In health every environmental change that displaces a biologic system from its mean steady state evokes appropriate countermeasures. Since the dynamic adjustments operating to reestablish a steady state involve many physiologic processes that proceed at different rates, one must define the relevant physiologic parameters for a given condition, and it is more precise to speak of a *nearly* steady state. On close examination a steady state is seen to contain many transient processes for which time is important in terms of fractions of a second.

An unsteady state is characterized by changing physiologic parameters in the course of transition from one nearly steady state to another. Unsteady states may result from breathing unusual gas mixtures, hyperventilation, hypoventilation, breath-holding, exercise, anesthesia, drugs, increasing apparatus dead space, and changes in posture or cardiac output. These causes may occur singly or in combination.

The present forms of terrestrial life have evolved on this rotating, revolving earth out of millions of generations of ancestry. It is not surprising, then, that all living organisms undergo continuous variations, or fluctuations, as does the geophysical environment with which they continuously interact. We are now in the process of discovering and describing the manifestations of this fundamental biologic phenomenon.

Some fluctuations contain no regularly recurring patterns of change with time and are termed *aperiodic*. In contrast, some relatively regular patterns of change repeat at nearly constant intervals; phenomena that recur with such regularity are termed *periodic*, or rhythmic, and can be analyzed in terms of amplitude, frequency, and phase. Some biorhythmic variations are linked to natural fluctuations of the geophysical environment such as the cycles of light and temperature, the ebb and flow of the ocean tides, and the annual rotation of the seasons. A host of periodic phenomena in animals and plants follow these periodic environmental changes. Many such oscillations have periods of approximately 24 hours and, accordingly, are termed *circadian* rhythms.

Biorhythmicity is also manifest as a variation of susceptibility to a variety of stressors, such as drug overdose, endotoxins, and high-intensity noise. Susceptibility is a function of the circadian system phase at the time the stress is applied. Indeed, experiments can be designed so that circadian system phase makes the difference between survival and death.

Biologic rhythms of large amplitude can be a source of considerable error in estimating mean values and normal ranges. Unfortunately, sampling at a fixed clock hour is not a sufficient precaution to control circadian rhythms as a source of variation in experimental studies.

Circadian rhythms persist even in coma and for several months after elimination of the most obvious time cues. However, during prolonged isolation the circadian system as a whole becomes desynchronized from the 24-hour clock (external circadian desynchronization).

Can a circadian rhythm, as some evidence suggests, desynchronize from other physiologic rhythms of the same organ system? What is the etiologic, diagnostic, and therapeutic significance of abnormalities of amplitude, period, or phase of physiologic rhythms? Certainly, we must consider the significance of physiologic rhythms in both health and disease.

ON TEACHING RESPIRATORY PHYSIOLOGY

The process of respiration is different in lower animals from that in mammals. In microscopic forms, such as protozoa, gas exchange involves only simple diffusion; a respiratory system does not exist. In insects, where the respiratory system is independent of the circulatory system, gases diffuse freely through a tracheal system that terminates in tracheoles in the deeper tissues. Coelenterates, fish, amphibia, and reptiles differ with respect to the coordination of their "ventilatory" and circulatory systems for the function of respiration. Birds have a unique ventilatory system in which a unidirectional flow of gas through the lungs is assisted by air sacs that fill and empty through the action of adjacent skeletal muscles.

The functions of respiration, circulation, electrolyte and water balance, metabolism, and body temperature are so interlocked that alterations of one evoke responsive adjustments in the others to establish a new dynamic steady state. When any such changes occur, respiration adjusts rapidly to metabolic demand, assuring the tissues an adequate supply of O_2 and removing excess CO_2.

Respiratory gas exchange produces arterial blood from mixed venous blood and is the essence of pulmonary function. The regulation of gas exchange to meet the changing *demands of the body* is the essence of respiratory physiology.

In health the mammalian cardiorespiratory system supplies O_2 to the metabolizing tissues of the body and removes excess CO_2 from them, maintaining optimal pressures of these two respiratory gases in the cells. This vital function is accomplished by the coordinated operation of two fluid pump systems—a blood circulatory system and a gas exchange system. The thorax is a variable displacement, variable frequency, air pump that moves air back and forth through the airways by active expansion followed by passive elastic recoil, thus presenting large volumes of inspired gas to large volumes of mixed venous blood. This air pump is devoid of valves and operates by creating a subatmospheric pressure. The right ventricle is a variable displacement, variable frequency, blood pump that drives the cardiac output in one direction through thin-walled capillaries in the alveoli of the lung. This blood pump has

valves and operates by creating a positive pressure. Ventilation is phasic, or intermittent, whereas lung perfusion is essentially continuous if pulsatile. In spite of the rather unlikely combination of flows, gas exchange is both efficient and well controlled. Inspired wetted gas moves into contact with moist warm respiratory surfaces convoluted within the lung. Here blood flow matches gas flow.

Respiration in air-breathing animals involves a set of coordinated, regulated physiologic processes. To appreciate the integrated function of the whole set, we must first understand the function of each component process. We will thus dissect the respiratory system into its component processes for presentation and study. However, as we will show, the functioning whole is somewhat greater than the sum of the functions of its separated parts because new functions are derived from the coordinated interaction of various components. The components that comprise the respiratory system include pulmonary ventilation, pulmonary circulation, ventilation/perfusion distribution, diffusion, transport of gases, and regulation of respiration.

Pulmonary ventilation. Ventilation is the process by which air is moved into the lungs toward the alveoli where gas exchange takes place. The muscles of breathing produce the intrathoracic pressure changes that move air into and out of the lung.

Pulmonary circulation. The pulmonary circulation supplies mixed venous blood to the pulmonary capillaries at the rate required for delivery of CO_2 and uptake of O_2 in the gas exchange region of the lung. Since the rate of pulmonary blood flow is normally determined by, and essentially equal to, cardiac output, it is under circulatory control. Thus, pulmonary circulation is as vital to respiratory physiology as pulmonary ventilation.

Ventilation/perfusion distribution. Respiratory gas exchange requires adequate rates of ventilation and perfusion (pulmonary capillary blood flow) and requires that these two flows be delivered to adjacent areas to minimize the diffusion impediment. If all ventilation went to the right lung and all circulation went to the left lung, respiratory gas exchange would not occur. Although the distribution of neither ventilation nor perfusion is ideal, mechanisms exist to minimize regional variation of ventilation/perfusion ratios. In the consideration of ventilation/perfusion problems, we cannot separate respiratory function from circulatory function.

Diffusion. Gases move by diffusion from regions of high pressure to regions of low pressure through membranes that separate alveolar gas from blood in the pulmonary capillaries. Equalization of gas pressure is achieved more quickly when the capacity for diffusion is large.

Transport of gases. Respiratory processes supply O_2 to the cells and remove the CO_2 produced by metabolism. Efficient transport and delivery of O_2 and CO_2 depend on the remarkably well-adapted properties of hemoglobin, the physical chemistry of blood, and the precise regulation of the systemic arterial circulation that perfuses the body tissues to maintain optimal respiratory gas tensions.

Regulation of ventilation. The central nervous system coordinates and regulates both ventilation and perfusion and, to some degree, their distribution in the lung. This function, together with adjustment of the systemic circulation, controls blood-gas transport and delivery. Ventilation changes efficiently to meet the demands of gas exchange throughout the wide range of conditions to which the body is exposed. Although we study each of the foregoing component processes separately, we must remember that efficient pulmonary gas exchange and circulatory transport and delivery are the result of coordination and regulation of all the foregoing processes.

On teleology. Teleology is a belief that natural phenomena are determined by an overall design or ultimate purpose in nature. As such, it is an aspect of the classic vitalism-versus-mechanism controversy. Because much of physiology appears to "make sense," we are tempted to think in terms of need and purpose. When scientists ask "Why?" they generally mean "How does it happen?" rather than "What is its purpose?" They avoid *teleology*, or *purpose*, as an explanation for natural events. Indeed, not every physiologic occurrence serves a useful purpose. Lack of purpose, however, does not imply lack of cause.

Goose pimples (cutis anserina) may, at one time, have kept furry animals warm, but this erection of skin papillae does nothing for modern man. It is likewise unrewarding to spend time worrying "What are hiccups for?" They are not "for" anything. There are wrong questions as well as wrong answers.

The word "function" is used by some to mean "purpose." If one asks, "what is the function of a yawn?" one is apparently assuming that because people yawn, yawning must serve some useful purpose. Yawning may be useful, but this is not guaranteed by the fact that people yawn.

If we think in terms of need and purpose, then we must conclude that the body makes mistakes. Scar tissue can impair function as well as localize infection; immune mechanisms can kill as well as protect. Books have been written about the "stupidity" as well as the "wisdom" of the body.

The remarkable adaptation of many molecules, processes, and mechanisms to the conditions of life is to be understood in terms of environment, mutations, biologic survival value, and natural selection. The natural selection of effective feedback control systems is the real reason that biologic phenomena appear to be purposeful. This appearance is also the chief argument for teleology. Thus, although teleology is an attractive projection of the mind, in this book we will ask "How?" rather than "Why?"

ON LEARNING RESPIRATORY PHYSIOLOGY

Medical students must learn and physicians must know respiratory physiology for proper diagnosis and effective treatment of broncho-pulmonary disease. With the advent of potent and effective therapeutic modalities—the result of advances in pharmacology and medicine—physicians, now more than ever before, have an obligation to understand the physiology of the body systems with which they deal. In the past, therapeutic impotence often made diagnosis academic so that comprehension of pathologic physiology was less a practical necessity. Today, however, it is necessary to know the meaning of alterations of blood-gas tensions, to understand the causes of change in expired gas composition, and to appreciate the factors affecting gas diffusion in the lung so that we can distinguish problems of ventilation/perfusion distribution from problems of diffusing capacity. Today it is useful to understand that spirometric measurements of flow rates and lung volume measurements can differentiate obstruction of airways from loss of lung elasticity. A knowledge of pathologic physiology is basic to the precise diagnosis of the cyanotic patient and is further essential for selection of proper treatment. Compassion is not enough. A good grasp of the material in this text is essential to physicians facing the questions, problems, and decisions of clinical medicine.

Each time we are introduced to a new field, we must learn a new vocabulary to communicate precisely with others in the field. As we learn mathematics, it is first necessary to become familiar with the symbols for addition, subtraction, multiplication, and division; then with those for exponents and logarithms; and later with those for the operations of differentiation and integration. Physics and chemistry require a new vocabulary and a new set of symbols for valences, atomic weights, and isotopes. It is not surprising therefore that there is a special terminology with definitions, abbreviations, and symbols for respiratory physiology. This terminology is generally consistent with that of chemistry, physics, and mathematics. Students must learn this basic vocabulary to comprehend this book as well as the literature of physiology. Table A-1 in the Appendix presents the system. We will define them again where they first appear in the text.

HISTORIC REVIEW

Respiratory physiology has developed enormously since Hippocrates (460-377 BC) first suggested that the main purpose of breathing is to cool the heart. Galen (130-201 AD) almost understood the circulation but continued to believe, as had Hippocrates, that breathing serves to cool the heart. His most significant teachings in respiratory physiology concerned diaphragmatic contraction and chest wall movement.

For centuries no advance was made in the understanding of respiratory physiology. Then, anatomists of the early Renaissance, such as Leonardo da Vinci (1452-1519), set the stage for further progress. Michael Servetus (1511-1553) found that blood passes from the pulmonary artery through the lungs into the pulmonary veins and that during this passage it becomes crimson. Soon thereafter it was realized that as blood passes through the lungs it takes up something from the air.

Jean Baptiste van Helmont (1577-1644) added acids to potash or limestone, collected the "air" thus produced, and observed that it extinguishes flame. He also knew that this "air" is the same as that produced in the process of fermentation and that present in the Grotto del Cane in Italy, a cave in which dogs died, whereas their erect masters survived. Van Helmont coined the word "gas" and named this "air" the "gas sylvestre." In this sense he discovered carbonic acid gas, or carbon dioxide.

William Harvey (1578-1657) described the relationship of the circulation to the lungs in his classic publication, *De Motu Cordis,* which appeared in 1628. Robert Boyle (1627-1691) observed that small animals die promptly in an evacuated chamber, from which he deduced that air contains a vital ingredient.

Joseph Black (1728-1799), a physician, made an important contribution to the chemistry of respiration through his studies of CO_2. Black discovered that when limestone or chalk is heated, a gas evolves as the substances lose weight and that the same volume of gas effervesces when these substances are treated with strong acid. He named this gas "fixed air" and knew that it would extinguish both flame and life. He also found that when limewater is exposed to air, a white precipitate of chalk slowly forms, suggesting that "fixed air" is a natural component of the atmosphere. Again, using limewater as a test, he proved that "fixed air" is produced when charcoal burns, in the fermentation of beer, and during the process of respiration. In 1754 Black published his M.D. dissertation entitled "Experiments on Magnesia Alba, Quicklime, and Some Other Alkaline Substances." He confirmed the metabolic production of "fixed air" by an experiment in 1764 in Glasgow, where he was a professor of chemistry. In an air duct in the ceiling of a church where 1,500 people congregated for a religious service for 10 hours, he dripped a solution of limewater over rags, producing a considerable quantity of crystalline lime ($CaCO_3$). Although from a chemical point of view Black did not characterize "fixed air" completely, he is generally given credit for the discovery of CO_2.

The next important steps were made by Joseph Priestley (1733-1804), who discovered oxygen, and Antoine Laurent Lavoisier (1743-1794), who overthrew the phlogiston theory and recognized the basic chemical similarity of respiration to combustion in the disappearance of O_2 and the appearance of CO_2. Lavoisier observed that animals succumb when confined in a sealed atmosphere as soon as they have absorbed or converted to "aeriform calcic acid" (CO_2) the greater part of the respirable portion of the air. Lazzaro Spallanzani (1729-1799) placed small animals in sealed tubes and measured the rates of O_2 consumption, CO_2 production, and the change of nitrogen volume. He also found that tissues excised from freshly killed animals and the skin and muscle of a recently deceased human being take up O_2 and give off CO_2, indicating that oxidation occurs in the tissues. In 1809 Allen and Pepys found that the volume of CO_2 produced is approximately equal to that of the O_2 consumed.

In 1837 Heinrich Gustav Magnus (1802-1870) improved the methods for blood-gas analysis. He made the first quantitative analyses of arterial and venous blood for O_2 and CO_2 content. He found that both venous and arterial blood contain carbonic acid, oxygen, and nitrogen and that there is more carbonic acid in venous than in arterial blood.

John Hutchinson (1811-1861) devised the spirometer, measured the vital capacity in both health and disease, and described the other subdivisions of the lung volume. Lothar Meyer (1830-1895) showed that blood oxygenation depends on atmospheric pressure. Paul Bert (1833-1886) first demonstrated that reduced inspired O_2 tension (hypoxia) causes hyperventilation, as well as the signs and symptoms of altitude sickness. His work, *La Pression Barométrique: Recherches de Physiologie Experimentale,* was published in 1878.

In 1867 Alexander Schmidt and Eduard Pflüger discovered that shed blood consumes O_2 and produces CO_2. In the same year Strassburg, Pflüger's student, measured the partial pressure of CO_2 in the tissues. In 1868 Pflüger began to study the role of O_2 and CO_2 in the regulation of pulmonary ventilation in dogs. Using improved methods of blood-gas analysis, he found that the arterial blood O_2 content of dogs breathing nitrogen decreased from a control level of 14 to 18 vol% to a level of 1 to 2 vol%, with resulting marked dyspnea. He also found that breathing a mixture of 30% CO_2 and 70% O_2 increased the arterial blood CO_2 content of dogs from a control level of 25 to 28 vol% to a level of 50 to 60 vol%, while only moderate dyspnea resulted. Although aware of the work of Dohmen, who reported enormous increases of tidal volume and moderate increases of breathing frequency during 10% CO_2 inhalation, Pflüger concluded that either CO_2 excess or O_2 lack stimulates breathing. However, he considered O_2 lack the quicker and stronger stimulus, not realizing that inhalation of 30% CO_2 depresses breathing. He also concluded that the normal carbonic acid content of blood excites the medulla oblongata.

In the early 1870s a disagreement arose between the laboratories of Pflüger and Carl Ludwig (1815-1895), which became known as the secretion-versus-diffusion controversy. Pflüger believed that simple diffusion accounts completely for the transfer of O_2 from alveolar gas to arterial blood, whereas Ludwig believed that the lungs pump O_2 from alveolar gas into the blood so that the oxygen pressure is higher in arterial blood than it is in alveolar gas. In the decades that followed, many respiratory physiologists studied this problem and took sides in the controversy.

In 1885 F. Miescher-Rüsch obtained the first quantitative evidence that the resting pulmonary ventilation rate is regulated primarily by carbon dioxide. Analyzing lung gas obtained by deep exhalation, he found an average value of 5.43% CO_2 (on a dry gas basis) in resting human subjects. During dyspnea produced by breathing gas mixtures containing CO_2, he found to his surprise that the CO_2 concentration of lung gas had risen to only 6.0% to 6.4%. He concluded that an increase of lung gas CO_2 concentration of less than 1% increases breathing. Because decreasing lung gas O_2 concentration by an amount greater than the increase of CO_2 concentration that stimulates breathing had no observable effect, Miescher-Rüsch deduced that CO_2 is the normal chemical stimulus for breathing.

Christian Bohr (1855-1911) constructed the first oxyhemoglobin dissociation curve for purified hemoglobin in 1886. Although the shape of this curve resembled a hyperbola (no values below 30% saturation), he later established its true sigmoid shape. G. V. Hüfner in 1890 was the first to consider the detailed shape of the oxyhemoglobin dissociation curve. In 1894 he measured the carbon monoxide capacity of oxyhemoglobin and, after making certain corrections, decided that 1 gm of hemoglobin combines with 1.34 ml of CO, although his value of 0.34% Fe for oxyhemoglobin implied 1.36 ml/gm. Both values are still used in some laboratories today to calculate the hemoglobin content of human blood from analytically determined O_2 or CO capacities.

In 1904 Bohr with K. A. Hasselbalch and A. Krogh discovered that adding CO_2 to blood drives O_2 out. This important effect, linking the processes of O_2 and CO_2 transport, is called the Bohr shift. Bohr's contributions are also honored in the terms *Bohr equation* (for calculation of respiratory dead space) and *Bohr integration* (a graphic integration procedure used to calculate the mean alveolocapillary diffusion gradient for oxygen). Hasselbalch made other contributions to our understanding of the acid-base chemistry of blood.

John Scott Haldane (1860-1936) also investigated the role of CO_2 in the regulation of pulmonary ventilation. In 1893 Haldane and Lorrain Smith observed that dyspnea occurs when the inspired CO_2 concentration in a closed chamber increases to a level of only 3%, whereas if O_2 concentration was reduced and CO_2 was removed, no effects were observed until O_2 concentration decreased to 14%. Working with John Gillies Priestley (1880-1941), Haldane developed a practical method of sampling alveolar gas that facilitated study of alveolar CO_2 concentration under a variety of experimental conditions. They showed that the resting pulmonary ventilation rate is normally regulated by CO_2, rather than by O_2. Haldane found that the partial pressure of CO_2 in alveolar gas remains relatively constant as barometric pressure varies from 646 to 1,260 torr, despite wide variation of ambient and alveolar O_2 pressure. He also observed that during inhalation of CO_2–enriched air, an alveolar CO_2 concentration increase of only 0.2% doubles alveolar ventilation rate and that breathing 5.5% CO_2 prevents posthyperventilation apnea. In addition to his many other contributions, Haldane developed the science of experimental human physiology. The work of Haldane, Priestley, and Yandell Henderson (1873-1944) demonstrated the importance of blood CO_2 tension, both as a normal stimulus to breathing and as a factor in maintaining respiratory homeostasis.

August Krogh (1874-1949) studied the distribution of capillaries in tissue, calculated coefficients for the diffusion of O_2 and CO_2 through tissue, and derived equations to describe tissue oxygen uptake. He designed a microtonometer for measuring the partial pressure of gases in blood, the tilting spirometer, the electric bicycle ergometer, a gas analyzer accurate to 0.001%, and an osmometer for blood plasma. In 1903 he showed that most of the O_2 used by the frog enters through the lung (short diffusion path), whereas most of the more readily diffusible CO_2 leaves through the moist skin. In 1910, with his wife Marie, he introduced the use of carbon monoxide into respiratory research. Application of the carbon monoxide technic increased knowledge of gas diffusion and uptake in the lungs and led to present clinical laboratory methods for measuring pulmonary diffusing capacity. Regarding the diffusion-versus-secretion controversy, the Kroghs proved experimentally that the process of diffusion alone can account for the transfer of O_2 and CO_2 between lung and blood. In 1910 they wrote, "The absorption of oxygen and the elimination of carbon dioxide in the lungs take place by diffusion and by diffusion alone." However, despite their conclusion, controversy continued as to whether the lungs secrete oxygen under certain conditions.

Joseph Barcroft (1872-1947) contributed to our understanding of the properties of hemoglobin, the oxyhemoglobin dissociation curve, blood-gas transport, the physiologic effects of altitude, the role of the spleen as a blood depot, fetal respiration and circulation in lambs, and initiation of the first breath. In a 6-day experiment performed on himself in 1919 at simulated high altitude (ambient P_{O_2} 84 torr) in a glass chamber, he found that an alveolar-arterial oxygen difference is maintained at all times, even during hypoxia and physical exertion. This experiment, together with his studies in the Andes during the winter of 1921 to 1922 at an elevation of 14,200 feet (4,328 M), demolished the secretion theory and established that pulmonary alveolocapillary oxygen transfer involves only the simple process of diffusion.

Lawrence J. Henderson (1878-1942) calculated the dissociation constants for oxygenated and deoxygenated hemoglobin, finding the former to be the stronger acid. He recognized that deoxygenation of hemoglobin binds the hydrogen ion of carbonic acid without change of blood pH and called this important physiologic mechanism the *isohydric change*.

Advances in the acid-base chemistry of blood clarified the relationship between CO_2 and blood acidity. In 1908 and 1909 Henderson applied the law of mass action to the $CO_2 - HCO_3^-$ system of blood and in 1909 Sorensen introduced the logarithmic pH notation for expressing hydrogen ion concentration. In 1917 Hasselbalch introduced the logarithmic version of the mass law expression known as the Henderson-Hasselbalch buffer equation. This equation interrelates the pH, CO_2 pressure, and total CO_2 content or bicarbonate ion concentration of blood plasma. In 1920 Henderson applied the Gibbs-Donnan equilibrium concept to blood, predicting the changes that occur in electrolytes and hemoglobin ions within the erythrocyte and in the surrounding plasma. In the same year M. H. Jacobs presented conclusive evidence that the uncharged CO_2 molecule can diffuse into the interior of tadpole cells, *Arbacia* eggs, and the petals of certain carnations, rendering them acid, whereas the charged H^+ enters the cell very slowly.

Donald D. Van Slyke contributed much to our understanding of respiration, metabolism, and quantitative clinical chemistry. To this day the Van Slyke manometric method remains a standard for analysis of blood gases in laboratories throughout the world. By 1928 knowledge of the steady-state reactions for carbon dioxide, oxygen, and electrolytes in blood was fairly complete as a result of intensive research by L. J. Henderson's group at Harvard and D. D. Van Slyke's group at the Rockefeller Institute.

During the 1920s and 1930s there was intensive study of the acid-base chemistry of blood, the biochemistry of CO_2, the interaction of CO_2 with oxyhemoglobin dissociation equilibria, the reaction of CO_2 with hemoglobin to form carbaminohemoglobin, blood CO_2 transport, and CO_2 hydration-dehydration reactions. The investigations of these two decades produced fundamental data on the biochemistry of blood, laid the foundations of clinical chemistry, and developed methods that were used in the following decade of clinical research.

Francis John Worsley Roughton (1899-1972) studied the kinetics of the reaction of molecular O_2 with deoxyhemoglobin to form oxyhemoglobin. With H. Hartridge, he developed the continuous flow rapid reaction method in which a solution of deoxyhemoglobin and a solution of O_2 were rapidly mixed and the streaming liquid observed at varying distances along an observation tube, the distance serving as a measure of the time elapsed since mixing. Having

shown that this reaction is rapid compared with the time an erythrocyte spends in a pulmonary capillary, Roughton turned to the problem of gas exchange in heterogeneous systems. He predicted the existence of a catalyst in blood that accelerates the reaction of CO_2 with H_2O to form carbonic acid. With N. U. Meldrum, he discovered the zinc-containing enzyme carbonic anhydrase in erythrocytes, which is essential to the unloading of CO_2 during the brief passage of venous blood through the pulmonary capillaries, and developed the theory of CO_2 transport in blood. He also showed that carbaminohemoglobin is formed by direct reaction of CO_2 with amino groups in the protein. Using recently developed knowledge of the structure of the hemoglobin molecule, he determined the dissociation constants of the active groups in the α and β chains and defined the interaction of CO_2 with 2,3-diphosphoglycerate. To evaluate the four Adair constants that describe the equilibrium of a tetrameric molecule, he developed accurate gasometric methods applicable to the extremes of the oxyhemoglobin dissociation curve, below 2% saturation and above 98% saturation, and found that the equilibrium cannot be fully described by a simple two-state model in which a single conformation change occurs after three ligand molecules have been bound.

Wallace O. Fenn (1893-1971) contributed greatly to our understanding of respiratory physiology by his studies of the mechanics of breathing, the pressure-volume relationships of lungs and chest wall, responses to breathing various gas mixtures, and responses to altitude. With Hermann Rahn he developed an important graphic synthesis, the O_2-CO_2 diagram, for displaying alveolar gas information.

In 1928 Werner Theodor Otto Forssmann performed the first cardiac catheterization, introducing a ureteral catheter into his own right atrium. This courageous experiment, for which he was reprimanded at the time, opened the way for studies of the human cardiopulmonary system that were previously impossible. Although contributions to knowledge of the cardiovascular system were great, cardiac catheterization also increased our understanding of human respiratory physiology. A wealth of information regarding cardiovascular pressures, cardiac output, and the pH and respiratory gas content of blood in health and disease resulted. The technic of cardiac catheterization was applied and extended in human subjects who had a variety of cardiopulmonary conditions for both diagnostic and research purposes by Andre Cournand and Dickinson W. Richards, who with Forssmann shared the Nobel prize for medicine-physiology in 1956.

Linus Pauling's discovery of sickle cell hemoglobin (Hb S), the cause of sickle cell disease, was the first step toward understanding the molecular biology of hemoglobinopathies. Following this important discovery, many other genetically determined abnormal hemoglobins were identified, some of which are associated with abnormalities of blood-gas transport. Pauling also applied the paramagnetic principle to oxygen analysis, an insight that resulted in a rapid dependable instrument for analysis of oxygen in mixture with diamagnetic gases.

Since the turn of the century, the scientific knowledge of respiratory physiology has grown almost exponentially. The rising flood of contributions challenges teacher and student alike to read, study, evaluate, and assimilate a wealth of new methodologies, data, information, theories, concepts, and models. The inexorable evolutionary expansion of physiology brings with it a number of problems. These include the dissemination and presentation of information, the proper role of computer technology, the emphasis due molecular biology as opposed to classic organ system biology, productivity as opposed to creativity, and the optimal balance of resources to be invested in basic as opposed to applied physiology. As we wrestle with these problems, it is encouraging to know that science is the first common enterprise of mankind. What is the future of the science of physiology?

CHAPTER 1

RESPIRATION AND METABOLISM

RESPIRATION AND VENTILATION

Biochemists and physiologists use the term *respiration* differently. When biochemists say respiration, they refer to the intracellular processes of hydrogen transport involving cytochromes and other enzymes. Physiologists use the term to mean those processes by which air is inhaled, O_2 is extracted from it by the blood and delivered to the tissues, and CO_2 is delivered from blood to lungs and then exhaled. This latter definition gives the context in which the term respiration will be used in this book.

The primary function of respiration is thus the exchange of gases, in which the mixed venous blood is arterialized by O_2 uptake and in which the CO_2 resulting from body metabolism is discharged. This exchange takes place at such a rate that the arterial blood O_2 pressure, CO_2 pressure, and pH remain within narrow limits throughout a wide range of physiologic conditions. The three fundamental respiratory processes involved in gas exchange are ventilation, diffusion, and circulation.

Four processes actively change respired gas—O_2 loss, CO_2 gain, saturation with water vapor, and temperature adjustment to $37°$ C. Unless the respiratory exchange ratio (R_E) is 1.0, the nitrogen concentration (on a dry gas basis) is *passively* increased or decreased. The respired gas washes intermittently into and out of the lungs in a discontinuous, but essentially exponential, process.*

---

*This is only one example of the many exponential processes in biology.

The lung presents a special situation with regard to its circulation and tensions of O_2 and CO_2. It is unique in that without circulation its oxygen tension (P_{O_2}) is greater and its carbon dioxide tension (P_{CO_2}) is less than are those of any other organ. Further, it is an organ that depends on wet gas as an air supply, has endogenous stores of substrate for nutrition, and lives for hours to days after excision from an experimental animal; hours are required to observe the effects of pulmonary artery ligation.

BASAL METABOLIC RATE

Metabolism includes all the simultaneously occurring *anabolic* (synthetic) and *catabolic* (degradative) biochemical processes in the animal body. The sum total of these processes is termed the *metabolic rate* and is expressed in terms of energy change per unit time. Metabolic rate thus includes a multitude of intermediary reactions. When there is no synthesis of either body substance (as during growth or repair) or products (such as milk or eggs), metabolic rate equals catabolic rate, because there is no *net* anabolism. If the body performs no outside work and does not change the total energy content of its reservoir of high-energy phosphate bonds, then catabolic rate equals the rate of heat production. The estimation of this rate by measurement of chemical changes in the body is termed *indirect calorimetry*.

Metabolic rate has been carefully studied. *Basal metabolic rate* (BMR) is the standard for comparison and is measured with the subject at rest and fasting, but not asleep. The term *basal* is arbitrary because during sleep, metabolic rate falls. The dimensions of metabolic rate are heat production units per unit time. However, the rate of O_2 consumption is more easily measured. Assuming 4.7 to 4.8* kcal/L of O_2 consumed permits conversion of the steady-state basal O_2 consumption to heat production units per unit time. In clinical practice this conversion is sidestepped by expressing BMR in terms of percent of predicted, or normal, rather than in absolute units.

Oxygen consumption varies with species, size, sex, age, hormonal factors, diet, temperature, activity, and season. The rate of O_2 consumption varies from tissue to tissue within the same organism and correlates appreciably with energy production. The rate of O_2 consumption by tissues or organisms is subject to both neural and hormonal influence and may adapt during exposure to changing environmental conditions. The bulk of O_2 is consumed by the mitochondria.

Metabolic rate is subject to many influences and regulatory mechanisms. Diverse factors such as cold acclimatization, body temperature, hormones, sedation, sleep, anesthesia, and certain chemical substances such as dinitrophenol and salicylates can exert significant effects. The BMR of human residents of very cold regions or cold-acclimatized animals may be 15% to 30% higher than the BMR before acclimatization or the BMR of the same species living in a temperate zone. A low level of oxidative metabolism, or aerobiosis, occurs during hibernation, hypothermia, and other states in which there is no lack of O_2 but rather a reduced requirement for it. The term *hypoxidation* has been proposed for these situations.

---

*The precise value of this conversion factor varies somewhat with the respiratory quotient. In a fasting animal catabolizing mainly fat and protein, heat production per liter of O_2 varies only from 4.7 (fat) to 4.8 (protein) kcal. For carbohydrate, such as starch, it would be 5.0 kcal. For calculation of heat production in a fasting state, use 4.7 kcal/L (STPD) of O_2 consumed, or 105 kcal/mole of O_2.

The rate at which different cells "live" varies enormously; one of the factors responsible for this variation is activity. The metabolic rate of resting muscle is quite low, whereas exercising muscle displays an extremely high rate. Conversely, the "level of living" of brain cells apparently varies little with thinking or mental activity; indeed, if thinking has a metabolic cost, it has yet to be measured. The lowest metabolic rates are found during sleep and anesthesia. Digestion of food involves heat-producing metabolic conversions, termed *specific dynamic action*. Specific dynamic action is large for protein (one may feel warm after a large protein meal), very slight for fats, and insignificant for carbohydrates.

One important physiologic homeostatic mechanism involves the pituitary and thyroid glands. In response to tissue needs the hypothalamic paraventricular nuclei elaborate a neurohumoral factor, thyrotropin-releasing hormone (TRH), that moves via the hypophyseal-portal vascular system to the adenohypophysis. The adenohypophysis then releases thyroid-stimulating hormone (TSH), which is carried by the general circulation to the thyroid gland. Thyrotropic hormone, in turn, acts on the thyroid gland, effecting release of the thyroid hormone, which reaches the body tissues through the general circulation, increasing metabolic rate.

BMR is widely used for clinical assessment of thyroid function. The test is of value when properly done and carefully interpreted. However, many factors besides thyroid function can influence the metabolic rate. Furthermore, the syndrome of hypothyroidism may result from a fault at any step in the thyroid regulatory cycle. It is quite possible to have marked hypometabolism with normal thyroid function. It is also possible for a completely athyrotic patient to register a normal BMR. Similarly, hypermetabolism does not necessarily mean hyperthyroidism.

The average young adult male consumes about 250 ml of O_2/min in a basal state. Women consume somewhat less, because of smaller size and a higher proportion of fat, which metabolizes at a considerably slower rate than lean tissue. Women live at an oxidative pace that is 5% to 10% slower than that of men. Oxygen consumption declines with age in both sexes, partly as a result of replacement of lean tissue with fat.

BMR declines continuously after the first few years of life. The BMR of children depends on size and body composition, but the rate per unit weight is higher than that of adults. Small children might be expected to be displaced along the log-log plot of metabolism per gram versus body mass toward small animals and to share with these a high metabolic rate per gram of tissue.

BODY VOLUME, SURFACE AREA, AND TEMPERATURE

The velocity of chemical reactions generally depends on temperature—the higher the temperature, the faster the reaction. For some reactions the speed is doubled when the temperature is raised 10° C or halved if the temperature is lowered 10° C. The same law appears to hold for biologic systems. If such a temperature change occurred in a whole animal, its Q_{10} (the change in metabolic rate for a 10° C change in temperature) would be 2.0. Actually, many animals show a Q_{10} closer to 3.0, since their metabolic rate drops to one third of normal if the body temperature is lowered 10° C. Hibernating mammals are able to live on a small fraction of the fuel they would normally use if their temperature remained high.

The rate of diffusion of molecules through water is a factor that effectively limits the size of living cells and thus determines the maximum possible distance of a cell from its capillary blood supply; in this sense it determines the structure of tissue. Fick recognized the analogy between the process of diffusion and heat transfer by conduction and first put diffusion on a quantitative basis, adapting the equation of Fourier. Diffusion in an isotropic* medium assumes that the rate of transfer of the diffusing substance through a unit area of a section is proportional to the concentration gradient measured normal to the section. Krogh estimated that a spherical organism of 1-cm radius, which uses 100 ml of O_2/kgm/hr, would need an ambient O_2 pressure of 25 atm, or 19,000 torr, to supply O_2 to its center by diffusion. He also calculated that such an organism cannot have a radius greater than 0.5 mm if it is to live by diffusion alone in water which is almost in equilibrium with air at 1-atm pressure.

Living cells produce heat as a by-product of the slow burning of food known as metabolism. This heat is liberated to the surroundings from the surface of the organism containing these cells. But if all cells produced the same amount of heat, large organisms would get hotter than small organisms because surface area does not increase at the pace of volume as organisms increase in size. For example, a cube that measures 1 cm on a side has a volume of 1 ml and a surface area of 6 cm^2, giving a volume/surface area ratio of 1:6; a cube 2 cm on a side has a volume of 8 ml and a surface area of 24 cm^2, giving a volume/surface area ratio of 1:3; a cube 3 cm on a side has a volume of 27 ml and a surface area of 54 cm^2, giving a ratio of 1:2. In general animals produce metabolic heat in rough proportion to their surface areas and not their volumes. The most widely used method for estimating the body surface area of human beings is the formula of DuBois:

$$BSA = 71.84 \times H^{0.725} \times W^{0.425}$$

where BSA is body surface area in square meters, H is body height in centimeters, and W is body weight in kilograms.

Two of the smallest groups of warm-blooded animals are shrews and hummingbirds. Both

---

*An isotropic medium is one whose diffusion properties are the same in all directions.

groups have low volume/surface area ratios, and both have very high metabolic rates. Animals belonging to the smallest species in each of these groups metabolize at rates so high that they generally cannot store enough fuel to last them overnight at these high rates. Each has a different solution to the problem. The shrew gets up periodically during the night to hunt for food; the hummingbird lowers its body temperature, thereby cutting the rate at which fuel is burned.

Whales and elephants produce far more heat than mice, but a gram of mouse tissue produces far more heat than a gram of elephant tissue. If one plots the logarithm of the heat produced per gram of tissue against the weight of the animal, all warm-blooded animals, including shrews, mice, rats, cats, dogs, man, horses, elephants, and whales, fall approximately on the same straight line. Thus the catabolic rate of homeotherms, from mice to elephants, shows a high positive correlation with body weight, which is seen best in a log-log plot of the two variables. The law that describes this relationship between body size and metabolic rate for interspecies comparison is as follows:

$$BMR = 70 \times W^{3/4}$$

where BMR is basal metabolic rate in kcal/day and W is body weight in kilograms.

OXYGEN CONSUMPTION AND CARBON DIOXIDE PRODUCTION
Oxygen uptake as opposed to consumption

A sprinter may run a 100-meter dash holding his breath. During this brief period he has essentially no O_2 *uptake*, although his O_2 *consumption* from lung and blood stores is high and his metabolic rate is still higher. A distance runner will consume less O_2 at the start than he will a few minutes later. During this transitional *unsteady state*, his O_2 consumption will not accurately reflect his metabolism. He gets a portion of his energy from anaerobic break-

down of glucose to lactic acid, but this *oxygen debt* will be paid off at the end of his run by hyperventilation, during which his O_2 consumption will exceed his metabolic rate. During a *steady state*, however, O_2 uptake is a measure of both O_2 consumption and metabolic rate.

Some O_2 diffuses through the skin into the blood. In a frog this is adequate to supply the metabolic requirement below a certain critical temperature. Not only are the frog's metabolism and, consequently, O_2 consumption decreased at a low temperature, but O_2 is more soluble in cold water than it is in warm, and hence is available in larger quantities. However, in dry-skinned man this *diadermic* breathing is apparently small enough to be neglected.

Carbon dioxide output as opposed to production

Every aerobic metabolizing cell consumes O_2 and produces CO_2. During a steady state, CO_2 output equals CO_2 production. However, the quantity of CO_2 stored in the body is large. Small changes in breathing can increase or decrease the level of CO_2 stores. When this occurs, the measured CO_2 output does not accurately reflect CO_2 production. Carbon dioxide is the most important acidic end product of metabolism. The lungs excrete about 13,000 mEq/day of carbonic acid, whereas the kidney excretes less than 100 mEq/day of sulfates, phosphates, and other fixed acids. Since the CO_2 production of an average man is about 200 ml/min, the lungs eliminate almost 300 L of CO_2 daily.

Respiratory exchange ratio as opposed to respiratory quotient

The metabolic respiratory quotient (R) is the molar ratio of CO_2 production to the corresponding O_2 consumption. During a steady state, this metabolic respiratory quotient can be calculated by dividing the CO_2 output by the O_2 uptake, because $R = R_S = R_E$.* The value of R depends on the kind of fuel being used by the metabolizing cells. If glucose is the only fuel, the following equations show that $R = 1.00$:

$$C_6H_{12}O_6 + 6\ O_2 \longrightarrow 6\ CO_2 + 6\ H_2O$$

$$R = \frac{CO_2\ production}{O_2\ consumption} = \frac{6\ CO_2}{6\ O_2} = 1.00$$

Fat contains relatively little O_2; thus more O_2 must be supplied to burn it. The metabolic respiratory quotient for fat therefore is low—about 0.70; the exact value depends on the particular fat that is burned. Protein has a metabolic respiratory quotient of slightly less than 0.80.

Rarely, if ever, does the entire body burn only one kind of fuel. Rather, a mixture of all three foodstuffs is metabolized, giving rise to metabolic respiratory quotient (R) values of 0.80 to 0.85 at rest. Early in the course of exercise the proportion of carbohydrate burned increases; this is reflected in an increased value for R. After prolonged heavy exercise, high proportions of fat are burned and rather low R values (below 0.80) result.

Unsteady states preclude accurate measurement of R by the usual methods. Oxygen uptake does not reflect O_2 consumption if an O_2 debt is being incurred or paid off. Carbon dioxide output does not reflect CO_2 production if body CO_2 stores are changing. In such unsteady states the ratio of CO_2 output to the O_2 uptake as determined by analysis of mixed expired gas is known as the respiratory exchange ratio (R_E). There are brief periods in which R_E climbs to values well over 1.0, for example, early hyperventilation, or falls to values below 0, for example, sudden breathing of a gas mixture low in O_2 and high in CO_2, so that O_2

moves from blood to lungs and CO_2 moves from lungs to blood. However, if metabolic activity and level of breathing are constant, R_E approaches R_S, although it may be many minutes before it truly reflects R_S.

The metabolic respiratory quotient does not change during unsteady states except in the case of exercise, when it rises. The respiratory exchange ratio, R_E, therefore usually reflects changes in the O_2 and CO_2 stores of the body. The CO_2 stores are large compared with the O_2 stores. The former are largely in the body tissues and change slowly, whereas the latter are nearly all in the blood and change quickly. During an unsteady state, therefore, changes in R_E simply reflect the rates of adjustment of CO_2 and O_2 stores.

EXERCISE AND METABOLISM

The waking hours of a person's day might be construed as being made up of three kinds of metabolism: basal, digestive, and exercise. If a young man whose basal O_2 consumption is 250 ml/min were basal for 24 hours, he would burn about 1,750 kcal/day. Actually, he consumes almost twice that number of kcal, or 3,000 to 3,500 kcal/day. Most of this difference is caused by varied levels of physical activity. Individuals employed in heavy work for many hours a day, particularly those working outside during cold weather, may consume two, three, or four times as much as the average young man on a 3,000-kcal diet.

Certain forms of physical exercise such as running, grade walking, swimming, or cross-country skiing may tax the exerciser to his limit. This limit, unsteady-state exercise in young men, has been measured in excess of 5 L (STPD) of O_2 uptake per minute, or in excess of 20 times basal. During spurts of maximal activity, this multiple must be presumed to be even higher, but since such spurts are highly unsteady states, the associated metabolic rates are difficult to measure.

What is the energy cost of descending stairs

---

*R_S is the steady state respiratory quotient. R_E is the respiratory quotient based on analysis of mixed expired gas. See Appendix, Symbols and abbreviations for respiratory physiology.

or of going downhill? Subjects who walk up a downward-moving escalator at a rate necessary to remain in the same place and who then walk down on an upward-moving escalator at the same rate find that the energy over and above that necessary for quiet standing is one third as great in walking down as it is in walking up the escalator. The same ratio should hold in climbing and descending stairs or mountains. Of the total energy expended in raising and lowering oneself against gravity, about 75% is attributable to climbing and 25% to descending. Another study shows that it is more economical to run up stairs than it is to walk up. The energy cost per unit time is greater in running up stairs, but the overall cost is less.

The physical work of the body may be classified into the various components of total metabolic rate as follows:

Internal, or invisible, work
  Basal metabolic rate
  Body position maintenance, if not recumbent or otherwise supported
  Body function, if in excess of basal
  Internal resistance to motion
External, or visible, work
  Work against gravity
    Effective, resulting in potential energy increase and measured as
      Body weight × vertical ascent
    Ineffective
  Accelerations and decelerations of body parts

Some investigators have argued, on theoretic grounds, that treadmill walking cannot simu-

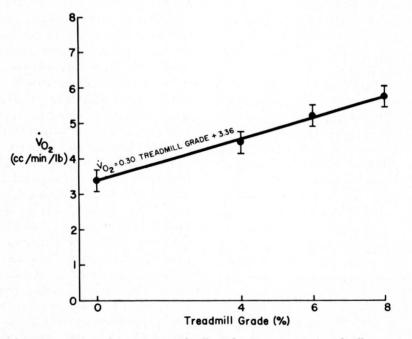

Fig. 1-1. Rate of oxygen uptake versus treadmill grade. Response to treadmill exercise in 10 healthy untrained Denver-acclimatized ($P_B = 623 \pm 5.8$ torr) young men after breakfast ad libitum. Mean ± standard deviation. All measurements made from eighth to tenth minutes of treadmill exercise. Treadmill belt speed was 2 mph (3.2 kph) in all studies. Percent grade as used here is sine of angle of inclination of treadmill multiplied by 100, giving the ratio of vertical ascent to belt travel or distance walked. (From unpublished data of N. B. Slonim.)

late mountain or hill climbing, because the exercising subject does not actually lift his weight against gravity; it is possible, by bending the knees while walking on a treadmill, to keep the eyes on a level with a particular point on an adjacent wall. However, actual experience on a hill and on a treadmill at the same grade with the same subjects shows that these two forms of activity are essentially equivalent. The percent grade of a treadmill is usually expressed as the sine of the angle of inclination multiplied by 100; thus at any given speed for any given time the distance walked is the belt travel (Fig. 1-1 and Table 1).

Minute volume of breathing, O_2 uptake, and heart rate all vary linearly with metabolic rate throughout a wide central range of exercise levels. The mechanism coordinating these physiologic parameters with the metabolic level is still unknown. The pumping ability of the heart normally limits cardiac output, and therefore O_2 uptake, during exhausting exercise. *Peak O_2 uptake* may be defined as the highest value obtained for rate of O_2 uptake as determined by measurement and analysis of mixed expired gas collected during the sixth minute of exhausting exercise.

Because this determination involves strenuous physical exertion, it is usually reserved for healthy, trained subjects. It is essential that a physician assure the health of subjects during

this most strenuous exertion. A common termination or endpoint with highly motivated subjects is abrupt collapse. Provision must be made to avoid injury in such event or in the event of syncope.

Various methods of determining peak O_2 uptake are used, and these differ with regard to exercise apparatus, duration of test, and approach to the limit. The treadmill, vertical ladder treadmill, and bicycle ergometer are all used as exercise apparatus. A common mistake is the failure to use a *low-resistance* breathing system in exercise studies; this point cannot be emphasized too strongly. The breathing system must be of uniform high caliber from the low-resistance respiratory valve all the way to the expired gas receiver.

The performance-limiting symptom of *healthy, trained* subjects is almost always weakness of the lower extremities. In no instance is dyspnea a performance-limiting factor. Syncope has been observed on rare occasion. Premature ventricular systoles are occasionally seen during exercise at heart rates in excess of 180 beats/min. Expiratory minute volume during exercise is customarily expressed at BTPS, but it is questionable whether either saturation or temperature equilibration is complete at high ventilatory rates. Because environmental conditions strongly affect exercise physiology and physical work capacity, it is advisable to record such simple environmental factors as barometric pressure, ambient temperature, and relative humidity. An appreciable correlation has been found between peak O_2 uptake and body surface area (correlation coefficient r = 0.70). In a study of 41 normal men, 25 to 45 years of age, an appreciable negative correlation was found between peak O_2 uptake and age.

METABOLIC LUNG FUNCTIONS

The metabolism of the lung supports a number of general as well as specific functions. The general functions include (1) performance of ex-

Table 1. Characteristics of 10 healthy untrained Denver-acclimatized young men who were subjects of the study shown in Fig. 1-1

	Age (years)	Height (inches)	Weight (pounds)	Body surface area (square meters)
Mean	23.9	70.7 (180 cm)	166 (75.3 kgm)	1.94
S.D.*	3.2	1.6 (4.1 cm)	17 (7.7 kgm)	0.10

*Standard Deviation

ternal work, including mechanical, osmotic, and electrical work, (2) the maintenance of gradients and unstable structures, and (3) the maintenance of lung temperature in its exposed situation. The specific functions include (1) maintenance and repair of structure, (2) smooth muscle contraction, including the normal tonus of bronchial smooth muscle, (3) ciliary activity, (4) phagocytic activity of alveolar macrophages, (5) synthesis of lipids such as pulmonary surfactant, (6) active transport, (7) nerve conduction, (8) synthesis of macromolecules such as proteins, DNA, and RNA, and (9) metabolism of prostaglandins.

Biochemical processes in the lung supply energy for various general and specific functions. In the lungs, as elsewhere, anaerobic glycolysis takes place in the cell cytoplasm, whereas the aerobic phase, which produces 13 times as much energy, occurs in the mitochondria. Ninety percent of the succinate oxidase in the lungs is in the mitochondria.

The lung itself has a relatively high metabolic rate, accounting for about 5% of the total body O_2 consumption at rest. Fetal lung tissue, in its intrauterine state of primary atelectasis, is characterized by high metabolic rate and low blood flow. Energy comes chiefly from two sources: blood glucose, which is quite dependent on the circulation, and fatty acids, which are less dependent on circulation. Thus, the lung is less sensitive to occlusion of its blood supply than, for example, the brain, which is almost completely dependent on glucose. Glucose deprivation has no significant short-term effect on the rate of O_2 consumption in the lung. The lung has a considerably more active hexose-monophosphate shunt than, for example, does the liver. As in other tissues, adenosine triphosphate (ATP) is the major immediate source of energy in lung tissue. A Pasteur effect, the diminution or abolition of glycolysis by oxygen, has been noted in rat lung slices, implying competition for adenosine diphosphate (ADP).

Standard tissue slice as well as homogenate technics are used to study the metabolism of lung tissue. It should be noted that tissue homogenation involves not only the loss of normal structural relationships but also denaturation and inactivation of biochemical substances, such as proteins. It is thus not surprising that calcium ions inhibit certain biochemical reactions in lung homogenates, but not in lung slices. Besides producing the lung lining fluids, including surfactant in the alveoli and mucus in the airways, the lung has metabolic activities of great physiologic importance that are not directly related to its respiratory function.

Since the discovery of surfactant, lung phospholipids have been known to be important for the mechanics of breathing. The lung is well adapted to synthesize phospholipids from a number of different substrates. A major substrate for oxidative metabolism in many body tissues is the lipid fraction of plasma termed *free fatty acids* (FFA). This fraction, consisting of long-chain fatty acids bound to serum albumin, comes from adipose tissue storage depots and is an important potential source of readily available energy. Lipogenesis from acetate is an active lung process. Whereas the liver incorporates a large fraction of FFA into triglyceride molecules, the lung converts them predominantly to phospholipids; of this, 85% to 90% goes into the lecithin component. Lipids absorbed from the gut are transported as chylomicra in the thoracic lymph duct to the venous circulation. In the pulmonary vascular bed lipoprotein lipases within or on the surface of capillary endothelial cells release fatty acids for oxidation by tissues, including the lung.

The lung synthesizes and metabolizes prostaglandins, a ubiquitous family of mediators derived from prostanoic acid, which have a broad spectrum of biologic activity. These products of arachidonic acid metabolism also exert powerful effects on the airway and pulmonary blood vessels. The lungs are a major metabolic site for synthesis, release, and degradation of prostaglandins. Most arachidonic acid products that affect bronchial smooth muscle are bronchoconstrictors, including the primary prostaglandins $F_{2\alpha}$ and D_2 and the thromboxanes. However, prostaglandins of the E series relax airway smooth muscle. Prostaglandins of the E and F series may play an important physiologic role in regulation of airway size and pulmonary blood flow. Prostaglandin A_1 escapes removal by the lung and is produced there as well as in other body sites. The lung does remove prostaglandins E_1 and F_2. These are metabolized rapidly, metabolic products appearing in pulmonary venous blood almost immediately, in contrast to the metabolism of biogenic amines, which are removed rapidly but metabolized slowly.

The lung also synthesizes, degrades, and removes many other substances from the bloodstream. For example, it removes 25% to 50% of the norepinephrine during a single passage, depending on the concentration of this biologic amine. Epinephrine and other closely related amines are removed less effectively from the pulmonary circulation. Another biologic amine, serotonin (5-hydroxytryptamine), is removed during a single passage even more efficiently than norepinephrine. An active transport system moves these mediators from the blood into the endothelial cells that line the pulmonary blood vessels, where they are metabolized. Norepinephrine is rapidly metabolized in the lung; serotonin is converted to 5-hydroxyindoleacetic acid (5-HIAA). There is also evidence that the lung removes bradykinin from the circulation and destroys it. However, histamine is apparently not metabolized in the lung.

Angiotensin is a hormone intimately involved in electrolyte balance and blood pressure regulation through its effect on aldosterone production in the adrenal cortex. Angiotensin I, a decapeptide, is converted to angiotensin II, an active vasopressor octapeptide, by angiotensin-converting enzyme (ACE) on the *surface* of the endothelial cells. The action is prompt and efficient, and the location obviates the problem of transporting a polypeptide across a membrane for activation.

Besides the active metabolic processes that remove substances from blood as it flows through the lungs, the capillary system also acts as a sieve, filtering out emboli and probably certain blood and bone marrow cells, such as megakaryocytes. Experimentally, some glass beads larger than 100 μm in diameter pass through the pulmonary circulation, although most are trapped in capillaries that have a diameter less than 10 μm. This supports the clinical observation that emboli 'of this size may pass through the lungs. These emboli probably pass through arteriovenous shunts whose varying size is regulated by neural or humoral factors not yet understood.

Breathing also plays a role in the regulation of water balance. Significant water loss occurs as air is saturated in the airways during inspiration. Water loss via this route is about 250 ml/day, increasing during fever and hyperpnea.

Many substances besides atmospheric gases pass readily across the pulmonary epithelium; hence, inhalation is an exposure that may result in significant absorption. Intoxication from inhalation of lead fumes is a clinical example of this fact. Inhalation anesthesia, on the other hand, makes clinical use of this phenomenon.

CHAPTER 2

LAWS DESCRIBING THE BEHAVIOR OF GASES

An understanding of the physical laws describing the behavior of gases is basic to the study of respiratory physiology. This knowledge is more important for the understanding of bronchopulmonary physiology than for any other organ system.

Ventilation and perfusion of the lung are governed by laws of physics, as are gas diffusion and gas transport. The fundamental importance and broad applicability of the physics of gases justify its early presentation in this book. Although this material is often relegated to an appendix, we place it here in continuity because we consider it both essential and integral to the subject matter of this field. Respiration concerns gases, and gases obey physical laws. Students of respiration cannot escape these laws. On the contrary, they must develop a working knowledge of them if they are to understand respiratory physiology. The time and effort spent in mastering this chapter are a necessary investment that will yield rich rewards. The following presentation is an elementary review of the kinetic concept of gases.

KINETIC THEORY OF GASES

Four statements comprise the kinetic theory of gases.

1. A gas that fills a container or occupies a space consists of an enormous number of minute discrete particles, or molecules, that have mass. Under the same conditions of pressure and temperature, all true gases (those fitting the kinetic theory of gases) contain the same number of molecules per unit volume. This is Avogadro's law (discussed in detail later in this chapter).

2. Gas molecules are in a state of ceaseless, high-velocity, random motion. Because they move and have mass, they have kinetic energy ($1/2 \, mv^2$). A gas, because of the incessant random motion of its individual molecules, completely fills all the available volume. At a given temperature all gases have the same kinetic energy. This means that there is an inverse relationship between mass and the square of velocity, their product being a constant at a given temperature.

3. As a further result of their motion, gas molecules continually collide with each other and with the walls of a container. They rebound from these collisions without loss of energy (decreased velocity) and may thus be regarded as perfectly elastic. At relatively low pressure the distance between gas molecules is large compared with their own size, and their attraction for each other is negligibly small; they do not attract their own or other molecular species. Thus, gas molecules exert force on each other only when they collide. Van der Waals' equation (see Appendix, Respiratory calculations) provides a correction for the interaction between molecules of real (non-ideal) gases.

4. The pressure (force per unit area) that a gas exerts is the summation of the impacts of its myriad, rapidly moving elastic molecules on

the confining walls of the container. The magnitude of the pressure depends on the average kinetic energy and concentration of the gas molecules (molecules per unit volume). As already indicated, at any given temperature the product mv^2 is the same for all gases; thus, at the same concentration, pressure is identical for all gases.

Although an oversimplification, the kinetic concept of an *ideal* gas, whose perfectly elastic, ceaselessly moving molecules neither occupy space nor attract each other, is useful in respiratory physiology. It predicts the behavior of *real* gases at low pressure, low concentration, or high temperature reasonably well and has facilitated the development of a set of physical laws that describe the behavior of *real* gases under ordinary ambient conditions. However, real gases deviate appreciably from ideal gas behavior as pressure and concentration increase and temperature decreases. Under these conditions the volume occupied by the gas molecules themselves becomes significant and the molecules attract each other appreciably, so that Van der Waals' forces are of more than theoretic importance. This is usually more relevant for calculations involving anesthetic gases than for respiratory gases.

The following laws describe the behavior of gases under ordinary conditions of pressure, temperature, and concentration in biologic as well as physical systems.

DIFFUSION AND GRAHAM'S LAW

Diffusion is the process by which matter moves from one part of a system to another as a result of random molecular motion. Fick derived equations termed his first and second laws that are mathematical statements of this process. At relatively low pressure, gas molecules move independently of each other; however, they collide continually and rebound elastically with no preferred direction—sometimes toward a region of higher, or sometimes lower, concentration. The motion of any single molecule can be described as a *random walk*. Although it is possible to calculate the mean square distance a gas molecule will travel in a given interval of time, it is impossible to predict in what direction it will move. Because there are more molecules in regions of higher concentration, random molecular motion results in a net transfer of molecules from regions of higher to regions of lower concentration. In the process pressure equalizes throughout the container. Diffusion in a mixture of gases is also a consequence of the continuous random movement of individual molecules and tends to rapidly equalize any local concentration differences that may exist. In certain ways diffusion is analogous to heat transfer by conduction—a process that also results from random molecular motion.

At any given temperature small molecules move faster, collide more frequently, and diffuse faster than large molecules. Since average kinetic energy, $\frac{1}{2}mv^2$, is the same for all gases at constant temperature, velocity increases as mass decreases. Graham's law states that the relative rates of diffusion of gases under constant conditions are inversely proportional to the square roots of the molecular weights of those gases.

Respiratory physiology involves both diffusion in gas mixtures and diffusion across membranes. Diffusion of gases across biologic membranes is affected by the solubility of the gas in the water of the membrane. This problem is discussed in Chapter 7 in the section on Pulmonary diffusing capacity.

AVOGADRO'S LAW

Avogadro's law states that equal volumes of different gases at the same pressure and temperature contain the same number of molecules. This is consistent with the product mv^2 being the same for all gases at a given temperature. A molecule of hydrogen, a very light gas, takes up as much space as a molecule of krypton, a heavy gas. This is the theoretic basis for the volumetric determination of the composition of gas mixtures. Avogadro's number, 6.02×10^{23}, is the number of molecules in a mole, or in a mass in grams of substance equal numerically to its molecular weight. No matter how heavy the gas, a gram molecular weight occupies a gram molecular volume, or 22.4 L (STPD), and contains Avogadro's number of molecules. This volume applies strictly to an *ideal* gas. The gram molecular volume of CO_2, a real gas, is 22.26 L (STPD). Loschmidt's number, 2.687×10^{19}, is the number of molecules of an ideal gas at $0°$ C and 760 torr that occupies a volume of 1 cc.

A further consequence of Avogadro's law is Gay-Lussac's law of combining volumes. If gases interact to form a gaseous product, the volumes of the reacting gases and the volumes of the gaseous products relate to each other in simple proportions, which can be expressed by small whole numbers.

BOYLE'S LAW

Boyle's law states that, at constant temperature, the volume of a given quantity (number of moles) of any gas varies inversely as the pressure to which that gas is subjected. For an *ideal* gas changing from pressure P_1 and volume V_1 to pressure P_2 and volume V_2 at constant temperature, $P_1V_1 = P_2V_2$. Since gas molecules create pressure by colliding with the walls of a container, compressing the volume of a gas increases the number of molecules per unit volume, the number of impacts per unit area of container wall, and thus pressure. For a given gas, pressure is a function of the number of impacts and the velocity of the gas molecules; at constant velocity (constant temperature) the change in pressure is proportional to the change in volume. At temperatures near their boiling points, the product of PV deviates from a constant. However, at room temperature or body temperature the physiologic gases (CO_2 and O_2) are so far from their boiling points that such deviation is negligible and can be ignored.

Boyle's law is widely used in respiratory physiology. It is important for understanding the pressure changes in the lungs during the breathing cycle. It is also the basis of the plethysmographic method for measuring the volume of gas that remains in the chest at the end of expiration, as will be explained in Chapter 4 in the section on Measurement of lung volume and its subdivisions.

CHARLES' LAW

Gas expands as it warms and shrinks as it cools. Charles' law, also called Gay-Lussac's law, states that the volume of a given mass of any gas, the pressure remaining constant, is directly proportional to the absolute temperature. Therefore, V = KT, where T represents absolute temperature. Thus the change in volume is proportional to the change in absolute, or Kelvin, temperature. If V_1 and V_2 are volumes of the same mass of gas at corresponding absolute temperatures, T_1 and T_2, then:

$$\frac{V_1}{V_2} = \frac{T_1}{T_2} \qquad (1)$$

On the absolute scale, mean respiratory tract temperature is $273° + 37°$ C = $310°$ K. If one breathes into a $6°$ C ($279°$ K) environment, one's breath volume shrinks one tenth as a result of the temperature drop (without consideration of the volume change caused by condensation of water vapor). Equations involving Charles' law are used to convert gas volumes measured at room temperature to the actual volume occupied by that gas saturated in the lungs at body temperature.

A phenomenon that can complicate gas volume measurement is the relationship of change in temperature to change in volume as pressure changes. When a gas is compressed (volume decreased), the temperature rises. This is called *adiabatic* heating. The effect is large enough to produce errors in the use of instruments, such as the body plethysmograph (Chapter 4).

GENERAL GAS LAW

The general gas law is a composite statement of the laws of Charles, Boyle, and Avogadro for an ideal gas:

$$PV = nRT \qquad (2)$$

where P is pressure, V is volume, n is the mass or number of molecules of gas, R is the gas constant (the numerical value of which depends on the units used to express the variables), and T is the absolute temperature. When pressure is expressed in atmospheres, volume in liters, and temperature in degrees absolute, the value of R is $0.082 \text{ L} \times \text{atmosphere} \times \text{mole}^{-1} \times \text{degree}^{-1}$. In respiratory physiology pressure is usually expressed as 760 torr; volume is 22.4 L (occupied by 1 mole of gas under standard conditions of temperature and pressure); temperature is 273° K (0° C); and the number of molecules is expressed as moles. When the equation is expressed in these units, the value of R is $62.36 \text{ L} \times \text{torr} \times \text{mole}^{-1} \times {}^{\circ}\text{K}^{-1}$.

Another form of the general gas law for an ideal gas permits calculations for changing conditions:

$$\frac{P_1 V_1}{T_1} = \frac{P_2 V_2}{T_2} \qquad (3)$$

where the subscript 1 indicates initial conditions of pressure, volume, and temperature, and the subscript 2 indicates the final conditions. This form of the general gas law is used to calculate volume corrections for gas measured under one set of conditions, for example, ambient temperature, but expressed under different conditions, for example, body temperature. Examples of this use are given toward the end of this chapter.

DALTON'S LAW OF PARTIAL PRESSURES

Barometric pressure is the pressure exerted by the weight of the gas in the atmosphere above the point of measurement. It varies with time as high or low pressure areas move through the atmosphere across the face of the earth; it decreases with altitude (Table A-4).

The average barometric pressure (P_B) at sea level is 760 torr—the weight of the atmosphere above balances a column of mercury 760 mm high in a sealed, evacuated tube.

The pressure of any particular gas, whether it is alone or in mixture with other gases, is termed *partial pressure* or *tension*. The partial pressure of a gas is the intensive factor on which its fugacity and chemical and physiologic actions depend. Respiratory physiologists use the capital letter P followed by the subscript chemical symbol of any gas to denote its partial pressure; thus the partial pressure of nitrogen is written P_{N_2}.

The partial pressure of a gas depends on the number of molecules of that gas in the given volume and on the temperature. It is completely independent of the presence of other gases that may be simultaneously present in the same volume. Dalton's law of partial pressures states that the total pressure exerted by a mixture of gases is equal to the sum of the separate or partial pressures that each gas would exert if it alone occupied the entire volume. This is expressed in the equation:

$$PV = V(P_1 + P_2 + P_3 + \ldots + P_n) \qquad (4)$$

For atmospheric air we can write:

$$P_B = P_{N_2} + P_{O_2} + P_{H_2O} + P_{CO_2} \qquad (5)$$

where P_B is the barometric or ambient pressure and the terms on the right side of the equation represent the partial pressures of nitrogen,* oxygen, water vapor, and carbon diox-

---

*The term *nitrogen* in respiratory physiology is often used to mean nonabsorbable, or "inert," gas. It usually includes small amounts of the rare gases such as argon, neon, and krypton (Table 2). The chemical and physiologic effects of "inert" gases cannot always be ignored. In gas chromatographic analysis, for example, argon is inseparable from oxygen; this may cause appreciable error. There is already considerable evidence that the "inert" gases are not inert in high concentration or chronic exposure. Nitrogen narcosis, xenon anesthesia, xenon combination with heme proteins, and the specific lethality of helium anoxia for various biologic systems are examples of the biologic effects of "inert" gases.

ide, respectively. The same equation describes the total pressure in alveolar gas, but the contributions of P_{H_2O} and P_{CO_2} are increased at the expense of P_{N_2} and P_{O_2}; the total alveolar pressure (P_A) is the same as that of atmospheric air (P_B).

It further follows that the fractional concentration of a gas in a mixture multiplied by the total gas pressure gives the partial pressure of the gas. Partial pressure = fractional concentration × total gas pressure. Thus we can obtain the partial pressure of O_2 in dry atmospheric air from its composition and the barometric pressure:

$$P_{O_2} = F_{O_2} \times P_B = \qquad (6)$$
$$0.2095 \times 760 \text{ torr} = 159 \text{ torr}$$

where F_{O_2} is the fractional concentration of O_2 in dry atmospheric air and P_B is barometric pressure.

The presence of water vapor in a gas complicates the calculation slightly. However, when total pressure is corrected for the contribution of water vapor and the concentration is expressed as the fraction of dry gas contributed by O_2, the same calculation can be used to estimate P_{O_2}:

$$P_{O_2} = F_{O_2} \text{ (dry)} \times (P_B - P_{H_2O}) \qquad (7)$$

An example of such use is the measurement of alveolar oxygen pressure ($P_{A_{O_2}}$). F_{O_2} must be measured in a dried sample of alveolar gas, and the applicable pressure must be atmospheric pressure minus P_{H_2O} at alveolar temperature (47 torr). Thus,

$$P_{A_{O_2}} = 0.16 \times (760 - 47) = 114 \text{ torr} \qquad (8)$$

WATER VAPOR PRESSURE

The words *vapor* and *gas* are often used interchangeably. However, vapor is more frequently used for a substance that, although present in the gas phase, exists as a liquid or solid at room temperature. Gas, on the other hand, is more frequently used for a substance that exists in the gas phase at room temperature. Thus, one speaks of water *vapor* but of nitrogen *gas*.

Vapor pressure is defined as the pressure exerted by the vapor phase of a liquid or solid in equilibrium with its own gas phase at a given temperature (allowing for interchangeability of the terms *gas* and *vapor*). For any given substance it is a function of temperature alone. The warmer a liquid, the greater its vapor pressure.

When a gas comes into contact with water, a process of equilibration begins in which water (and all species of gas or vapor molecules) achieves a predictable, calculable distribution between the gas and liquid phases of the system. Water molecules evaporate into the gas until the rate at which they leave the liquid phase is equal to the rate at which they return from the gas phase. The rate at which the water molecules evaporate is a function of temperature, and the water vapor pressure in the gas phase at equilibrium is also a function of temperature. *The partial pressure of water vapor in a gas phase that is in contact and equilibrium with liquid water is a function of temperature alone and does not depend on the pressure as long as total pressure exceeds water vapor pressure.* Alveolar gas is saturated with water vapor at about 37° C; its water vapor pressure is thus always 47 torr as long as ambient pressure exceeds 47 torr.

Fig. 2-1 shows the exponential relationship between temperature and water vapor pressure and gives a table of values for the range of physiologic interest. This relationship is also termed the *absolute humidity curve*. Absolute humidity is the mass of water vapor present in a unit volume of the atmosphere; it is usually expressed in grams per M^3 or in terms of water vapor pressure. The absolute humidity of alveolar gas at respiratory tract temperature is 47 torr ($P_{H_2O} = 47$ torr).

Relative humidity is the ratio of the quantity of water vapor actually present in the atmo-

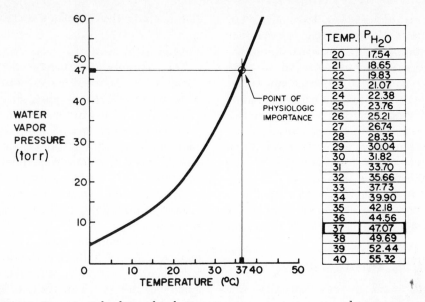

TEMP.	P_{H_2O}
20	17.54
21	18.65
22	19.83
23	21.07
24	22.38
25	23.76
26	25.21
27	26.74
28	28.35
29	30.04
30	31.82
31	33.70
32	35.66
33	37.73
34	39.90
35	42.18
36	44.56
37	47.07
38	49.69
39	52.44
40	55.32

Fig. 2-1. Exponential relationship between water vapor pressure and temperature.

sphere to the quantity that would saturate the atmosphere at the existing temperature. It is also the ratio of the actual water vapor pressure to the water vapor pressure that would be required to saturate the atmosphere at the existing temperature. If at a certain temperature the P_{H_2O} of a gas is 40 torr and the relative humidity is 100%, then relative humidity would be 50% at a P_{H_2O} of 20 torr but only 10% when P_{H_2O} is 4 torr. If the air cools but the water vapor pressure remains the same, relative humidity increases until the air reaches the temperature at which the relative humidity is 100%. This temperature, the *dew point,* is the temperature at which condensation of water vapor in the air occurs.

Air is rarely completely dry, and gas within the body is always very damp. This dampness, or water vapor, occupies a portion of the gas phase and therefore is a portion of the total gas pressure. Water vapor obeys Dalton's law, exerting a pressure that is independent of the pressure of the other gases present. For this reason the ambient pressure must be cor-

rected for water vapor pressure (P_{H_2O}) *before* dry gas pressures are calculated. At sea level on an average day the barometric pressure is 760 torr. The total pressure of all gases in the lung expressed on a dry gas basis is therefore 760 torr − 47 torr = 713 torr. If analysis of a sample of alveolar gas shows 5.60% CO_2 (dry gas basis) and if the corresponding barometric pressure is 760 torr, then alveolar CO_2 pressure is calculated as follows:

$$P_{ACO_2} = F_{ACO_2} \times (P_B - P_{AH_2O}) \qquad (9)$$
$$P_{ACO_2} = 0.056 \times (760 \text{ torr} - 47 \text{ torr}) =$$
$$40 \text{ torr}$$

where F_{ACO_2} is the fractional concentration of carbon dioxide in the alveolar gas, P_B is the barometric pressure, and P_{AH_2O} is the alveolar water vapor pressure. Note that fractional concentration of the gas on a *dry* basis is multiplied by total *dry* gas pressure. Note also that in using the value 47, we assume normal respiratory tract temperature.

When water evaporates to form its vapor,

heat energy is required to accomplish this change of state. This phenomenon, *evaporative cooling*, is of physiologic importance in temperature regulation by insensible water loss and panting. Latent heat of vaporization is the quantity of heat necessary to change a gram of liquid to its vapor without change of temperature and is expressed in calories per gram.

The Joule-Thomson effect is the cooling that occurs when a compressed gas expands in such a way that no external work is done. This cooling is inversely proportional to the square of the absolute temperature. It is the corollary of adiabatic heating, discussed earlier in this chapter.

DISSOLVED GAS AND HENRY'S LAW

Henry's law states that the quantity of a slightly soluble gas that dissolves in a liquid at a given temperature is almost directly proportional to the partial pressure of that gas in the gas phase. This statement holds only for gases that do not react chemically with the solvent. After chemical combination with a solvent or reaction with another solute, the chemically combined gas no longer contributes to partial pressure of the dissolved gas in physical solution. Henry's law therefore does not apply to the total uptake of such gases as CO_2 or NH_3, but only to that portion remaining in physical solution.

At equilibrium the rate at which gas molecules leave the liquid is equal to the rate at which they enter the liquid. Gas in the liquid phase also has a partial pressure that is defined as equal to the partial pressure of the gas in the gas phase at equilibrium. Under equilibrium conditions the partial pressures of gas in the gas phase and gas in the liquid phase are equal. Any change in the partial pressure of the gas, whether in the liquid or in the gas phase, produces a corresponding change in the other phase until equilibrium is reestablished.

The solubility of a gas is the ratio of concentration of gas in the solution to its concentration in the gas phase above it. The *concentration* of dissolved gas must be carefully distinguished from its *partial pressure*.

The solubility of a gas depends also on temperature. As temperature increases, solubility decreases. It is readily observed that bubbles of air come out of solution and form on the container wall before heated water is brought to a boil. Likewise, if a glass of cold water is removed from a refrigerator, bubbles form on the sides of the glass as it warms to room temperature. Air is more soluble in cold water (in the refrigerator) than it is in warmer water (at room temperature).

The total volume of a gas that dissolves in a given volume of liquid depends not only on the partial pressure of the gas but also on the solubility of the gas in the liquid. This relationship is expressed mathematically in Henry's law:

$$\frac{\text{Volume of dissolved gas}}{\text{Volume of liquid}} = P \times C_s \qquad (10)$$

where P is the partial pressure of the gas and C_s is the coefficient of solubility. The numerical value of the coefficient depends on the units in which it is expressed. The Bunsen solubility coefficient, commonly used in the physical sciences, is expressed in liters (STPD) of dissolved gas per liter of liquid at 1 atm of gas pressure. In biologic sciences the solubility of a gas in body fluids is usually expressed in volume percent*/mm Hg gas pressure (vol%/torr). The differing solubility of gases in a liquid is illustrated by comparing the solubility of O_2 dissolved in blood plasma (0.003 vol%/torr) with that of CO_2 (0.063 vol%/torr), a 21-fold difference.

To determine the partial pressure of a gas in a liquid, it is necessary to measure the concen-

---

*It is conventional to express the amount of gas in blood in volume percent. Volume percent, abbreviated *vol%*, is the volume in milliliters (STPD) of a gas dissolved in 100 ml of blood.

tration or pressure of the gas in an equilibrated gas phase. This is commonly done by allowing a small bubble of gas to remain in contact with a relatively large volume of the liquid (for example, blood) at constant temperature until equilibrium with respect to gas tensions has been achieved. Partial pressure of the gas in the equilibrated gas bubble can then be determined.

The partial pressure of a gas is a measure of its tendency to escape from a system and is usually expressed in torr. Gas pressure is one of the factors that determines the availability, or effective "local concentration," of gas molecules for physicochemical reaction. The biomedical effects of any gas are thus a direct function of its *partial pressure*, not its *concentration*. Within a given system, pressure and concentration are related parameters and must *both* be considered in analyzing the dynamics of biomedical gas effects. Gas concentrations alone without simultaneous data for ambient pressure, or total gas pressure, are generally insufficient for biomedical purposes; a biomedically useful description of a gas must include either the partial pressure of that gas or the information necessary to calculate it. Henry's law is essential for understanding blood-gas transport, movement of gases in body fluids, and physiologic responses to varying inspired gas concentrations.

LAWS RELATING TO GAS FLOW
Biophysical components of resistance to breathing

Resistance means opposition to motion. Because motion involves friction, resistance occurs in any part of the respiratory system that moves or in which air movement occurs. Resistance to breathing involves the dynamic forces required to initiate and maintain gas flow through the airways during the breathing cycle. Total respiratory resistance consists of airway resistance plus pulmonary tissue resistance plus chest wall resistance, but this section is limited to a discussion of the physics related to the resistance to gas flow in the respiratory system. Gas flow during breathing is opposed by inertial forces, viscous resistance, and airway resistance.

Inertial forces. A force must be applied to a gas to start it in motion or, once the gas is in motion, to change its velocity or direction. The force required to overcome this inertia is related to the mass of the gas and to the acceleration imparted. Physiologically, inertia is a negligible fraction of the resistance to breathing.

Viscous resistance. The viscous component of resistance to breathing is caused by tissue friction during inspiration and expiration. In healthy subjects viscous resistance is approximately 20% of the total resistance to breathing. The larger resistance component is related to friction between gas molecules, which resists air movement in the airway passages.

Airway resistance. The airway component includes friction between the gas molecules and the walls of the airways plus the internal friction between the gas molecules themselves (viscosity). In subjects at rest it constitutes the remaining 80% of total respiratory resistance.

Viscosity (internal friction) is the resistance within a fluid to flow (change of shape) and is expressed in *poises*, or dyne $\times$ second $\times$ cm^{-2}. Kinematic viscosity is the ratio of viscosity to density and is expressed in CGS units called *stokes*. When flow is laminar, we may visualize viscosity as the result of friction between adjacent concentric layers of flowing gas. As gas molecules from the slower moving outer layers diffuse laterally into the faster moving inner layers, the inertia of the slower molecules retards the latter. This random lateral exchange of molecules accounts for the phenomenon of gas viscosity. It also explains why it takes a driving pressure to maintain gas flow and why gas viscosity, contrary to that of liquids, increases with temperature, since more lateral movement occurs at higher temperature.

Laminar and turbulent gas flow patterns

As gas flows slowly and steadily through a straight, smooth, rigid, large-caliber, cylindric tube, a laminar (streamlined) flow pattern develops. Friction between the gas molecules and the wall of the tube retards the outer layer of gas, while this layer in turn retards the gas layer next inside. Thus we may think of concentric layers of gas flowing parallel to the wall of the tube at linear flow rates that increase toward the center. Such a laminar flow pattern has a parabolic velocity profile.

Turbulent gas flow

When the molecules of gas flowing through a tube reach a critical *linear* velocity, the character of flow changes. Concentric layers no longer slide smoothly over adjacent layers, and the orderly laminar flow pattern degenerates into eddy currents and turbulence. Gas now tends to advance along the tube at the same velocity at the center as it does at the periphery. This transition from a laminar flow pattern to chaotic turbulent flow is a function of density, linear flow velocity, viscosity, and tube radius.

Density multiplied by velocity expresses momentum, whereas diameter divided by viscosity relates to viscous forces. The flow regime of a flowing fluid thus depends essentially on a ratio of inertial effects to viscous forces. This ratio is described by Reynolds' number, N_R. When inertial effects increase to a critical level, resulting in an increased N_R, instability results and the flow pattern degenerates into chaotic turbulence.

Effect of gas density on flow

The density of a gas changes in proportion to the absolute pressure. Increasing gas density favors turbulence, requiring increased driving pressure to maintain the same gas flow. The density of respired gas decreases with altitude and may also change greatly when artificial breathing mixtures are administered or in artificial chamber atmospheres.

With decreased gas density there is less turbulence associated with any given rate of gas flow and, in addition, less driving pressure is required for any turbulent flow that may be present. This effect of density is of considerable practical importance in the performance of tests of ventilatory capacity at altitude. For example, at the modest elevation of 1 mile (mean $P_B = 625$ torr) the predicted values for tests of ventilatory capacity are estimated to be from 8% to 15% greater than at sea level.

Mixtures of 80% helium–20% oxygen have been used to reduce the work of breathing in patients with diffuse obstructive bronchopulmonary disease. It is interesting that this mixture decreases work by decreasing density, but increases work by reason of slightly increased viscosity. However, the *net* effect is decreased work during quiet breathing, but especially at higher ventilatory rates.

MECHANICAL ENERGY BALANCE*

The relationship between driving pressure and airflow for a given gas can be characterized by the use of an equation called the *mechanical energy balance:*

$$P_i - P_o = \Delta P = \rho \frac{\dot{V}^2}{2} \left[\frac{1}{A_o^2} - \frac{1}{A_i^2} \right] + \Sigma\lambda \quad (11)$$

where P_i is inflow pressure, P_o is outflow pressure, ΔP is driving pressure, ρ is gas density, $\dot{V}$ is airflow rate, A_o is exit cross-sectional area, A_i is entrance cross-sectional area, and $\Sigma\lambda$ is sum of the serial mechanical energy losses caused by frictional or viscous effects.

This energy balance describes the effect of airways and gas composition on the airflow that results from a given driving pressure. Changes of gas composition alter gas density and viscosity effects, and changes of airway dimensions or shape alter frictional effects on gas flow.

The first term on the right side of the equa-

---

*This discussion of airflow resistance is more complete than some students need. However, it may be useful to students who have an interest in physics and engineering.

tion expresses the effect of differences between entrance and exit cross-sectional areas on the kinetic energy of the system. It can be ignored in this application because the airflow rate during breathing is not great enough to produce a large kinetic energy effect. This leaves the more simple equation:

$$\Delta P = \Sigma \lambda \qquad (12)$$

The equation is deceptive in its apparent simplicity, since the remaining term on the right side represents a complicated function of the physical properties of the gas, the geometry of the airway passages, and the gas flow rate. The first consideration in defining $\Sigma \lambda$ is whether the flow is partly turbulent or totally laminar.

Reynolds' number, N_R, provides a criterion for determining whether flow is laminar or turbulent:

$$N_R = \frac{4 \dot{V}}{\upsilon \pi d} \qquad (13)$$

where N_R is Reynolds' number, $\dot{V}$ is airflow rate, υ is kinematic viscosity = viscosity/density, π is 3.1416, and d is diameter of passageway (cm).

If proper units are used for the terms, they cancel, leaving N_R as a dimensionless number. When $N_R < 2,000$ for flow in a smooth-bore tube, the flow pattern is laminar (streamline). For laminar flow the mechanical energy losses are defined by Poiseuille's law:

$$\lambda_\ell = \Delta P = 8 \times N \times \left(\frac{L}{\pi r^4}\right) \times \dot{V} \qquad (14)$$

where λ_ℓ is mechanical energy loss for laminar flow of gas (dynes/cm^2), ΔP is driving pressure (dynes/cm^2), N is gas viscosity (poises, or dynes $\times$ sec $\times$ cm^{-2}), L is length of passageway (cm), r is radius of passageway (cm), and $\dot{V}$ is airflow rate (ml/sec).

The driving pressure required to move air through a smooth, nonbranching tube of constant diameter is a function of gas viscosity and flow rate and of the length and radius of the tube. To put some of these units in a more familiar perspective, a pressure of 1 cm H_2O is equal to 980 dynes/cm^2 and the viscosity of air is about 1.9×10^{-4} poise (dynes $\times$ sec $\times$ cm^{-2}). These physical characteristics of the gas and of the passageway can be combined with the other constants (8 and π in the equation) to provide another single constant, K_ℓ, for a given system:

$$\Delta P = K_\ell \dot{V} \qquad (15)$$

This equation states that as long as airflow is laminar there is a linear relationship between ΔP and $\dot{V}$. The constant, K_ℓ, is determined by the characteristics of the gas and the geometry of the passageway.

When $N_R > 2,000$, turbulent flow develops and the relationship between ΔP and $\dot{V}$ is sharply changed. This type of flow involves random bulk mixing of the gas in the passageway, and streamline flow cannot exist. The mechanical energy loss for turbulent flow in a smooth, straight tube of uniform cross-sectional area leads to the equation:

$$\lambda_t = \Delta P = \frac{4L}{d} \left(\rho \frac{v^2}{2}\right) f \qquad (16)$$

Where λ_t is mechanical loss for turbulent flow, v is velocity of airflow, and f is the Blasius friction factor, which equals $0.0791 \times N_R^{-0.25}$. The equation can be simplified by expanding the friction factor and putting it in a form that presents airflow rate instead of velocity:

$$\lambda_t = \frac{0.24 \, L \times \rho \times 0.75 \, N \times \dot{V}^{1.75}}{d^{4.75}} \qquad (17)$$

The physical characteristics of the gas (ρ and N) and the geometry of the airway (L and d) can also be combined into a new constant, K_t. Hence, the mechanical energy loss for turbulent flow in a smooth airway is:

$$\Delta P = K_t \dot{V}^{1.75} \qquad (18)$$

For conduits not hydrodynamically smooth, which branch, converging for flow in the opposite direction, and change directions abruptly and have continuously varying cross-sectional areas, engineering considerations suggest that the actual mechanical energy losses are increased because of a higher degree of turbulence in the air stream. Under this condition the Blasius friction factor is not applicable because N_R becomes larger and f becomes smaller, until it is of no importance. Under these conditions, the mechanical energy loss is proportional to the square of the flow:

$$\Delta P = K_{t(e)} \dot{V}^{2.0} \qquad (19)$$

The mechanical energy losses described by the equations relating driving pressure to some function of airflow rate occur simultaneously throughout the airway, including the nasal passages, trachea, bronchi, bronchioles, and terminal airways. Thus, flow at a given point in the airway will be laminar or turbulent, and the geometry of the airway affects the level of turbulence so it may or may not be enhanced. Because the total pressure drop is the sum of all series pressure differences, the pressure drop through the total airway can be related to flow:

$$\Delta P = (\Sigma K_\ell) \dot{V} + (\Sigma K_t) \dot{V}^{1.75} + (\Sigma K_{t(e)}) \dot{V}^2 \qquad (20)$$

Most respiratory physiologists assume that a simplified form known as Röhrer's equation adequately describes the relationship in the airway passages. Röhrer's equation is:

$$P = K_1 \dot{V} + K_2 \dot{V}^2 \qquad (21)$$

where K_1 represents (ΣK_ℓ) and K_2 represents $[\Sigma K_{t(e)}]$.

The sizes of K_1 and K_2 express the relative contributions of laminar and turbulent flow to the mechanical energy loss (resistance to airflow in the airways). Since they are affected by the geometry of the airways at a given airflow velocity (flow rate), it follows that changes in the geometry of the airways, for example, bronchoconstriction, are reflected in changes in K_1 and K_2 and therefore in the relationship between ΔP and $\dot{V}$ at that flow rate.

A measure of the energy loss resulting from airflow in the airway passages is expressed as airway resistance, R_{aw}. This includes the resistance of airflow through the nose during nose breathing, though R_{aw} is more commonly measured during mouth breathing and reflects the resistance to airflow below the pharynx (larynx, trachea, bronchi, bronchioles, and terminal airways). R_{aw} is defined as $\Delta P/\dot{V}$ at a given airflow rate (usually 0.5 L/sec in adults). Thus, $R_{aw} = \Delta P/\dot{V} = K_1 + K_2 \dot{V}$. Because the relative contributions of laminar and turbulent flow are affected by airflow velocity, the relationship between pressure and flow through a given system is changed if the flow rate is altered. On the other hand, if gas composition remains constant, for example, humidified air at body temperature, changes in R_{aw}, or the value of $\Delta P/\dot{V}$ at a given flow rate, reflect changes in the effective geometry of the airway passages, such as diameter. This results from alterations in the constants, K_1 and K_2, in Röhrer's equation.

PHYSICAL PRINCIPLES APPLIED TO AIRWAY RESISTANCE CALCULATIONS

The fluid mechanical analogy for Ohm's law for electricity (resistance = voltage/current) is expressed for airway resistance as:

$$R_{aw} = \frac{\Delta P}{\dot{V}} \qquad (22)$$

where R_{aw} is expressed in cm $H_2O \times L^{-1} \times sec^{-1}$, ΔP in cm H_2O, and $\dot{V}$ in L/sec. Of course, R_{aw} is different at different airflow rates, depending on the values of K_1 and K_2 (see previous section); hence, the flow rate must be specified if any comparison with normal standard values is to be meaningful.

As in the electric analog, series resistances are additive. For example, the total resistance to the movement of air into and out of the lungs is the sum of upper and lower airway resistances. In fact, there are three series resistances that to some degree contribute independently to R_{aw}. They include nasal airway resistance, R_n, resistance to airflow through the larynx, R_{lar}, and lower airway resistance, R_a. Thus, total resistance to airflow to and from the lung during normal breathing is:

$$R_{tot} = R_n + R_{lar} + R_a \qquad (23)$$

The airway passage consists of parallel circuits as well as series resistances, so equations for parallel resistances must be used for an accurate, comprehensive description of mechanical energy losses.

Parallel passages exist in the nose, where the right and left nasal airways are separated by the nasal septum. Parallel passages also exist in the lung, beginning with the right and left main bronchi. The parallel pathways are multiplied by more than 20 generations of branching airways, each of which gives rise to additional parallel pathways for airflow and therefore to multiple parallel resistances.

As with electric analogs, parallel resistances can be summed only by using the reciprocal of resistance, or conductance. Thus,

$$\frac{1}{R_{tot}} = \frac{1}{R_r} + \frac{1}{R_\ell} \qquad (24)$$

where R_{tot} is total airway resistance (cm H_2O $\times$ L^{-1} $\times$ sec^{-1}), R_r is resistance on the right side (either right bronchus or right nares), and R_ℓ is resistance on the left side, parallel to R_r (either left bronchus or left nares, depending on R_r).

The equation can be manipulated to calculate the resistance of two parallel circuits:

$$R_{tot} = \frac{R_r \times R_\ell}{R_r + R_\ell} \qquad (25)$$

For the combined resistances to be meaningful, they must be measured at the same flow rates. This is easier to control with the combination of series resistances and can be done by measuring the partitioning of airway resistance simultaneously in the same breath. That is, by measuring ΔP across the nose and the larynx during a breath in which flow rate is measured, R_n and R_{lar} can be correctly measured at the

same flow rate and therefore can be legitimately summed. On the other hand, it is difficult to measure the partitioning of flow between parallel pathways. Flow through right and left nares can be measured either simultaneously or sequentially with the correct equipment, but no practical way exists (other than by bronchial intubation) to accurately measure the partition of flow between the right and left lobes of the lungs. Thus, some of the theoretic errors associated with measuring R_{aw} cannot be avoided, although it is usually calculated on the basis of ΔP and total $\dot{V}$, without reference to parallel pathways in the airways serving the lungs. This causes no problem unless there is a disproportionate change in the geometry of the airways that changes the partition of flow between them.

As already indicated, it is possible to measure ΔP (driving pressure) across the nasal airways and across the larynx, but no *direct* method is available for measuring the ΔP between the alveoli and any point above them, including the atmosphere, which would be required for a simple calculation of lower airway resistance. Instead, an indirect method is used to estimate alveolar pressure. It applies Boyle's law to the change of alveolar volume (measured with a body plethysmograph) that results from compressing and expanding gas in the lung during the process of breathing. This will be discussed in more detail in Chapter 4 but is presented here to indicate that, although the measurement of R_{aw} appears to be a simple procedure, it is actually complicated because of the difficulty in measuring ΔP, which is essential for the calculation of R_{aw}.

CALCULATIONS RELATING TO GAS VOLUME

From the general gas law, $PV = nRT$, it is apparent that if we specify the conditions of pressure, volume, and temperature, then the number of gas molecules or mass of a gas, n, is implied (R is a known constant). As a corollary, to specify a certain number of gas molecules, or mass, the volume of gas must be measured simultaneously with its temperature and pressure. As Avogadro's hypothesis indicates, when the temperature is 273° K and pressure is 760 torr, a volume of 22.4 L contains 1 mole of gas, or 6.02×10^{23} molecules (Loschmidt's number $\times$ 22,400). The general gas law also permits a comparison of volume measurements made in different environments.

As presented earlier, if the mass (number of molecules) of a gas does not change, PV/T is a constant. This permits calculation of the volume change that accompanies a known pressure or temperature change. An example of such a calculation will demonstrate its use.

The *vital capacity* is a measure of the volume of air that can be expelled from the lungs by maximal effort after a maximal inspiration. The expired gas is collected in a spirometer and is near room temperature at the time of the volume measurement. However, it is more relevant to express the vital capacity in terms of the volume change in the lungs. Is there a significant change in the volume of expired gas as a result of its temperature decrease from, for example, 37° C in the lung (V_{BTPS})* to 25° C in the spirometer (V_{ATPS})?* Charles' law can be used to show that the volume decreases by a

factor of $\dfrac{273° + 25°}{273° + 37°} = \dfrac{298°}{310°} = 0.961$, or about

4%, as a result of the 12° C temperature decrease. The measured volume would need to be increased by about 4% to correct for only the cooling effect on the volume of gas expelled from the lungs when measured in a spirometer.

But the expired gas was saturated with water vapor at 37° C, and some of the water vapor condensed as the temperature fell to 25° C in the spirometer. The water vapor pressure required to saturate gas at 37° C is 47 torr, whereas the water vapor pressure required to

*See Appendix, Symbols and abbreviations for respiratory physiology.

saturate gas at 25° C is about 24 torr. In gas volume calculations it is easier to use partial pressure changes than fractional concentration changes because the volume change in turn alters the fractional concentration of the remaining components. However, a volume change does result from a change in the water vapor concentration, and it can be calculated. If we assume that the total (barometric) pressure was 755 torr, the fractional concentration of water vapor would fall from 47/755 = 0.0623 at 37° C to 24/755 = 0.0318 at 25° C. The decrease of F_{H_2O} was therefore 0.0305. Of course, since the total volume decreased by 3%, the amount of water vapor decreased by an additional 3% (because its concentration was fixed at F = 0.0318), and this caused a real loss of about 3.14% in the total volume of expired gas resulting from water vapor condensation.

In gas volume calculations this effect is expressed more simply as a proportionate change in the total dry gas pressure. Thus, $P_B - P_{H_2O}$ (at a given temperature)/$P_B - P_{H_2O}$ (at a different temperature) defines the volume change that results. In this example $\dfrac{755 \text{ torr} - 47 \text{ torr}}{755 \text{ torr} - 24 \text{ torr}} = \dfrac{708 \text{ torr}}{731 \text{ torr}} = 0.9685$, which is the volume change resulting from water vapor condensation at the temperatures indicated. Thus, the volume in the spirometer would need to be increased by 3.15% to correct for the volume lost as a result of moisture condensation from the expired gas as it cools in the spirometer.

These two correction factors can be applied separately to the measured spirometer volume to calculate the volume change in the lung during the vital capacity test. However, if the general gas law is applied directly to the problem, a general equation can be developed for the conversion of the volume under one set of conditions to the volume under any other set of conditions.

Consider the initial gas condition to be ambient temperature (25° C) and pressure (755

Table 2. Normal composition of clean dry atmospheric air near sea level*

Constituent gas and formula	Content (percent by volume)	Content variable relative to its normal	Molecular weight†
Nitrogen (N_2)	78.084	—	28.0134
Oxygen (O_2)	20.9476	—	31.9988
Argon (Ar)	0.934	—	39.948
Carbon dioxide (CO_2)	0.0314	‡	44.00995
Neon (Ne)	0.001818	—	20.183
Helium (He)	0.000524	—	4.0026
Krypton (Kr)	0.000114	—	83.80
Xenon (Xe)	0.0000087	—	131.30
Hydrogen (H_2)	0.00005	?	2.01594
Methane (CH_4)	0.0002	‡	16.04303
Nitrous oxide (N_2O)	0.00005	—	44.0128
Ozone (O_3)	Summer: 0-0.000007	‡	47.9982
	Winter: 0-0.000002	‡	47.9982
Sulfur dioxide (SO_2)	0-0.0001	‡	64.0628
Nitrogen dioxide (NO_2)	0-0.000002	‡	46.0055
Ammonia (NH_3)	0-trace	‡	17.03061
Carbon monoxide (CO)	0-trace	‡	28.01055
Iodine (I_2)	0-0.000001	‡	253.8088

*From U.S. standard atmosphere, Washington, D.C., 1962, U.S. Government Printing Office, p. 9.
†On basis of carbon-12 isotope scale for which $C^{12} = 12$.
‡The content of this gas may undergo significant variations from time to time or from place to place relative to the normal indicated for it.

torr), saturated with water vapor ($P_{H_2O} = 24$ torr at 25° C), and the second condition to be at body temperature (37° C) and pressure (755 torr), saturated with water vapor ($P_{H_2O} = 47$ torr at 37° C). For the dry gas volume:

$$\frac{V_2 P_2}{T_2} = \frac{V_1 P_1}{T_1} \tag{26}$$

$$V_2 = \frac{V_1 P_1}{T_1} \times \frac{T_2}{P_2} = V_1 \times \frac{T_2}{T_1} \times \frac{P_1}{P_2} \tag{27}$$

$$= V_1 \times \frac{273 + T_2° C}{273 + T_1° C} \times \frac{P_B - P_{H_2O} @ T_1}{P_B - P_{H_2O} @ T_2} \tag{28}$$

$$= V_1 \times \frac{273 + 37}{273 + 25} \times \frac{755 - 24}{755 - 47} \tag{29}$$

$$= V_1 \times \frac{310}{298} \times \frac{731}{708} = V_1 \, 1.04 \times 1.032 \tag{30}$$

$$V_{BTPS} = 1.073 \times V_{ATPS} \tag{31}$$

The same equation can be used to convert gas volume under any set of known conditions to any other set of known conditions.

In calculations that involve O_2 uptake or CO_2 output, it is customary to convert the gas volumes measured under ambient conditions, saturated, to STPD conditions—standard temperature (0° C), standard pressure (760 torr), and dry ($P_{H_2O} = 0$). The same equation can be used, with proper substitution for ambient conditions:

$$V_{STPD} = V_{ATPS} \times \frac{273°}{273 + T° C} \times \frac{(P_B - P_{H_2O} @ T° C)}{760} \tag{32}$$

The reader who is not clear about the derivation of each of the terms in the equation should develop it in the manner shown here for conversion from V_{ATPS} to V_{BTPS}.

HOMOGENEITY AND COMPOSITION OF ATMOSPHERIC AIR

The composition of our atmosphere has changed greatly since the earth was formed $4\frac{1}{2}$ billion years ago. However, the rate of change has always been exceedingly slow until recently. Certain pollutants are now regularly present in detectable and increasing concentration. Local or regional abnormalities of atmospheric composition have developed around centers of pollution.

We pollute the air we breathe with impunity. We dump enormous quantities of wastes into it as if it were a gigantic sewer. We are truly the *effluent* society. Within the relatively short space of several generations we will convert the carbon in fossil fuels, which were half a billion years in the making, into CO_2.

For the present, Table 2 describes the generally homogeneous gaseous composition of our atmosphere from sea level up to an altitude of about 60,000 feet (18 km).

Table 3 shows the change in composition of

Table 3. Changes of composition of air in the lungs

Component	$F_{atmospheric}$*	$F_{alveolar}$*	$F_{expired}$*
N_2 (inert)	0.786	0.749†	0.767‡
O_2	0.209	0.136	0.167
CO_2	0.000	0.053	0.040
H_2O	0.005§	0.062‖	0.026¶

*Fractional concentration *(not dry)*.
†Volume increase caused by saturation with H_2O.
‡Composition change caused by condensation of H_2O and dilution of alveolar gas with dead space gas (inspired air).
§Assumes 25% to 30% relative humidity.
‖Assumes saturation at 37° C.
¶Temperature effect on P_{H2O}.

the major air components when air is breathed. Inert gas (N_2) changes concentration passively, as a result of saturation and condensation of water vapor and changes in the amount of CO_2 and O_2 added to or removed from air in the alveoli. Expired gas composition differs from that of alveolar gas because of temperature difference and dilution with inspired air in the airway (anatomic dead space).

CHAPTER 3

DEVELOPMENT AND FUNCTIONAL ANATOMY OF THE BRONCHOPULMONARY SYSTEM

LUNG FUNCTION IN UTERO

Most organs, including the heart, kidneys, and liver, begin to function early in fetal life and gradually develop up to the time of birth. This is also true for the nonventilatory functions of the lung. The lung has vigorous metabolic activity in utero, an essential prenatal activity that prepares the fetus for the process of breathing after birth.

The production of fetal lung liquid begins early in fetal development, and its composition changes during fetal life. The exact site of production remains unknown but probably involves most of the lung. This is not surprising if we consider that the epithelial tissue that forms the lung derives from the foregut, which also produces and secretes fluid.

Early in development, lung liquid serves only to fill the developing airway spaces. During the last trimester type II alveolar epithelial cells contribute to the production of a lung liquid, the composition of which is more complex than a simple plasma ultrafiltrate. Electrolyte pumps are active, and surfactant is synthesized. Surfactant material, present in lung lining fluid, lowers surface tension and is of great importance for breathing. Lamellar inclusion bodies are present within type II cells after about 20 weeks of intrauterine life. These bodies are present before the production of surfactant, a compound of dipalmitoyl lecithin and a specific apoprotein, both of which are produced by type II cells. When surfactant is released into the alveoli, it spreads over the hypophase, which is rich in mucopolysaccharides and lipids and serves to store surfactant. During later fetal development there is normally well-regulated production and release of surfactant. This storage assures that, after the lungs expand and the lung liquid spreads out over the surface of the alveoli and airways, there is enough surfactant to reduce surface tension and permit normal lung function.

Besides production of lung fluid, other metabolic lung activity includes removal and degradation of certain biologic materials produced in the body. Although during fetal life the total output of the right ventricle does not flow through the lungs during each cycle, it does after birth. The lungs are strategically located to function as a biologic filter. Such lung activities occur in utero well before birth.

EMBRYOLOGIC DEVELOPMENT

The epithelial structure of the lung begins as an outgrowth of the primitive foregut during the third week of gestation (3-mm embryo). The anterior wall of the primitive tube develops a longitudinal bulging ridge that pinches off from the main tube, except at the cephalic end.

The parallel tubes then separate, producing the esophagus posteriorly and the trachea and bronchial tree anteriorly. Through a process of budding, branching, and advancing, the subdivisions of the lung form.

The phases of lung development are defined as follows. The *embryonic period* covers the first 5 to 6 weeks of embryonic life, including the early phases of creation and development of the lung. During this period ten principal branches of the bronchial tree develop on the left and eight develop on the right; they will become the familiar lobar and segmental lung units. The *pseudoglandular period* lasts until the 15th or 16th week and includes the period of bronchial development. The lung consists of a network of connective tissue with an actively proliferating bronchial mass. At this stage the lung appears glandular, and columnar epithelium lines the airways. Since the lung is not really glandular, the term pseudoglandular is used for this developmental period. The *canalicular period* lasts from the 16th to the 24th or 26th week. During this time the primitive bronchioles branch farther, and there is a relative decrease in the amount of connective tissue. The lung becomes obviously lobular and more vascular. The epithelium that lines the airways flattens and thins. Toward the end of this period type I and type II alveolar lining epithelia appear, and capillaries protrude into the epithelium, sometimes forming potential areas of thin capillary-airway interface. As this process continues, there is a proliferation of areas that could maintain gas exchange if required. From the 24th or 26th week to term the final stage, or *terminal sac period*, of fetal lung development occurs. The duct system extends; surface area of the spaces increases by formation of saccules. Capillaries line the walls, some projecting into the saccule lumen.

There is controversy over whether or not alveoli are present at birth. Some investigators have reported alveolar wall intersections at term in the human being, although they are not present in many laboratory animals. Some alveoli are probably present at birth, perhaps 15 to 25 million, but most alveoli develop during the months after birth. Regardless of the exact time of their appearance, alveoli continue to develop during infancy and childhood.

There is also disagreement concerning the time when alveolar multiplication ceases. It is generally agreed that the most rapid replication occurs in the immediate postnatal period. However, some believe that the adult number of alveoli (about 300 million) are present by the end of the first year of life, whereas others believe that alveolar multiplication continues at a gradually decreasing rate until somatic growth stops. The most common estimate is that alveolar multiplication ceases at about 8 years of age, after which the number of alveoli remains constant for many years.

STRUCTURE OF THE BRONCHOPULMONARY SYSTEM

The lungs are somewhat conical in shape and have an apex, a base, and three surfaces (Fig. 3-1). The cardiac fossa and the hilum are on the mediastinal surface. The hilum is a triangular depression containing lymph nodes where bronchi, blood vessels, and nerves enter to form the root of the lung. The diaphragmatic surface of the lung is concave.

The weight of the lungs depends on the amount of blood and other fluids they contain but averages 1,110 gm for the adult male and 900 gm for the female. The right lung accounts for about 55% of total lung weight and function. The right lung has upper, middle, and lower lobes, whereas the left lung has only an upper and a lower lobe. However, the left upper lobe has an upper division comparable to the right upper lobe and a lower, lingular division comparable to the right middle lobe.

The visceral pleura that surrounds the pulmonary lobes is a stable membrane that overlays a separate *limiting membrane* of the lung. The limiting membrane and the pleura somewhat restrict lung expansion.

The pleura consists of two layers: a thin del-

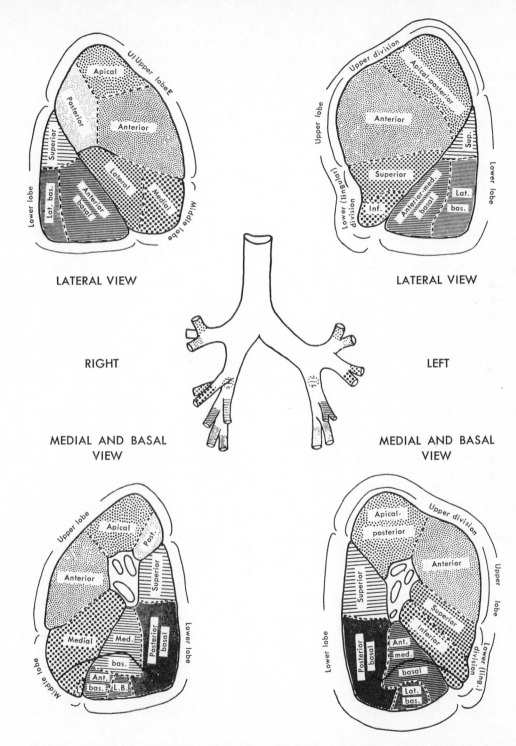

Fig. 3-1. Nomenclature of the bronchopulmonary segments according to Jackson and Huber. Bronchial branches are named for the pulmonary segments they supply. (From Huber, J. F.: J. Nat. Med. Ass. **41**:54, 1949.)

icate sheet of elastic and collagenous fibers under which is a separate layer of dense elastic and collagenous tissue. The dense layer stabilizes the visceral pleura. Lymphatic channels and blood vessels, including a rich capillary network, lie below the visceral pleura.

The parietal pleura lines the inner surface of the thoracic cage. It is separated from the visceral pleura by a thin layer of liquid, the volume of which is probably less than 10 ml. This liquid is probably an ultrafiltrate of plasma from the parietal (thoracic) pleura. It lubricates the surfaces, minimizes friction, and facilitates changes of lung shape as the lung adjusts to changing thoracic shape during breathing. The liquid is normally removed by the lymphatic system beneath the visceral (lung) pleura. When the rate of pleural fluid formation exceeds the rate of removal, liquid accumulates in the space between the two pleural surfaces (intrapleural space) and a *pleural effusion* results. Because the right and left visceral and parietal pleurae are entirely separate, a pleural effusion may exist on the right, on the left, or bilaterally.

The tracheal cartilages form incomplete rings that are deficient posteriorly, where they are replaced by smooth muscle. The right main stem bronchus, wider and shorter than the left, is about 2.5 cm long; it follows the direction of the trachea more closely than does the left main stem bronchus. The left main stem bronchus, smaller in caliber but longer than the right, is nearly 5 cm long; it also diverges from the direction of the trachea at a greater angle than does the right main stem bronchus. Because of the verticality of the right main stem bronchus and its larger diameter, aspirated foreign bodies lodge more commonly in the right lung. The angle between the two major bronchi is somewhat larger in the female.

The right middle lobe bronchus is of relatively small caliber and length and sometimes bends sharply near its bifurcation. It is surrounded by a collar of lymph nodes draining both middle and lower lobes and thus particularly subject to obstruction, recurrent infection, and atelectasis. Such partial or complete collapse of the right middle lobe is clinically termed *middle lobe syndrome* and, on occasion, requires surgical resection, or lobectomy.

The right and left main stem bronchi divide into lobar bronchi and these, in turn, subdivide by irregular dichotomy through 23 generations, finally arborizing into terminal bronchioles (0.6 mm in diameter), respiratory bronchioles (0.4 mm in diameter), alveolar ducts, atria, alveolar sacs, and alveoli. To describe this arborization, generations of airways are given a numerical order, beginning with the trachea as 0, and ending with the most peripheral airways. The first four orders of bronchi and their corresponding pulmonary segments are named according to position, providing a reference for roentgenographic, bronchoscopic, and physical findings. The smallest named units of lung structure are the bronchopulmonary segments, of which there are ten on the right and eight on the left. The Jackson and Huber terminology for the bronchopulmonary segments is widely used.

The first 16 orders of bronchi merely conduct air and are supplied by the bronchial, rather than the pulmonary, arteries. Moving distally through the airway, there is a progressive loss of cartilage, mucus-secreting elements, and cilia. At order 11, cartilage disappears, and the airway is called a *bronchiole*. From this order on, radial traction of the lung (peribronchial radial traction) maintains airway patency. Scattered alveoli appear at the 17th through 19th generations, which are thus called transitional airways. The *terminal bronchioles* within the lung lobule, with a total cross-sectional area of 180 cm^2, are the last fully epithelialized and ciliated air passages. Alveoli increase, and at order 20 their mouths form the entire wall of the airway, which is now called the *alveolar duct*. Although some alveoli arise directly from *respiratory bronchioles*, most arise from the alveolar ducts, which give rise either to single alveoli or to *al-*

veolar sacs containing two or more alveoli. Since the cross-sectional area of the trachea is 2.5 cm^2 and that of the alveolar sacs (not alveoli) is 11,800 cm^2, the cross-sectional area of the airway increases by a factor of 4,720 from trachea to alveolar sacs.

The *primary lobule* is the basic unit of bronchopulmonary structure. It consists of all the airways and air spaces arising from a single terminal bronchiole, including the respiratory bronchiole, alveolar ducts, alveolar sacs, and dependent alveoli with their blood vessels. There are about 23 million primary lobules in the human lung. The primary lobule is the fundamental unit of gas exchange.

The *secondary lobule* is that volume of lung bounded by connective tissue septa, which arise from the pleura and extend into the lung. The septa vary in size but are in the form of irregular polyhedra 1 to 2.5 cm in diameter. A secondary lobule contains 30 to 50 primary lobules.

The autonomic nerve supply of the bronchopulmonary system consists of branches from the vagi and sympathetics that form anterior and posterior plexuses at the lung hila and supply the bronchi and blood vessels.

The lung has two different circulatory systems. The pulmonary circulation serves the gas-exchange function; the bronchial circulation supplies the bronchi and bronchioles as far as the distal end of the terminal bronchioles, as well as certain other structures, such as lymph nodes. The pulmonary arteries accompany the bronchi as they arborize and finally terminate in a dense alveolar capillary network. The pulmonary veins arise mainly from alveolar capillaries and to a lesser extent from capillary networks of the alveolar ducts, bronchioles, and pleurae. Small veins coalesce into larger veins that generally follow an intersegmental course rather than that of the arteries and bronchi. Two large veins finally emerge from each lung to empty into the left atrium of the heart.

The bronchial circulation consists of relatively small systemic arteries that arise from the aorta, accompany the bronchi, and drain mainly into the pulmonary venous system. However, two bronchial veins form at the roots of the lungs, the right draining into the azygos vein and the left into the highest intercostal, or accessory hemiazygos, vein.

Small pulmonary arteries (not arterioles) divide into capillaries at the level of the respiratory bronchioles and alveoli. These capillaries form a dense network, the basic element of which is a short cylindric tube. Each capillary segment adjoins from two to four adjacent segments, forming a hexagonal three-dimensional structure, which is continuous through the secondary lobules. The internal capillary diameter is about 8 μm and the average length is about 10 μm. Total capillary blood volume is about 140 ml, and the total surface area is about 70 M^2, about the same as that of the total alveolar surface. Pulmonary capillaries in the lung base, which have high transmural pressures, bulge into the alveolar spaces, whereas during quiet sitting or standing those at the top of the lung lie flat within the alveolar walls. Pulmonary venules arise from the capillaries of the alveolar septa, the pleura, and the bronchial artery. In the healthy lung the bronchial and pulmonary systems anastomose only by way of the capillaries; capillaries of the bronchial circulation anastomose with those of the pulmonary circulation at the level of the respiratory bronchioles. However, the pulmonary artery alone supplies the respiratory bronchioles, the alveolar ducts, and the alveoli.

Microanatomy of the alveolocapillary region

The alveolar parenchyma consists of the alveoli and pulmonary capillaries. The alveolar walls contain a dense network of capillaries and reticular, collagenous, and elastic fibers. The alveolar septum consists of a connective tissue space supporting alveolar capillaries and containing collagen and elastic fibrils, fibroblasts, and occasional leukocytes and histiocytes.

Small holes, or stomata, are present in the alveolar septa of most mammals. These discontinuities are called the alveolar *pores of Kohn.* They are 3 to 13 μm in diameter, depending on alveolar volume (degree of lung inflation). The pores are located between, and usually surrounded by, capillaries. They are present in the alveoli of most adults but are not present in infant lungs. It has been suggested that they are the sites previously occupied by septal phagocytes, but this is speculation; the origin of the pores remains unknown.

Alveolar duct ectasia is a change associated with aging that consists of enlargement of the lumina of alveolar ducts, with a broadening and a decrease in depth of their subtending alveoli. The terminal alveoli also show broadening, decrease in depth, and enlargement of their mouths. These changes are greatest in the apices of the lung and are found in approximately 50% of individuals 60 to 80 years of age, more than 85% of those older than 80 years of age, but are not found in subjects less than 30 years of age.

The existence of the *alveolocapillary membrane,* just below optical microscopic visibility, was first demonstrated by means of the electron microscope, which also revealed its intimate structure. The normal alveolocapillary membrane consists of five layers (Figs. 3-2 to 3-5): (1) *pulmonary surface epithelium,* a continuous, exceedingly thin (0.1 to 0.5 μm) layer of squamous epithelium that lines the alveoli, (2) superficial reticulin basement membrane, a framework with elastic fiber network and little collagen, (3) ground substance, (4) capillary reticulin basement membrane, and (5) capillary endothelial cell.

The pulmonary surface epithelium is a continuous membrane perforated only in places by cells desquamating into the alveolar spaces; it is also directly continuous with the epithelium of the terminal bronchioles. The superficial reticulin basement membrane of the alveolar wall is continuous with the basement membrane of the bronchiolar basement epithelium supporting the pulmonary epithelium. The capillary

reticulin basement membrane supports the capillary endothelium and is continuous with the basement membrane beneath the endothelium of larger pulmonary blood vessels.

The cells observed in normal pulmonary alveoli may be classified into seven distinct categories. The first category comprises alveolar epithelial cells, which form the pulmonary surface epithelium, also termed small, type A, or type I. The attenuated cytoplasm of this alveolar epithelial cell displays little or no affinity for histologic dyes. These squamous cells are incapable of phagocytosis.

The second category is a second type of cuboidal alveolar epithelial cell of definite morphology, termed large, type B, or type II cells (Fig. 3-4). They have almost no phagocytic activity. They occur singly and usually contain interesting cytoplasmic osmiophilic lamellar inclusion bodies, which produce the surfactant that reduces surface tension at the alveolar interface. Type II cells may extend completely across an alveolar septum to border on two adjacent alveolar air spaces. Type II alveolar epithelial cells normally occur in a ratio of about 1:1 with type I cells.

A third category of cells is the pulmonary alveolar macrophages, large migratory cells measuring up to 12 μm in diameter, which are present in moderate numbers within the alveoli. The combined volume of all the alveolar macrophages in the lungs is about equal to that of the thyroid gland. In contrast to alveolar epithelial cells, alveolar macrophages have a strong affinity for a variety of histologic dyes. As the name implies, alveolar macrophages have pseudopods, exhibit ameboid motion, and are highly phagocytic. They change shape by means of cell membrane surface forces, microtubules, and actin microfilaments. They are involved in pulmonary defense and clearance, ingesting viable and nonviable foreign particles that have eluded the cough reflex and the mucous escalator, as well as scavenging endogenous debris. Pulmonary cleansing mechanisms

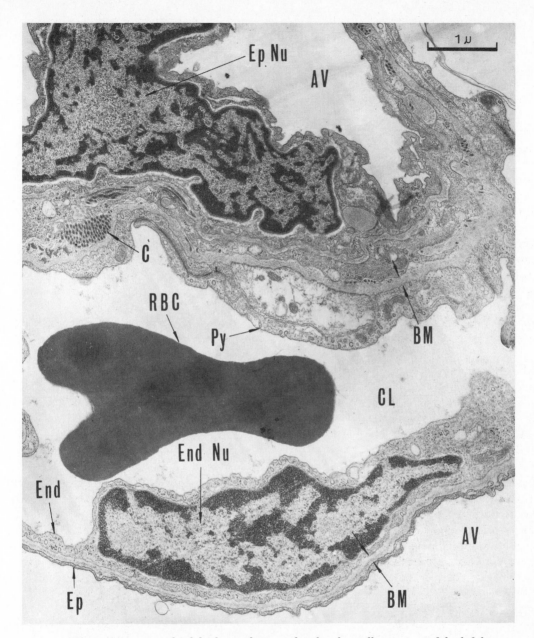

Fig. 3-2. Electron micrograph of the lung, showing the alveolocapillary region of the left lower lobe of a healthy 35-year-old man. *AV,* Alveolar space; *BM,* basement membrane; *CL,* capillary lumen; *C,* collagen (in cross section); *END,* endothelial cytoplasm; *End Nu,* endothelial nucleus; *Ep,* epithelial cytoplasm; *Ep Nu,* epithelial nucleus; *Py,* pinocytic vesicle; *RBC,* red blood cell. (Courtesy A. E. Vatter, Department of Pathology, Webb-Waring Institute, University of Colorado Medical Center, Denver, Colo.)

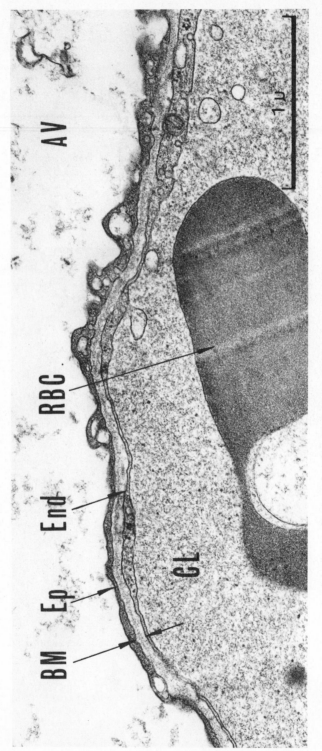

Fig. 3-3. Electron micrograph of the lung, showing the alveolocapillary region of the left lower lobe of a healthy 35-year-old man. *AV,* Alveolar space; *BM,* basement membrane; *CL,* capillary lumen; *End,* endothelial cytoplasm; *Ep,* epithelial cytoplasm; *RBC,* red blood cell. (Courtesy A. E. Vatter, Department of Pathology, Webb-Waring Institute, University of Colorado Medical Center, Denver, Colo.)

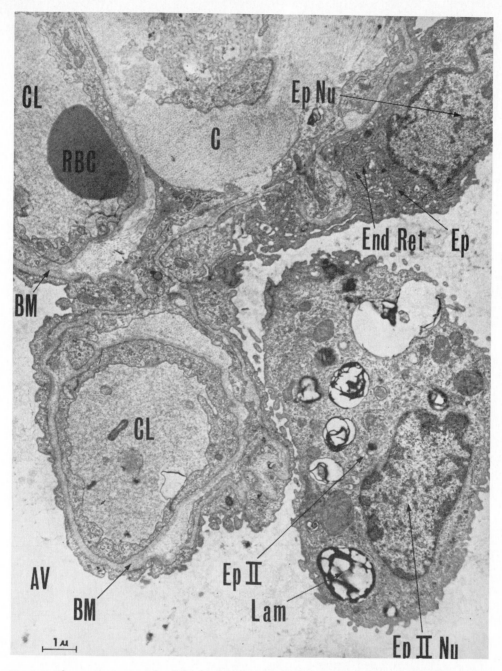

Fig. 3-4. Electron micrograph of the healthy human lung (specimen from the left lower lobe of a 74-year-old man), showing alveolocapillary structures with large epithelial (type B, type II) cell containing cytoplasmic lamellar bodies. *AV,* Alveolar space; *BM,* basement membrane; *CL,* capillary lumen; *C,* collagen; *End Ret,* endoplasmic reticulum; *Ep,* epithelial cytoplasm; *Ep Nu,* epithelial nucleus; *Ep II,* cytoplasm of alveolar epithelial cell, type II; *Ep II Nu,* nucleus of alveolar epithelial cell, type II; *Lam,* lamellar body; *RBC,* red blood cell. (Courtesy Robert L. Hawley, Mercy Institute of Biomedical Research, Denver, Colo.)

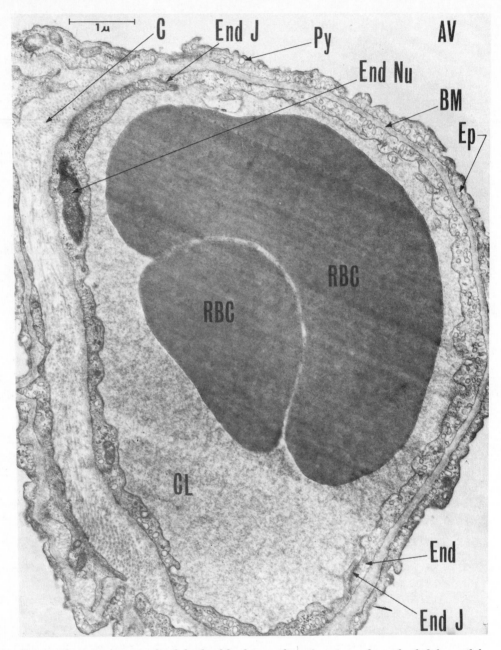

Fig. 3-5. Electron micrograph of the healthy human lung (specimen from the left lower lobe of a 74-year-old man), showing erythrocyte in a pulmonary capillary. *AV,* Alveolar space; *BM,* basement membrane; *CL,* capillary lumen; *C,* collagen; *End,* endothelial cytoplasm; *End J,* junction of two endothelial cells; *End Nu,* endothelial nucleus; *Ep* epithelial cytoplasm; *Py,* pinocytic vesicle; *RBC,* red blood cell. (Courtesy Robert L. Hawley, Mercy Institute of Biomedical Research, Denver, Colo.)

continually remove alveolar macrophages, transporting them with their ingested foreign material up the tracheobronchial tree by ciliary action of the mucous escalator, where most of this material is swallowed; however, some enter lymphatic channels, through which they move to regional lymph nodes.

Alveolar macrophages respond to certain stimuli. For example, heparin induces migration of macrophages from pulmonary capillaries across the alveolocapillary membrane and into alveolar spaces. Bacille Calmette Guérin (BCG) vaccine increases macrophage metabolism even before phagocytosis occurs. After ingestion lysosomal enzymes within the macrophage digest the engulfed material. Under certain conditions these enzymes are then released with large amounts of prostaglandins produced at the time. Macrophages release prostaglandins in response to microorganisms, BCG, and asbestos, but not latex. There is evidence that under certain circumstances activated macrophages damage the lung.

Macrophages ingest but cannot kill certain microorganisms, for example, *Mycobacterium tuberculosis,* nor can they destroy certain particles. In certain diseases, alveolar macrophages ingest materials, becoming foam cells, dust cells, or heart failure cells. Tobacco smoke also produces morphologic changes in the macrophage, including enlargement, brown inclusions, loss of surface ruffles, and pits. Living alveolar macrophages are obtained for study in nearly pure form by saline washing (bronchoalveolar lavage) of animal lungs.

The four remaining categories include the endothelial cells that line the pulmonary blood capillaries, fibroblasts, histiocytes or septal macrophages (rare in normal lung), and migratory leukocytes, which are normally present. Both granulocytic and lymphocytic cells leave the blood capillaries by diapedesis and enter the interstitial tissue of the alveolar septum. They penetrate the superficial reticulin membrane to pass between the pulmonary epithelial cells into the alveolar spaces, from which they are continually removed by pulmonary cleansing mechanisms via the airway. These cells are thus present in normal bronchial secretions. The lung is a heterogeneous organ with respect to cell type; the study of individual cell types presents appreciable problems.

AIRWAY DYNAMICS
Airway caliber changes

The part of the respiratory tract lying within the chest cavity is subject to intrathoracic pressure. During inspiration gas in the airway is at less than atmospheric pressure, and intrapleural pressure is even less. The resultant transmural (transpulmonary) pressure difference distends the airway (passive dilation). During expiration the reverse occurs. Intrapleural pressure increases more than airway pressure and the resulting reversal of transmural pressure difference compresses the airway (passive constriction), increasing airway resistance.

During spontaneous breathing there is synchronous rhythmic fluctuation of bronchomotor tone, the airways actively dilating during inspiration and actively constricting during expiration.

As the lungs inflate during inspiration, lung elasticity exerts radial traction on intrapulmonary airways, increasing their caliber. During expiration the reverse occurs. Hence, airways dilate during inspiration and constrict during expiration. Because airflow rate is a function of the fourth or fifth power of the airway radius, depending on the flow regime, even small changes of airway caliber affect flow considerably.

Airway caliber decreases during asphyxia. Asphyxia, the combination of hypoxia and hypercapnia, both of which dilate airways, is usually associated with discharge of epinephrine from the adrenal medulla, also a bronchodilating influence. A deep breath is perhaps the most potent bronchodilator known.

The sympathetic neuron-effector junction in the airways is composed of the nonmyelinated termination of a postganglionic sympathetic neuron and the adjacent effector cell that it innervates. The adrenergic neuron synthesizes the catecholamine norepinephrine (the principal neurohumoral transmitter), stores it in small granules, and releases it in response to appropriate stimuli, such as nerve impulses or certain drugs. Epinephrine dilates the airway through an inhibitory action; this action is blocked by dichloroisoproterenol.

Laryngeal irritation reflexly constricts the airways. The afferent nerve fibers of this reflex are subepithelial in location and decrease in frequency from the larynx down to the respiratory bronchioles. Both afferent and efferent limbs are vagal. Stimulation of these subepithelial nerve fibers produces cough as well as bronchoconstriction. Laryngeal irritation increases total lung resistance, decreases anatomic dead space, but does not change lung compliance significantly; this suggests constriction of large conducting airways. Electric stimulation of cervical efferent vagus nerves causes similar changes.

The initial condition of the airways is an important variable because a given change in caliber produces a larger effect when the airways are initially small. The synthetic drug, isoproterenol, the prototype beta-adrenergic stimulator, is a widely used and potent bronchodilator; it is administered as both oral and sublingual tablets and by aerosol inhalation. Isoproterenol reverses vagal cholinergic reflexes. Rarely, the inhalation of pure isoproterenol precipitates severe bronchospasm; the mechanism of this paradoxic reaction remains unknown.

Histamine stimulates cough receptors by an autonomic reflex. Histamine inhalation produces a reaction resembling an asthmatic attack. Besides stimulating the reflex cholinergic bronchospasm, histamine acts locally to produce smooth muscle contraction. Injection of histamine into the pulmonary circulation decreases lung compliance, slightly increases total lung resistance, but does not decrease anatomic dead space, suggesting constriction of peripheral lung units. Anatomic studies, showing predominant constriction of the alveolar ducts, confirm this conclusion.

Serotonin (5-hydroxytryptamine) produces bronchoconstriction as well as increased pulmonary arterial pressure. Serotonin-secreting tumors (carcinoids) are sometimes misdiagnosed as asthma.

The inhalation of tobacco smoke causes both bronchoconstriction and bronchodilatation, as well as constriction of the bronchial arteries. These reactions are partly caused by the ganglionic effects of nicotine but also involve local stimulation of vagal and sympathetic bronchopulmonary reflexes. Injection of nicotine into the bronchial artery produces acute bronchoconstriction, contralateral bronchoconstriction by vagal reflex, and vasoconstriction of the bronchial arteries, possibly through sympathetic nervous action. Heparin is reported to reverse cigarette smoke–induced airway constriction.

The airways of patients with chronic diffuse obstructive bronchopulmonary disease, especially asthmatic patients, are hyperreactive to a variety of stimuli. Asthmatic patients frequently suffer severe bronchoconstriction following inhalation of dusts, cold air, and performance of routine tests of ventilatory capacity, such as the maximal voluntary ventilation or forced expired vital capacity. The intensity of this reaction may equal that of their response to potent irritants. Airway resistance of asthmatic patients commonly decreases during mild to moderate physical exertion but increases in the immediate postexercise period. A careful medical history can often elicit such a sequence. Propranolol, a potent beta-adrenergic blocking agent, is contraindicated in asthma.

Airway reactivity to various stimuli is an insufficiently studied variable that probably plays a role in the pathogenesis of chronic diffuse obstructive bronchopulmonary disease.

Airway water loss

Osmotically, the skin behaves as if it were a 9% or 10% salt solution. Fingertips wrinkle in sea water (about 3.5% salt) as the superficial cells swell with the water they absorb but do not pass on into the circulation. When relative humidity is below about 92%, water is lost insensibly from the skin to the air. However, when humidity is above this level, the skin is "drier" than the air and there is a water gain. Paradoxically, this insensible gain may occur at the same time that there is a sweat loss.

Unlike skin, the upper airways do not behave osmotically as a strong salt solution. Their water vapor tension is so slightly reduced that they could maintain about 99.5% relative humidity in adjacent quiet air. Contrary to views presented in older physiology texts, there is virtually no water loss from the lungs of normal mammals; the warm, wet upper airways lose water as they saturate the stream of inspired gas before it reaches the lungs.

The amount of water lost from the airways depends on air temperature. On a cold winter day, even a cold nose adds some water to the inspired air. A warm trachea adds still more water as the air column descends to warmer and warmer tracheal levels, and more air comes into contact with the wet airway walls. By the time the inspired air reaches the lower end of the trachea, it has come very close to respiratory tract temperature and is about 99.5% saturated with water vapor. Since the fluid lining the alveolar walls is not distilled water but contains dissolved materials, this fluid wets the inspired air no further.

During expiration warm, wet alveolar gas flows past airway walls of progressively lower temperature. As this gas cools, it deposits moisture on these walls, including the cooler membranes of the nose, which may even drip as a result of this condensation. The wet stream of expired gas leaves the body at a temperature only slightly above that of the nose, but its water content is 100% of the maximum absolute humidity for that temperature. Much of this water appears as a small cloud as it condenses in the cold winter air.

As water evaporates during inspiration, it removes heat from the airway (evaporative cooling), but expiration with its attendant condensation returns a portion of this heat. The heat of vaporization varies with temperature but, in the winter example given, should be between 575 and 595 cal/gm of water evaporated or condensed.

PULMONARY CLEARANCE MECHANISMS

It is indeed remarkable that the normal lower respiratory tract is almost sterile, since bacterial contamination by inspired air and aspiration of upper respiratory tract secretions are common occurences. The ability of the lower respiratory tract to dispose of inhaled particulate matter involves the mechanisms of phagocytosis and ciliary activity. In peripheral lung, where the epithelium is devoid of cilia, alveolar macrophages and rich lymphatic networks trap and dispose of the small inhaled particles that impinge on the respiratory surfaces.

There is evidence that these mechanisms are impaired by cigarette smoke inhalation and by the use of alcohol (ethanol). *Staphylococcus aureus* is rapidly cleared from the lungs of mice after implantation by a precise aerosol system; the clearance curve is quantitative and exponential. It is also known that bacterial pathogens can be isolated from the bronchial secretions of patients with chronic bronchitis during periods of apparent well-being, suggesting that antibacterial factors effective in the normal bronchial tree are impaired in chronic bronchitis.

The mucous escalator

The total output of bronchial secretions in the healthy adult human being is estimated to be 100 ml daily. Normal bronchi contain two types of mucus-producing glands: the surface goblet cells, which react to irritation or chronic inflammation, and the submucosal glands, which are mixed serous and mucous. The latter respond to vagal stimulation with increased mucous output. The submucosal bronchial glands atrophy after pulmonary denervation.

The composition of normal mucus is 95% water, 2% glycoprotein, 1% carbohydrate, less than 1% lipid, and 0.03% DNA. The glycoproteins, which average 1-million molecular weight, are coiled polypeptide chains with saccharide side-chains. Sputum glycoproteins increase the viscosity of mucus and serve as a protective lining and lubricant. Sputum viscosity can be decreased by hydration, increasing pH, increasing ionic strength, proteolytic enzymes (including papain, trypsin, and chymotrypsin), neuraminidase, and by rupture of S-S linkages, as with acetylcysteine, iodine, or iodinated tyrosine. The neutral and acid mucopolysaccharides have been distinguished and analyzed. Bronchial glands produce two types of sialomucin and two of sulfomucin. All four types of acid glycoproteins are present in the mucus of adults, but only sulfomucin is present in that of infants and children up to 4 years of age.

The protective function of the respiratory cilia is well established. Each ciliated epithelial cell bears approximately 275 cilia, and each cilium has nine peripheral and two central fibers anchored to basal corpuscles. Nerves do not supply the ciliated cells; their control mechanism remains unknown. The beat of the cilia, one after another, is rapid, coordinated, and unidirectional, continuously propelling a sheet of mucus (mucous blanket) from the lower respiratory tract upward toward the oropharynx at a rate of approximately 0.33 mm/sec or 2 cm/min. Here the mucus with its entrapped cells and inhaled particles, such as pollens and infectious particles, is eliminated by expectoration or by swallowing into the stomach, where normal gastric acidity and digestive processes render the material harmless.

The mucus produced by the goblet cells and mucous glands floats on a watery subphase layer of unknown origin. Cilia do not beat within the layer of viscous mucus but rather in the low viscosity watery medium, stroking the undersurface of the mucus. The physicochemical properties of this watery fluid affect the ciliary beat in a manner that remains unknown.

Mucociliary clearance, or transport, is effected by the mucous escalator. This function is optimal at normal P_{O_2}, whereas both hyperoxia and hypoxia impair it. Clearance is stimulated by cough and adrenergic bronchodilator drugs, such as epinephrine; it is impaired by drying, for example, by heated but unhumidified indoor air during the winter, and by certain pollutants, such as cigarette smoke.

The mucous blanket plays an important role in protecting the lower airways and alveoli from infection. Antibacterial action has been attributed to enzymes and immunoglobulins found in these secretions. Lysozymes destroy the walls of bacteria and kill the organisms. Other enzymes have also been identified. IgA is the principal immunoglobulin found in normal mucous secretions. Deficiency of such immunoglobulins may contribute to the predisposition of some individuals to recurrent respiratory infections.

COUGH

Cough is an extreme example of high resistance to expiration. The cougher inspires, closes the glottis, performs a Valsalva maneuver, and then suddenly opens the glottis. The enormous transmural pressure collapses the lower trachea. The cartilaginous rings encircle two thirds to three fourths of the trachea; the balance is made up of soft tissue, or the pars membranacea. As air is expelled during cough, this soft tissue invaginates into the tracheal lumen, creating in cross section a crescent moon shape. This "barrel," the trachea, forms itself around the "bullet," the bolus, preventing air from escaping around it and thus conserving the full force of the explosive expiration for expulsion of the bolus.

Cough is a cholinergic vagal reflex, the receptors for which are located mainly in the upper airway. Although the nature of the cough receptors is not completely clear, they are thought to be *mechanoreceptors*. Airflow velocity in the upper airways is probably a critical factor; when these airways constrict to such a degree that airflow velocity exceeds a certain threshold, cough receptors are stimulated, initiating the reflex. The rate of change of stimulus intensity is an important factor in producing cough.

Mechanical, chemical, or physical stimuli initiate the cough reflex. Bronchoconstriction and cough are produced by inhalation of sulfur dioxide (SO_2), inert dust particles 1 to 6 μm in diameter, such as charcoal, citric acid, histamine, and cold air. Transient stretch of the airways is a potent stimulus to cough. Airway constriction caused by mechanical stimulation of the upper airways or by the mucus, edema, and irritation accompanying upper airway infections also stimulates the cough reflex. Stimulation of the external acoustic meatus may also produce cough, a fact that is sometimes of clinical value.

After acute tracheobronchial infections airway reactivity increases transiently; this increase is blocked by the parasympatholytic drug, atropine. Age decreases the sensitivity or increases the threshold of the cough receptors.

Cough serves an important protective function. It clears the airways of secretions that increase airway resistance and removes obstructing foreign matter (secreted or inhaled), thus improving the distribution of inspired gas within the lungs. Because healthy individuals rarely cough, frequent or persistent cough is always a symptom of clinical importance.

Antitussive (cough-suppressing) drugs serve the important purpose of minimizing cough after thoracic or abdominal surgery, when coughing would be painful or even dangerous, and after certain types of eye surgery, when unnecessary movement or transient venous pressure increases should be avoided. Antitussive drugs that have a mild or transient effect are often useful in suppressing cough from acute respiratory tract infections, allowing the patient to rest. However, overzealous use of antitussive agents can be hazardous. Cough may be needed to clear the airways. Potent antitussive drugs should be used only after considering the consequences of depressing airway reactivity and bronchopulmonary reflexes, and used then only with caution.

AIRWAY REACTIVITY

The airway reacts, actively or passively, to a variety of circumstances. The passive reactions are purely mechanical responses to changing transmural pressure. To understand the active responses of the airway, one must know the physiology of its nerve and blood supply. Vagal and sympathetic efferent pathways innervate the conducting airways; sympathetic innervation is relatively less important than parasympathetic innervation. The pulmonary circulation perfuses the peripheral lung units, including terminal bronchioles and alveolar ducts, while the bronchial circulation perfuses conducting airways. Experimentally, bronchial artery injection of a substance being tested for possible airway effect provides better distribution of the test material than aerosol inhalation.

CHAPTER 4

LUNG VOLUME AND ITS SUBDIVISIONS

The lung volume and its subdivisions are basically anatomic measurements; however, alterations in either absolute or relative size may reflect the effects of cardiopulmonary disease. The standard terminology for lung volume and its various subdivisions, or compartments, is given in Fig. 4-1. The term *volume* refers to one of the four primary (nonoverlapping) subdivisions of the total lung capacity; the term *capacity* refers to one of the four lung compartments that is measured by tests of pulmonary function. Each capacity consists of two or more primary volumes. Most of the lung subdivisions are measured from *resting midposition*—the respiratory level of a resting subject who is neither inspiring nor expiring—the thoracic forces tending to expand the chest balance, the lung forces tending to contract it. Midposition defines the volume of gas in the lungs at the end of a spontaneous expiration.

LUNG VOLUMES

Tidal volume (V_T) is the volume of gas added to and then removed from the lungs with each breath; it is usually 500 to 600 ml. Tidal volume comprises the volume entering the alveoli (350 to 450 ml) plus the volume remaining in the airway (150 to 175 ml) per breath. It increases in parallel with increased metabolic rate (O_2 consumption and CO_2 production), for example, in exercise. During mild to moderate exercise V_T increases largely through an increase in the volume of gas in the lungs at the end of inspiration (at the expense of inspiratory reserve volume). During heavy exercise V_T increases further through a decrease in the volume of gas in the lungs at the end of expiration (at the expense of expiratory reserve volume).

Tidal volume in liters multiplied by breathing frequency in breaths per minute gives total pulmonary ventilation rate, $\dot{V}_E$, which is expressed in L (BTPS)/min.

Expiratory reserve volume (ERV) is the maximum volume of gas that can be expired at the end of a spontaneous expiration (from resting midposition); it measures reserve expiratory capability. Expiratory reserve volume reflects thoracic and abdominal muscle strength, thoracic mobility, and the balance of elastic forces that determine midposition at the end of spontaneous expiration.

Residual volume (RV) is the volume of gas that remains in the lungs at the end of a maximal expiration; it is the minimum volume of gas that the lungs can contain if both lungs and thorax are intact. It reflects the balance of elastic forces of lung and thorax, muscle strength affecting expiratory reserve volume, and the volume of extrapulmonary structures in the chest, for example, heart and blood vessels.

Inspiratory reserve volume (IRV) is the maximum volume of gas that can be inhaled at the end of a spontaneous inspiration; it is the reserve available for increasing tidal volume. If midposition does not change, IRV decreases as tidal volume increases. Inspiratory reserve volume reflects the balance between lung and chest elasticity, muscle strength, thoracic mobility, midposition, and tidal volume.

LUNG CAPACITIES

Besides division into the four primary lung compartments, the lung volume is also divided into four *capacities*. Although such a term seems logical, it is not customary to speak of an "expiratory capacity." Measured or calculated by standard technics, three of the capacities provide clinically useful information on the effects of various cardiopulmonary diseases.

Inspiratory capacity (IC) is the maximum volume of air that can be inhaled from midposition and comprises V_T plus IRV. Midposition is a more reproducible level than is the peak of spontaneous inspiration; hence IC is used more commonly than IRV.

Functional residual capacity (FRC) is the volume of gas remaining in the lungs at the end of a spontaneous expiration when lungs and chest are in midposition; it comprises ERV plus RV. During expiration and the ensuing respiratory pause, arterial blood O_2 content decreases as CO_2 content increases. Although detectable with a normal FRC, these fluctuations are small and often ignored. A small FRC results in larger respiratory fluctuations of arterial blood-gas composition as gas exchange proceeds during the period between successive inspirations. Conversely, a large FRC buffers the change of alveolar gas composition in response to changes of alveolar ventilation, inspired gas composition, or metabolic rate. For example, with increased FRC and initially high alveolar P_{CO_2}, either increased alveolar ventilation rate or increased time is required to produce the same decrease of P_{CO_2} as with a normal FRC. The rate at which lung gas composition stabilizes after an abrupt change in the composition of the breathing mixture depends on FRC, breathing frequency, tidal volume, and dead space.

Vital capacity (VC) is the maximum volume of gas that can be exhaled after the deepest possible inspiration. It consists of three subdivisions: IRV, V_T, and ERV. Vital capacity limits the increase of V_T during maximal ventilatory effort. Although the term vital capacity is de-

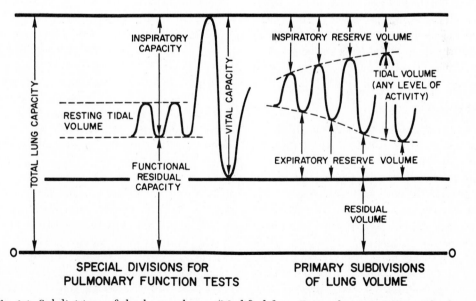

Fig. 4-1. Subdivisions of the lung volume. (Modified from Pappenheimer, J. R., and others: Fed. Proc. **9:**602, 1950.)

fined in this way unless further qualified, there is frequent clinical use for *inspiratory vital capacity*. This term is defined as the maximum volume of gas that can be inhaled after the fullest possible expiration. Although expiratory and inspiratory vital capacities are essentially equal in health, inspiratory vital capacity may be appreciably larger in patients who have diffuse obstructive bronchopulmonary disease.

In 1846 Hutchinson devised the first spirometer and described the compartments of the lung volume. He measured the VC of 2,000 healthy males and of patients with various chest diseases, recognizing that VC increases with height and decreases with age. The average VC of males is larger than that of females; a small difference related to sex remains after correction for difference of body size. However, the two populations overlap. The VC of young adults is roughly proportional to lean body mass.

Total lung capacity (TLC) is the maximum volume of gas that the lungs can contain; it is the sum of IC and FRC as well as the sum of VC and RV. However, TLC is not the volume of air available for gas exchange, nor is it a measure of ventilatory capacity. Conditions that change the component lung *capacities* also affect the TLC.

CHANGES IN LUNG VOLUME AND ITS SUBDIVISIONS

When a standing subject lies down in the supine position, the lung volume and its subdivisions change as blood shifts into the thorax and the weight of the abdominal viscera moves the hemidiaphragms toward the head. Vital capacity usually decreases slightly as a result of increased intrathoracic blood volume, although in some cases there is no measurable change. Application of tourniquets to the lower extremities prevents this decrease. Fig. 4-2 shows the expiratory shift of the resting midposition. Functional residual capacity decreases with ERV as IRV and IC increase. Relative to TLC the lungs are about one-half inflated during quiet breathing in the upright position but only about one-third inflated in the supine posture. Standing on one's head exaggerates these differences. Conversely, standing erect causes a descent of the abdominal viscera and allows the hemidiaphragms to assume a more inspiratory position; FRC and ERV increase at the expense of IRV since V_T is not greatly affected.

The pulmonary circulation contains 500 to 600 ml of blood, a volume that fluctuates slightly during the respiratory cycle. During inspiration there is a slight increase of thoracic blood volume, and during expiration an equal decrease. A forced inspiratory effort (Müller maneuver) or forced expiratory effort (Valsalva maneuver) against a closed glottis produces much larger changes in blood volume. After deep inspiration a forced expiratory effort against the closed glottis squeezes out a volume of blood, leaving room for further inspiration during the next (immediate) inspiratory effort. Such a Valsalva maneuver can increase vital capacity by 200 to 300 ml.

Age changes the lung volume and its subdivisions. As elastic lung recoil diminishes, the resting midposition shifts in the direction of inspiration. This increases FRC, and RV to a lesser degree. The thoracic cage stiffens with age and chest mobility decreases. The greater FRC and decreased chest distensibility limit IC. Thus, VC decreases slightly with age.

The ratio of residual volume to total lung capacity (RV/TLC) has considerable clinical significance; it is usually expressed as a percentage. Normal values range from 15% in young individuals to about 30% in the aged. Many writers give a value as high as 50% for older subjects; however, in our opinion this high value is the result of failure to distinguish between the effects of age and disease. Note that a change of the RV/TLC ratio may reflect a change of either RV or TLC, or both, and that proportionate change of both numerator and denominator in the same direction results in no change of the numeric value of the ratio.

The lung volume and its subdivisions may be

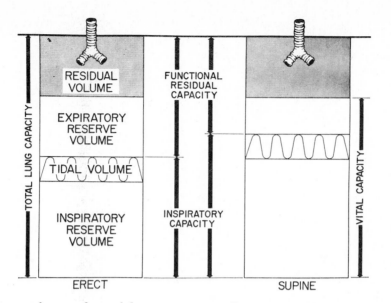

Fig. 4-2. Lung volume and its subdivisions. Diagram illustrates the importance of body position.

very abnormal in patients who have bronchitis-emphysema syndrome. Residual volume may increase by a factor of 2 or 3, and TLC may be 150% or more of that predicted. Since RV increases proportionately more than TLC, the ratio RV/TLC also increases; this ratio may reach 70% in severe cases.

Conditions producing pulmonary fibrosis and lung stiffness, such as tuberculosis, silicosis, and certain viral pneumonias, characteristically reduce TLC and RV, although RV may increase. Thoracic deformity, whether congenital or acquired, reduces TLC and VC. A high proportion of patients who have severe thoracic deformity suffer from chronic alveolar hypoventilation, a condition that usually terminates in cardiopulmonary failure. Since no word existed meaning a condition of reduced thoracic volume, Slonim has proposed the neologism *stethomeiosis*.

MEASUREMENT OF LUNG VOLUME AND ITS SUBDIVISIONS

Since the lung volume and its subdivisions are essentially anatomic compartments within

the chest, their size is expressed in terms of gas volumes at body temperature, ambient pressure, and saturated with water vapor (BTPS). When they are measured or calculated by having a subject exhale into an external container or apparatus that is cooler than body temperature, the exhaled gas volume shrinks and loses water vapor. Such externally measured gas volumes are converted to volume at BTPS.

Some of the subdivisions, or compartments, of the lung volume are measured with a special gas volume recorder termed a *spirometer*. A commonly used type of spirometer is shown in Fig. 4-3. This instrument has a pen that writes on a rotating drum, inscribing a cartesian plot of spirometer gas volume versus time. When gas is blown into the spirometer, the bell rises, lowering the pen that is suspended over a pulley. As gas is inhaled from the spirometer, the bell falls, raising the pen. As a result of the pulley, inspiration produces an upward, and expiration a downward, deflection on the spirographic record. Using the spirometer bell factor (the volume of gas per unit linear dis-

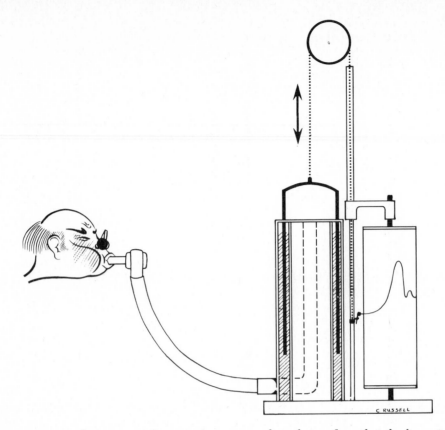

Fig. 4-3. A type of spirometer. Spirometers measure the volume of gas that the lungs inhale and exhale, usually as a function of time. They are used to measure the volume changes and flow rates of spontaneous breathing and various breathing maneuvers.

placement, usually in ml/mm), we can calculate volume changes and thus V_T, IRV, ERV, and VC. A variety of spirometers are available for clinical use. The Stead-Wells, a widely used spirometer, has the pen attached directly to the bell. This reverses the volume tracing so that inspiration is indicated by a *downward* excursion and expiration by an *upward* excursion of the pen.

Spirometers also measure the capacity for dynamic changes of lung volume; that is, they measure the volumetric flow rate of gas into and out of the lung. The forced expiratory spirogram (Fig. 4-4) is a useful clinical tool for the evaluation of pulmonary function.

Loss of ventilatory capacity is of two types: (1) reduced volume of gas that can be moved per breath (restrictive loss) and (2) reduced maximal flow rate of gas during a breath (obstructive loss). Restrictive loss occurs in patients who have diminished lung or chest wall elasticity—the result, for example, of pulmonary fibrosis. Obstructive loss occurs in patients who have diffuse airways obstruction—the result, for example, of asthma or bronchitis-emphysema syndrome. Analysis and interpretation of the spirogram are discussed in Chapter 17.

FRC, RV, and TLC cannot be measured with a spirometer because these compartments

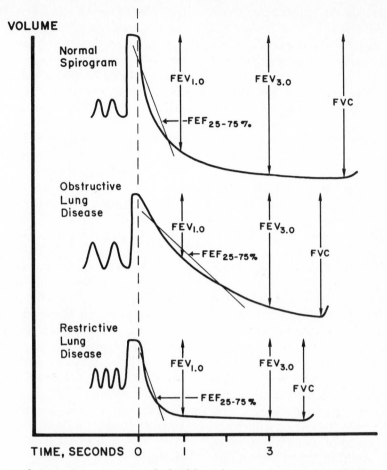

Fig. 4-4. Forced expiratory spirogram of a healthy subject (top), a patient with chronic diffuse obstructive bronchopulmonary disease (middle), and a patient with restrictive ventilatory impairment (bottom).

contain gas that cannot be expelled from the lungs. Any of three indirect methods can be used to calculate them. The closed-circuit method involves the dilution of an inert, insoluble, foreign gas (usually helium) as it mixes with the gas in the lungs. The subject breathes into a sealed spirometer system of precisely known volume, containing a known initial concentration of helium. As the gas in the spirometer mixes with the gas in the lungs, helium concentration in the spirometer circuit gradually decreases to a new level. The volume of O_2

taken up by the subject from the spirometer during the test is either replaced by continuous O_2 inflow or otherwise corrected. The CO_2 exhaled into the spirometer is removed by absorption. The following equation is then used to calculate the volume of gas in the lung at the beginning of the test:

$$V_L = \left(V_{Sp} \times \frac{He_{initial}}{He_{final}} \right) - V_{Sp} + C$$

where V_L is the initial lung volume, V_{Sp} is the spirometer volume, $He_{initial}$ is the initial concentration of helium in the spirometer, He$_{final}$ is the final concentration of helium in both lung and spirometer, and C is a correction factor that cancels the apparent change of gas volume in the lungs caused by N$_2$ "excretion" and helium absorption. The calculated gas volume must be converted from the basis of ATPS to BTPS. When this method is used, the initial lung volume is usually FRC, from which ERV is subtracted to obtain RV, or to which IC is added to obtain TLC.

In bronchospirometry a special endobronchial catheter separates the gas flows and volumes of the two lungs, permitting individual measurement of lung volumes, ventilation, and O$_2$ uptake. Normally, the right lung accounts for 55% and the left lung for 45% of volume, ventilation, and gas exchange.

The open-circuit nitrogen wash-out method for determining functional residual capacity* involves measuring the N$_2$ concentration in a sample of alveolar gas, washing out the lung N$_2$ with O$_2$, and measuring the quantity of N$_2$ that was contained in the lung volume (FRC). The subject is connected to a one-way breathing system while in the resting midposition and begins to breathe pure O$_2$. The mixed expired gas is collected for a period of 7 minutes or more, depending on the expected rate of lung mixing. All the N$_2$ must be washed out during the collection period. At the end of the wash-out period, a final alveolar gas sample is taken for measurement of the N$_2$ concentration. From the volume of expired gas and its N$_2$ concentration, we can calculate the total volume of N$_2$ that was washed out of the lungs during the period of O$_2$ breathing. Using the difference between the initial and the final alveolar N$_2$ concentration and the volume of N$_2$ washed out of the lungs, we can calculate the lung volume in which that N$_2$ was contained (FRC). A correction is made for the volume of N$_2$ brought to the lungs by the blood from body stores during the wash-out period.

A third method of measuring FRC uses a body plethysmograph, or "body box." The subject is placed within a gas-tight chamber of about 600 L, slightly smaller than a telephone booth, and breathes fresh air through a communication to the outside. After temperature and humidity within the chamber have stabilized, the subject compresses the gas in the lungs by blowing against a pressure transducer that blocks the breathing line. The resulting volume changes within the sealed box produce corresponding pressure changes within the box that are sensed by a second pressure transducer and recorded for each effort. The pressure decreases in the gas-tight box as a result of compressing air in the lungs according to Boyle's law, PV = K. The volume calibration procedure consists of introducing a known volume of air into the sealed box with the subject inside and measuring the resulting pressure change. The sensitivity of the system (Δ ml/Δ cm H$_2$O pressure) is used together with the pressure change that results from lung gas compression to calculate the change of lung volume during the lung compression maneuver. The measured volume and pressure changes within the lung, together with the known initial ambient pressure, permit calculation of the total thoracic gas volume (V$_{TG}$) and FRC.

The first two methods, closed-circuit helium dilution and open-circuit nitrogen wash-out, measure *communicating* gas volume in the lungs, that is, the lung gas that can mix with the breathing mixture. By contrast, the body plethysmograph measures *total* intrathoracic gas volume, including gas that is and gas that is not in communication with the alveoli. Thus, the body plethysmographic measurement includes any *intraabdominal* gas that is present in the intestines or stomach. This gas is measured because it also is compressed by the ex-

---

*For further discussion of the open-circuit nitrogen wash-out method, see Chapter 17.

piratory effort against the transducer during the test.

Total thoracic gas volume, as measured in the body plethysmograph, is usually the same or slightly larger than FRC measured by the helium dilution or nitrogen wash-out methods. However, in chronic diffuse obstructive lung disease in which there is air trapping, in conditions in which there are regions of very slow gas mixing, or in pneumothorax, there may be considerable difference between V_{TG} and FRC. This possibility must be considered in the clinical interpretation of FRC measurement.

CHAPTER 5

BREATHING PATTERNS AND VENTILATION

Breathing is the alternate inspiration and expiration of air into and out of the lungs. *Ventilation* is the volume of air moved into or out of the lungs per unit time and is calculated as the product of breathing frequency (f) and tidal volume (V_T). Our definition of breathing does not include the process of gas exchange essential for effective breathing.

PATTERNS OF BREATHING

Several patterns of breathing are sufficiently significant and distinctive to be designated by special terms and discussed as entities. Certain abnormal patterns of breathing are described at the end of Chapter 13.

Eupnea is normal spontaneous breathing of which we are usually unaware. Ventilation satisfies metabolic demand. The frequency of breathing, f, at rest is 13 to 17 breaths/min, with a V_T of about 500 to 600 ml (BTPS). Normal resting pulmonary ventilation rate (minute volume of breathing) is thus about 7.5 L (BTPS)/min.

Hyperpnea is the increased pulmonary ventilation that matches an increased metabolic demand. For example, muscular exercise increases pulmonary ventilation by increasing both f and V_T. As a healthy trained subject exercises more and more intensely, pulmonary ventilation rate increases initially more by contributions from increased V_T than by contributions from f; later, increases of f contribute proportionately more.

Hyperventilation also describes increased pulmonary ventilation but refers to ventilation that *exceeds* metabolic requirements. Hyperventilation is defined variously in terms of total pulmonary ventilation, alveolar ventilation, or alveolar P_{CO_2}. It may be produced by thoracic reflexes, conscious voluntary effort, or psychogenic factors (for example, hysterical hyperventilation). In the healthy subject, alveolar hyperventilation decreases arterial blood P_{CO_2} and increases arterial blood P_{O_2} slightly; hyperpnea does not.

Hypoventilation means underventilation in relation to the metabolic rate. For example, a total pulmonary ventilation rate of 8 L (BTPS)/min may be adequate at rest but constitutes hypoventilation during even mild exercise. Like hyperventilation, hypoventilation is defined in terms of total pulmonary ventilation, alveolar ventilation, or alveolar P_{CO_2}. Hypoventilation always increases alveolar P_{CO_2} and, when the inspired gas is air, is the only condition that does this. Hypoventilation is only one of several conditions that decrease arterial blood P_{O_2}. In bronchopulmonary diseases causing uneven distribution of inspired gas, some lung regions may be hyperventilated, whereas others are hypoventilated.

Tachypnea is increased rate, or frequency, of breathing; it does not necessarily imply a change of total pulmonary ventilation. If total pulmonary ventilation does increase, tachypnea may occur with either hyperpnea or hyperventilation; if total pulmonary ventilation decreases because of concomitant decrease of tidal volume, tachypnea may actually occur with hypoventilation.

Dyspnea is difficult or labored breathing. It is defined as the uncomfortable subjective awareness of the desire for increased breathing. Dyspnea is thus a symptom, not a sign. Clinically, it is usually associated with increased work of breathing as, for example, in chronic diffuse obstructive lung diseases. However, it is also experienced by patients who have congestive heart failure or psychogenic hyperventilation. Curiously, it is not directly related to chronic hypoxemia and hypercapnic acidosis. It is likely that a healthy trained subject does not experience true dyspnea even during the most extreme physical exertion, possibly because such exertion is not associated with the subjective component of anxiety.

Orthopnea refers to dyspnea that is experienced only in recumbency (usually supine) and is promptly relieved by assuming an upright position. Clinically, orthopneic patients usually have one of several conditions: congestive heart failure, severe asthma, severe lung failure, or occasionally severe anxiety. Orthopnea is remarkably absent in most patients who have bronchopulmonary diseases, including chronic obstructive lung diseases even when associated with cor pulmonale. The upright position relieves lung congestion in the cardiac patient and provides a mechanical advantage for making optimal use of the accessory muscles of respiration, decreasing pulmonary blood volume and increasing vital capacity in asthmatic patients and those with lung failure.

Apnea is the absence or cessation of breathing, usually in the resting midposition. It connotes temporary cessation with the expectation that breathing will resume spontaneously. Apnea occurs during swallowing and sleep, after hyperventilation, as a result of trauma, and sometimes at birth. If breathing does not resume, the condition is termed *respiratory arrest*.

DEAD SPACE

It was realized in the 19th century that the last portion of each inspired breath does not reach the alveoli where gas exchange takes place. The volume of the *anatomic dead space* was estimated from postmortem casts of the respiratory tract. Anatomic dead space is the volume of all the non–gas-exchanging airways from the nose (or mouth during mouth-breathing) down to the respiratory bronchioles and alveoli.

The concept that a portion of the inspired air is delivered to alveoli in which gas exchange is incomplete, thus adding an *alveolar dead space* to the ineffective portion of each V_T, developed in the 1930s. The sum of these two volumes— the *physiologic* dead space—defines the portion of each inspiration that does not equilibrate with gas pressures in the pulmonary capillary blood.

In any lung there exists a broad spectrum of alveoli having different ventilation and blood flow relationships. Thus, some alveoli are hypoventilated while others are hyperventilated with respect to the ventilation required to accomplish gas exchange and equilibrate alveolar and arterial blood-gas pressures. Despite this spectrum, dead space is calculated as if alveoli were either optimally ventilated and perfused (complete equilibration) or not perfused at all (no gas exchange). Thus, V_D is a *theoretic* or *virtual*, rather than *actual*, volume—the volume of inspirate that would return to the atmosphere unchanged if all air undergoing *any* gas exchange achieved complete equilibrium with pulmonary end-capillary blood.

Calculation of anatomic dead space

If all the CO_2 expelled from the lungs comes only from alveolar gas (none is considered to come from dead space air), the rate of CO_2 production can be calculated from either alveolar or expired gas analysis:

$$\dot{V}_{CO_2} = F_{E_{CO_2}} \times \dot{V}_E = F_{A_{CO_2}} \times \dot{V}_A \qquad (1)$$

The same relationship exists for a single breath. Converting the relationship to one for V_T gives:

$$F_{E_{CO_2}} \times V_T = F_{A_{CO_2}} \times (V_T - V_D) \qquad (2)$$

Rearranging the equation:

$$F_{A_{CO_2}} \times V_D = (F_{A_{CO_2}} \times V_T) - (F_{E_{CO_2}} \times V_T) \qquad (3)$$

$$F_{A_{CO_2}} \times V_D = V_T (F_{A_{CO_2}} - F_{E_{CO_2}}) \qquad (4)$$

The equation can be used to calculate $F_{A_{CO_2}}$ if V_D is known or to calculate V_D if $F_{A_{CO_2}}$ is known. It was developed by Bohr in the 19th century to calculate $F_{A_{CO_2}}$ from an assumed value for dead space. However, in 1905 Haldane found that the composition of alveolar gas is relatively uniform (within the limits of his analytic ability), and he used the Bohr equation to calculate dead space after measuring expired gas and alveolar CO_2 concentrations and V_T. If the gas concentration of inspired air is measured and substituted in equation (5) below, the equation for dead space can be generalized and applied to any gas (G) taken up or given off in the lungs:

$$V_D = V_T \times \frac{F_{A_G} - F_{E_G}}{F_{A_G} - F_{I_G}} \qquad (5)$$

where G is the gas used to measure anatomic V_D.

The Fowler technic for measuring anatomic V_D is a graphic method based on analyzing a rapidly responding CO_2 concentration curve and relating the pattern of change to the ex-

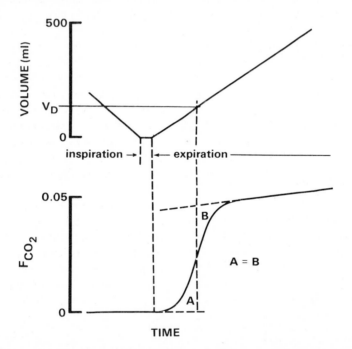

Fig. 5-1. Diagrammatic illustration of the Fowler method for measuring anatomic dead space. The lower tracing is a record of expiratory F_{CO_2} and the upper tracing is a record of tidal volume (V_T). The vertical dashed line bisecting the sigmoid portion of the F_{CO_2} curve represents the theoretic front that would be seen if all dead space (nonequilibrated) air were expelled first, followed only by alveolar (completely equilibrated) gas. The front is defined as the vertical line located where area A equals area B. The volume of expired gas coinciding with this theoretic front equals anatomic dead space (V_D) and is measured on the V_T record.

pired volume (Fig. 5-1). The curve has three phases, reflecting (1) expiration of dead space air that has the composition of inspired air (assumed to contain no CO_2 if air is breathed), (2) a sigmoid transition from dead space air to alveolar gas because of variable pathway lengths and longitudinal mixing of alveolar and dead space gas during expiration, and (3) a CO_2 plateau representing alveolar gas concentration. At rest, the plateau usually has a slight positive slope related to some nonuniformity of alveolar gas composition and shifts in the evenness of regional lung emptying. In patients who have certain lung diseases, the plateau may be so uneven that the method is unreliable for estimation of anatomic V_D.

Physiologic dead space is calculated from measurements of P_{CO_2} in mixed expired gas and arterial blood. Arterial blood P_{CO_2} is assumed to be equilibrated with the alveolar gas in each region of the lung; hence, an arterial blood sample represents mean alveolar P_{CO_2}. The $P_{a_{CO_2}}$, which is assumed equal to $P_{A_{CO_2}}$, is compared with the P_{CO_2} of mixed expired gas $(P_{E_{CO_2}})$. The P_{CO_2} of the expired gas which is saturated with water vapor at lung temperature is calculated as follows:

$$P_{E_{CO_2}} = F_{E_{CO_2}} \times (P_B - 47) \tag{6}$$

where P_B is the barometric pressure and 47 is the water vapor pressure in torr for air saturated at 37° C. Substituting CO_2 pressures for fractional concentration in equation (5), and assuming that inspired P_{CO_2} is 0, gives the equation for physiologic dead space:

$$V_D = V_T \times \frac{(P_{a_{CO_2}} - P_{E_{CO_2}})}{P_{a_{CO_2}}} \tag{7}$$

Factors affecting anatomic dead space

Size of subject. Radford predicted anatomic V_D from body weight; for a subject of normal stature, V_D in milliliters approximately equals body weight in pounds. However, V_D does not parallel body weight in obesity and it is probably a poor estimate of V_D in children. A better estimate is based on body height, a relationship that holds from birth to adulthood.

Age. Anatomic V_D increases slightly with age. This change probably reflects loss of elasticity and increased lung volume, rather than a direct effect on the larger airways.

Position of the head. In conscious subjects, the V_D is increased by extending the neck and pushing the jaw forward. With the neck flexed and the chin depressed, anatomic V_D can be reduced to about half the value of the former position. Unfortunately, airway resistance is highest in the head positions that provide the smallest V_D; thus, effects on ventilation are not predictably related to head or jaw position.

Drugs. Anatomic V_D increases after vagotomy or administration of ganglionic blocking agents. Bronchoconstrictor agents decrease V_D. Histamine has a direct effect on the airway muscle, but some drugs, such as neostigmine, act only through vagal pathways and do not affect the increased V_D that follows vagotomy. Anesthetic agents alter V_D according to their general effect on the autonomic nervous system. For example, V_D increases during halothane anesthesia but is decreased by the anesthetic gas nitrous oxide.

Breathing pattern. Changes of breathing pattern strongly affect anatomic V_D. Increasing tidal volume increases V_D. The greater end-inspiratory lung volume causes a greater distending pressure (transpulmonary pressure increases) that stretches the elastic airways as well as the lung. A V_D increase of about 20 ml accompanies each 1-L increase of end-inspiratory lung volume above normal.

Changing breathing frequency also has a significant effect on the measured anatomic V_D. Frequency (or flow rate) changes affect the measured value in several ways. Increasing frequency increases measured V_D. A decrease in the time available for longitudinal movement of alveolar gas into the airway after the end of inspiration contributes to the effect. Besides diffusion of gases, the oscillatory action resulting from the heartbeat mixes alveolar gas with airway dead space air. This effect is more pronounced at low flow rates and during periods when breath is held. During oscillatory mixing, alveolar gas pressure remains in equilibrium with that in the pulmonary capillaries, $F_{A_{CO_2}}$ remains high, and a decreased V_D is calculated.

At high breathing frequencies, particularly when V_T and airflow velocity are high, there may be insufficient time for equilibration of gases between inspired air and alveolar gas before expiration begins. Thus, alveolar gas composition may fluctuate, and the first portion of alveolar gas to be expired may resemble a mixture of inspired (dead space) air and alveolar gas (low CO_2 concentration).

The measurement of anatomic V_D is also complicated by laminar flow in the airways. The velocity profile of laminar gas flow in a tube is parabolic; thus, a central tongue of alveolar gas reaches the mouth early during expiration (the phenomenon reverses during inspiration). Particularly with the Fowler graphic technic, this phenomenon can produce an error if the slow expiration of dead space air from distal airways is mistaken for the slope of the alveolar plateau.

It is important to recognize the effect of anatomic V_D on alveolar ventilation, since V_D can vary greatly. For example, during rapid breathing the measured V_D can become increasingly large and can even exceed anatomically feasible limits with very rapid breaths. It can also be smaller than anatomically feasible if measured after a breath-hold period or during very slow breathing.

It is well known that certain patients whose V_T is less than their anatomic V_D are able to ventilate their alveoli and animals that pant in hot environments have tidal volumes considerably less than anatomic V_D. This occurs because of high air velocity in the center of the airway and the longitudinal parabolic front of the inspired air column. Hence, some alveolar ventilation occurs even with small tidal volumes, and gas exchange proceeds with what would appear to be zero alveolar ventilation based on V_T and V_D calculations.

Factors affecting alveolar dead space

Alveolar dead space is the difference between physiologic and anatomic dead space. It is thus that portion of the inspired gas that reaches the alveoli but does not undergo gas exchange. This is primarily the result of underperfusion of the affected alveoli. Alveolar V_D is too small to be measured in healthy subjects, particularly young people, but can become large enough to interfere with alveolar ventilation in patients who have certain lung diseases, even though total pulmonary ventilation is high.

Most alveolar dead space changes result from abnormal ventilation–blood flow relationships in the affected alveoli; it results from ventilation of underperfused lung regions. As explained in a later section, there is nonuniform distribution of both ventilation and perfusion, the distribution of perfusion being the more uneven. When maldistribution is severe enough, alveolar dead space increases.

In pulmonary arterial hypotension, the uppermost lung regions are poorly perfused. Thus, alveolar dead space increases in hemorrhagic blood loss, head-up tilt, and elevated airway pressure in the upright position (for example, positive end-expiratory pressure ventilatory assistance to a seated subject). On the other hand, recumbency decreases alveolar dead space because lung perfusion is more even and more closely matched to the distribution of ventilation in that body position.

Increased dead space accompanies pulmonary embolism, an occlusion of a branch or branches of the pulmonary artery. Some clinicians consider a V_D to V_T ratio of 60% or more one of the criteria for diagnosis of pulmonary embolism, but many false positives occur in patients who have circulatory failure. Obstruction of regional vessels by masses or external forces also increases dead space. Inadequate perfusion of ventilated lung regions occurs in destructive lung diseases and in those disturbing distribution of ventilation and/or blood flow.

Dead space terminology

There is general agreement on the use of the term anatomic dead space; however, some people prefer the term *total* or *effective* dead space to *physiologic* dead space. The reasoning follows: when physiologic dead space exceeds anatomic dead space appreciably, the difference is largely pathologic. The conventional term physiologic dead space includes the pathologic alveolar dead space that results from disease, the alveolar dead space that results from ventilation/perfusion mismatching, and the anatomic dead space.

ALVEOLAR VENTILATION

Alveolar ventilation, also termed *effective ventilation*, is the volume of fresh air introduced into the gas-exchanging regions of the lung per minute. At the end of expiration the conducting airways are filled with alveolar gas, a volume of gas that returns to the alveoli at the beginning of the next inspiration but cannot participate further in gas exchange because it has already done so. The *effective* volume of each inspiration is thus tidal volume minus dead space volume. Total pulmonary ventilation rate, or minute volume of breathing, is the product of volume per breath and breaths per minute. For total ventilation rate (volume expired per minute):

$$\dot{V}_E = V_E \times f \qquad (8)$$

For dead space ventilation rate:

$$\dot{V}_D = V_D \times f \qquad (9)$$

For alveolar ventilation rate:

$$\dot{V}_A = \dot{V}_E - \dot{V}_D = (V_E - V_D) \times f \qquad (10)$$

Dead space ventilation rate is the difference between total ventilation rate ($\dot{V}_E$) and alveolar ventilation rate ($\dot{V}_A$). Since only small dead space changes occur as a result of V_T changes (about 3% of the V_T change), an alteration of dead space ventilation associated with a changing breathing pattern is largely the result of a change of f. If V_T remains unchanged, dead space ventilation rate increases with f.

There is almost a linear relationship between f and $\dot{V}_D$. Over a considerable range a certain percentage change of f produces a similar change of $\dot{V}_D$. If f doubles, for example, from 13 to 26, then $\dot{V}_D$ also approximately doubles. With a normal (unchanged) V_T of 500 ml and a V_D of 150 ml, $\dot{V}_E$ would increase from 6.5 L/min to 13.0 L/min and $\dot{V}_D$ would parallel that change, increasing from 1.95 L/min to 3.9 L/min. $\dot{V}_A$ would also double, increasing from 4.55 L/min to 9.1 L/min.

On the other hand, if $\dot{V}_E$ doubles as a result of increasing V_T rather than f, the effect on $\dot{V}_A$ is somewhat different. If V_D remains unchanged (consider it to be unaffected by the increase of V_T) and if f remains constant at 13 L/min, then when V_T doubles, $\dot{V}_E$ also doubles, from 6.5 L/min to 13 L/min, but $\dot{V}_D$ remains constant at 1.95 L/min. As a result, V_A *more* than doubles, increasing from 4.55 L/min to 11.05 L/min.

In pulmonary disease the response to a change of $\dot{V}_A$ is a change of either V_T or f, depending on the condition. Chronic obstructive bronchopulmonary disease increases expiratory airway resistance and the work of breathing. In this situation, the most *economical* way to increase $\dot{V}_A$ is for V_T to increase and breathing frequency to remain as low as possible. By contrast, in pulmonary fibrosis, characterized by stiff lungs that require increased energy for inflation, airway resistance is not increased and a more economical pattern of breathing is an increased f with V_T as small as possible.

The ventilation equation

During a steady state of the circulation and ventilation, the rate of metabolic CO_2 production is constant and equals the rate of CO_2 elimination (without a change in the body stores of CO_2). CO_2 production is the product of $\dot{V}_A$ and $F_{A_{CO_2}}$, as shown in equation (1). $F_{A_{CO_2}}$ can be converted to $P_{A_{CO_2}}$ in the same way as shown in equation (6) for expired gas:

$$P_{A_{CO_2}} = F_{A_{CO_2}} \times (P_B - 47) \qquad (11)$$

Solving this equation for $F_{A_{CO_2}}$ and substituting for $F_{A_{CO_2}}$ in equation (1):

$$\dot{V}_{CO_2} = \frac{P_{A_{CO_2}}}{(P_B - 47)} \times \dot{V}_A \qquad (12)$$

$$\dot{V}_{CO_2} \times (P_B - 47) = P_{A_{CO_2}} \times \dot{V}_A \qquad (13)$$

If metabolic rate does not change, $\dot{V}_{CO_2}$ is relatively constant, and the product $P_{A_{CO_2}} \times \dot{V}_A$ is a constant:

$$P_{A_{CO_2}} \times \dot{V}_A = K \text{ (for constant } \dot{V}_{CO_2}) \qquad (14)$$

Thus, $P_{A_{CO_2}}$ and $\dot{V}_A$ are reciprocals. Assuming no change in $\dot{V}_{CO_2}$, if a subject hyperventilates to such a degree that $\dot{V}_A$ doubles, $P_{A_{CO_2}}$ is re-

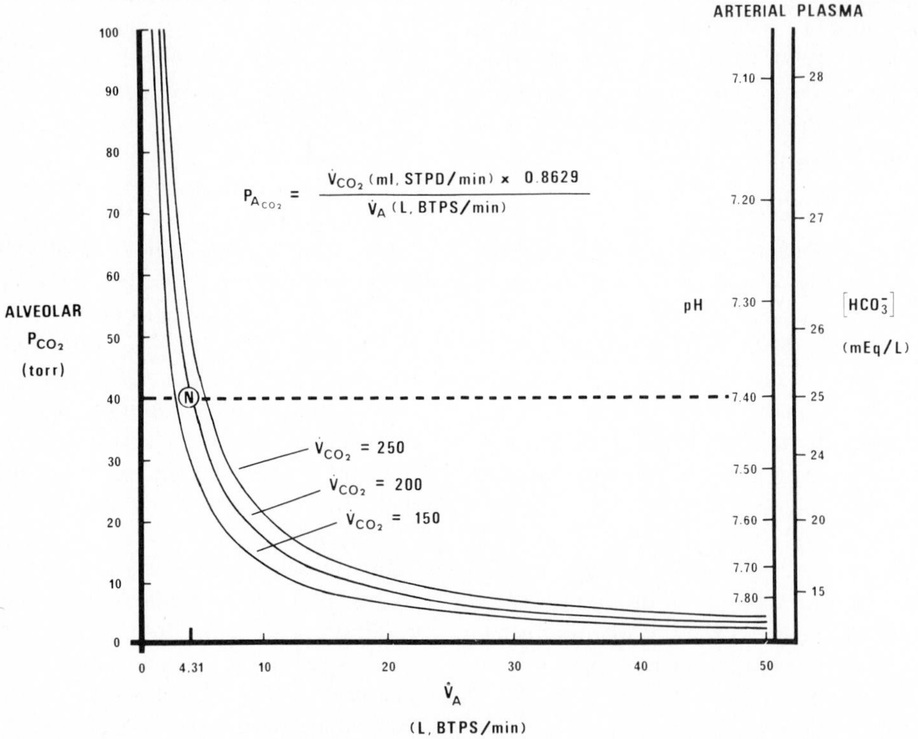

Fig. 5-2. Alveolar P_{CO_2} as a function of alveolar ventilation rate. This graph shows the constancy of the product $\dot{V}_A \times P_{A_{CO_2}}$ when CO_2 output ($\dot{V}_{CO_2}$) is constant. The rectangular hyperbolic relationship also shows how greatly $P_{A_{CO_2}}$ is affected by changing $\dot{V}_A$. If regional $P_{A_{CO_2}}$ does not change with changing $\dot{V}_A$, then regional CO_2 output ($\dot{V}_{CO_2}$) is proportional to $\dot{V}_A$.

duced to half. If the subject hypoventilates so that $\dot{V}_A$ is halved, $P_{A_{CO_2}}$ doubles. This relationship is shown graphically in Fig. 5-2 and can also be seen in Fig. 11-2 by comparing ventilation ratio with P_{CO_2}. Because in health alveolar and arterial blood P_{CO_2} are equal, the effect of acute P_{CO_2} changes on arterial plasma pH and bicarbonate ion concentration can be shown on the right vertical axes of Fig. 5-2.

Since the ratio of CO_2 production to oxygen consumption during a steady state is defined as R_s, CO_2 output equals CO_2 production and oxygen uptake equals O_2 consumption:

$$R_s = \frac{\dot{V}_{CO_2}}{\dot{V}_{O_2}} \text{ and } \dot{V}_{CO_2} = \dot{V}_{O_2} \times R_s \qquad (15)$$

If R_s is known and $F_{A_{CO_2}}$ and $\dot{V}_A$ can be measured, R_s can be combined with the ventilation equation for calculation of O_2 consumption:

$$\dot{V}_{O_2} = \frac{\dot{V}_A \times P_{A_{CO_2}}}{R_s (P_B - 47)} \qquad (16)$$

It is more convenient to use $\dot{V}_E$ (which must be measured to calculate $\dot{V}_A$ anyway) and to measure $F_{E_{CO_2}}$ from the collected expired gas (expressed as a fraction of *dry* gas):

$$\dot{V}_{O_2} = \frac{\dot{V}_E \times F_{E_{CO_2}}}{R_s} \qquad (17)$$

Since $\dot{V}_{O_2}$ is always expressed in terms of STPD, it is necessary to correct $\dot{V}_E$ for temperature and pressure before making the calculation. Because $F_{E_{CO_2}}$ is expressed on a dry gas basis, a correction for water vapor pressure is not necessary. The correct equation for calculation of O_2 consumption based on expired gas measurements is:

$$\dot{V}_{O_2} \text{ (STPD)} = \frac{\dot{V}_E \text{ (BTPS)} \times F_{E_{CO_2}}}{R_s} \times \qquad (18)$$
$$\frac{273 \times P_B}{(273 + T° C) \times 760}$$

CHAPTER 6

MECHANICS OF BREATHING

THE BREATHING CYCLE

Ventilation is a periodic phenomenon in which a volume of fresh air enters the lungs and undergoes gas exchange, after which an approximately equal volume of gas (called the tidal volume, or V_T) composed of mixed inspired air and alveolar gas is exhaled into the atmosphere. The beginning of the breathing cycle is considered to be the start of inspiration from the resting expiratory level, when a volume of gas defined as functional residual capacity (FRC) is in the lungs. The period of the cycle, measured in seconds, is defined as the interval between successive inspiratory maneuvers. The inverse of the period is the breathing frequency (f), expressed in breaths per minute (rather than fractions of breaths per second, which would result if units for the period were retained).

Total pulmonary ventilation rate (expiratory), or $\dot{V}_E$ (liters per minute), is the product of V_T (milliliters per breath) and f (breaths per minute) divided by 1,000 (a conversion from milliliters to liters):

$$\dot{V}_E = f \times \frac{V_T}{1,000} \qquad (1)$$

$\dot{V}_E$ varies less than either f or V_T, which means that a general reciprocal relationship exists between the two determinants of ventilation. When f is high, V_T tends to be smaller; when V_T is large, f tends to be smaller.

Breathing involves a smooth transition between inspiration, expiration, and the pauses between, but our discussion at this point will treat each of them individually in order to present a clear description of the mechanics of breathing. Their integration into a smooth breathing pattern and regulated ventilation is described in Chapter 13.

ANATOMIC BASIS FOR LUNG VOLUME CHANGE

The volume of the thorax can increase in three dimensions: vertical, lateral, and anterior-posterior (a-p). Although the vertical diameter varies most, because of movement of the hemidiaphragms, the lateral and a-p diameters ordinarily increase together and result in volume changes that can amount to as much as 40% of total lung volume change, depending on the body position (standing, sitting, or supine) or the level from which the lung volume change is measured (from maximal expiration or from FRC). Thus, changes of thoracic volume in all directions are important for inducing lung volume changes.

The upper portion of the thorax is somewhat irregularly conical, sloping forward, with the insertions of the ribs on the sternum lower than their origins on the spine. These upper ribs can rotate around a transverse axis that elevates their anterior ends, thus lifting the sternum. This elevation increases the a-p dimension of the thorax and is called the "water pump handle" effect. The lower ribs share little in the increase of the a-p dimension because they have less downward direction from origin to insertion.

All mobile ribs (from the second to the 10th) have a second axis of rotation around the lateral dimension described from their origin on the spine to their insertion on the sternum (the 11th and 12th ribs do not insert on the sternum and do not rotate). Since the middle of the rib lies below the line of rotation, a lateral rotation causes their elevation and an outward movement of the rib cage. This increased lateral dimension caused by lifting of the ribs is called the "water bucket handle" effect.

The diaphragm forms a muscular lower margin of the thorax. It normally functions as a continuous unit, but the right and left halves have their own innervation and each is served by its respective phrenic nerve. Interference with impulse transmission in one phrenic nerve affects only that hemidiaphragm. For these reasons it is often necessary to speak of the two *hemidiaphragms.*

The hemidiaphragms are tendinous in the center, but muscular at the periphery. They are inserted along the lumbar vertebrae and muscles of the back, on the lower ribs laterally and on the xiphoid process of the sternum anteriorly. The hemidiaphragms are strikingly domed, with the muscle fibers oriented almost vertically near the insertion. Their central tendons therefore are pulled downward during contraction, increasing the vertical dimension of the thorax. To be consistent with the analogy for other dimensional changes in thoracic size, this increased length of the thoracic cavity might be called the "bicycle pump handle" effect.

INSPIRATION

The processes just described for increasing the dimensions of the thorax in all three directions occur during inspiration. The external intercostal muscles are largely responsible for increases in both the a-p and the lateral directions because of the shape of the ribs and the oblique orientation of these muscles between the ribs. The diaphragm is of course responsible for expansion in the longitudinal dimension.

During hyperpnea or dyspnea the auxiliary muscles of inspiration come into play. Contraction of the scalene muscles elevates the upper ribs, which also lifts the rest of the thorax. The sternocleidomastoid muscles elevate the sternum. Although other muscle groups might assist in vigorous inspiratory efforts, these two groups are more commonly considered to be the auxiliary muscles of inspiration. When ventilation is increased greatly, other muscles related to the pharynx, larynx, and nasal passages come into play, reducing resistance to airflow and thereby allowing high levels of ventilation.

EXPIRATION

Expiration is usually passive. A continuous "braking" action caused by a sustained but reduced inspiratory muscle tone slows expiration and smooths the transition between inspiration and expiration. Inspiratory muscles relax completely only near the end of expiration. Only when expiration is vigorous because of hyperpnea or difficult because of obstruction is expiratory force increased by activating expiratory muscle groups. The internal intercostal muscles have an oblique orientation opposite to that of the external intercostals. This orientation is such that contraction tends to move the ribs closer together and rotate them downward, thereby reducing both the a-p and lateral dimensions of the thorax. (Interchondral interosseous muscles are also included as internal intercostal muscles.) These muscle groups are of considerable importance when the diaphragm is paralyzed and during coughing.

The abdominal muscles can also contribute to active expiration when it is needed. Abdominal muscles ordinarily include the external oblique, rectoabdominal, internal oblique, and transverse abdominal muscles. Their contraction increases abdominal pressure by depressing the lower ribs, flexing the trunk, and flattening the abdomen. This pushes the diaphragm upward and assists in forced expiration. The effect is to accelerate the expiratory flow rate and to decrease the end-expiratory lung volume by moving the diaphragm farther upward into the thorax than would occur if expiration were entirely passive.

RELAXATION FORCES

Both lungs and chest wall have elasticity, and in the intact thorax each is deformed by the elastic pull of the other. If removed from the enclosing chest wall, the lungs contract to a much smaller size; freed from the opposing elastic force of the lungs, the chest expands to a larger volume. When lungs and chest wall are in normal relationship, with their pleurae in contact and no external force applied, the resting lung volume reflects the balance between these two opposing elastic forces, the FRC (Chapter 4).

Because the elastic forces of lungs and chest wall oppose each other, the interface between visceral and parietal pleurae (potential intrapleural space) is at subatmospheric ("negative") pressure. If this intrapleural interface develops a communication with the outside air or with intrapulmonary gas, gas moves into the "negative" intrapleural pressure region, creating an actual intrapleural space, or pneumothorax.

It is reasonable to ask why air (or a component of respiratory gas) does not respond to the "negative" pressure and diffuse into the intra-

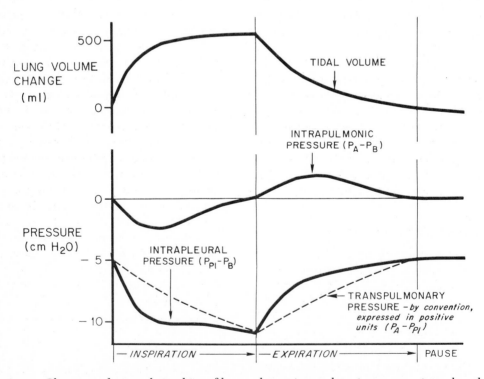

Fig. 6-1. Changes and interrelationships of lung volume, intrapulmonic pressure, intrapleural pressure, and transpulmonary pressure during a breathing cycle.

pleural space. The total pressure of gases in equilibrium with the tissues (and the potential spaces associated with those tissues) is less than atmospheric, so a reverse pressure difference exists. Gas pressure in tissues is actually less than the pressure in the intrapleural space. This can be explained on the basis of the shape of the O_2 dissociation curve and the CO_2 dissociation curve of blood. This is discussed in detail in Chapter 10.

Breathing and body position both change intrapleural pressure. With the trunk erect, gravity pulls the abdominal contents down, pushing out the abdominal wall. The hemidiaphragms descend, and the volume of the chest cavity increases. During recumbency, gravity pulls the abdominal contents toward the head, decreasing the volume of the chest cavity and increasing intrapleural pressure.

The idealized relationships among lung volume change and intrapulmonic, intrapleural, and transpulmonary pressures for a normal spontaneous breathing cycle are shown in Fig. 6-1. It is important to recognize that intrapulmonic and intrapleural pressures are measured and expressed as differences from atmospheric (barometric) pressure. Transpulmonary pressure is, by convention, expressed in *positive* units as the difference between alveolar and intrapleural pressures. It is superimposed on the intrapleural pressure scale in Fig. 6-1 to demonstrate its relationship to intrapleural pressure.

RELAXATION PRESSURE CURVE

If a subject inhales moderately, closes the glottis, and relaxes the respiratory muscles, the pressure in the lungs exceeds atmospheric pressure; inflation increases the elastic recoil of the lung and decreases the opposing elastic force of the chest wall. If the subject inhales more deeply, closes the glottis, and relaxes, intrapulmonary pressure increases still further. However, if the subject exhales completely, closes the glottis, and relaxes, intrapulmonary

pressure is subatmospheric; the deflationary elastic force of the lung is now less than the inflationary elastic force of the chest. A plot of an infinite number of such relaxation pressures against their corresponding lung volumes gives the *relaxation pressure curve* (Fig. 6-2).

The pressure at every point on this curve is the resultant of the elastic forces exerted by the lung and those exerted by the chest wall. At about 70% vital capacity the chest is the size it would assume if there were no lung elasticity pulling it in; at this volume* lung elasticity is solely responsible for the relaxation pressure. Above 70% vital capacity lung and chest forces are no longer antagonistic but operate additively to give the relaxation pressure curve.

MAXIMUM PRESSURE CURVES

The relaxation pressure curve results from passive elastic forces of the lung and chest. However, it is only part of a larger picture that includes maximum inspiratory and maximum expiratory pressure curves (Fig. 6-3). These maximum curves indicate the limits within which ventilation must occur. We commonly exert maximum or submaximum expiratory pressure against a closed glottis (Valsalva maneuver) while straining at stool, during childbirth, or while lifting. The maximum expiratory pressure attainable varies with the lung volume at which the pressure is exerted. The larger the initial lung volume, the greater the pressure that can be exerted; the smaller the initial lung volume, the more subatmospheric ("negative") is the maximum inspiratory pressure (Müller maneuver). Obviously, further inspiratory efforts are without effect at full inspiration, just as further expiratory efforts are without effect at full expiration.

---

*The chests of patients who have lost lung elasticity approach this volume, acounting for the barrel-chest appearance of such individuals and their large functional residual capacity values. In extreme ectomorphs this effect is more difficult to observe because the barrel chest resembles the normal-sized chest of average individuals.

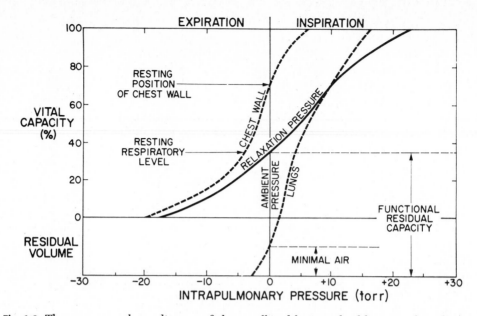

Fig. 6-2. The pressure-volume diagram of chest wall and lungs in healthy man: the relaxation pressure curve. The relaxation pressure curve (solid line) of the chest wall and lungs is the sum of its two components: the elasticity of the chest wall and diaphragm (dashed line on left), and the elasticity of the lungs (dashed line on right). The relaxation pressure curve crosses the ambient pressure or 0 axis where lung elasticity exactly balances chest wall elasticity, thus indicating the resting respiratory level and defining the functional residual capacity. At about 70% of the vital capacity, relaxation pressure results entirely from lung elasticity. At that level the lung curve intersects the relaxation pressure curve, and the chest wall curve crosses the ambient pressure on 0 axis, thus indicating the resting position of the chest wall. Minimal air is defined by the level at which the lung curve intersects the ambient pressure, or 0, axis. (Redrawn from Rahn, H., Otis, A. B., Chadwick, L. E., and Fenn, W. O.: Am. J. Physiol. **146:**161, 1946.)

The maximum pressure curves are the resultant of active muscle forces (external intercostals and diaphragm during a Müller maneuver; internal intercostals and abdominal muscles during a Valsalva maneuver) and the passive elastic forces of the lung and chest. By subtracting the relaxation pressure curve from the maximum expiratory pressure curve, we obtain a length-tension diagram for the respiratory muscles.

The great pressure, usually exceeding 100 torr for a maximum Valsalva maneuver, impedes systemic venous return to the right heart. If continued longer than 10 or 15 seconds, cardiac output and consequently cerebral blood flow diminish greatly and unconsciousness may occur.

COMPLIANCE

Compliance is a measure of the distensibility of the chest and/or lungs—the ease with which lung volume is changed. It is expressed in units of liters (BTPS) of lung volume change per centimeter H_2O pressure change. Greater compliance means a larger volume change per unit pressure change.

For calculating *lung* compliance (C_L) we use

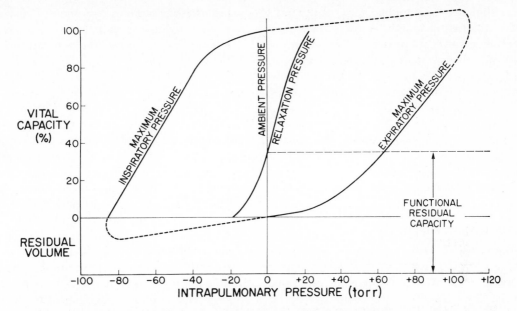

Fig. 6-3. The pressure-volume diagram of chest wall and lungs in healthy man. On the vertical axis 100% capacity represents maximum inspiration, and 0% vital capacity represents maximum expiration at ambient or 0 intrapulmonary pressure. The diagram shows the pressures that are developed passively (relaxation pressures) and those that can be developed actively (maximum pressures) at various lung volumes. When the lung is maximally expanded with high intrapulmonary pressure (dashed line in right upper corner), there is danger of lung rupture. When intrapulmonary pressure is lowest (dashed line in left lower corner), there is extreme dilation of blood vessels and danger of hemorrhage. (Redrawn from Rahn, H., Otis, A. B., Chadwick, L. E., and Fenn, W. O.: Am. J. Physiol. **146:**161, 1946.)

transpulmonary pressure, the pressure difference (ΔP) across the lung. It is the difference between alveolar pressure and intrapleural pressure.

Alveolar pressure cannot be measured directly during ventilation, but it is the same as mouth pressure when the glottis is open and no air is flowing (Fig. 6-1). Therefore, under those conditions, intrapleural pressure is equal to transpulmonary pressure. The measurement of intrapleural pressure (and $\Delta P_{p\ell}$) is discussed in a later section of this chapter.

Compliance of the total thorax (C_{th}) is calculated from the static pressure required to maintain a given volume change from FRC. It

is accomplished by voluntarily producing a measured lung volume change (either inspiring or expiring from the resting midposition), then measuring the airway pressure change required to passively maintain the thorax at its new volume. Fig. 6-2, with intrapulmonary pressure on the horizontal axis and lung volume (percent vital capacity) on the vertical axis, shows that a larger pressure change is required to produce a given volume change in the combined system than in either lungs or chest wall alone.

Compliance of the bronchopulmonary system is a measure of its elasticity, the resistance to deformation (strain) produced by an applied force (stress). Truly elastic bodies have a linear relationship between applied force and resulting deformation, or length (Hooke's law). If we substitute change in pressure for change in force and change in volume for change in length, a pressure-volume curve for the bronchopulmonary system can be plotted. This elasticity curve is the relaxation pressure curve (Fig. 6-2), a measure of the *static* compliance of the system. Bronchopulmonary diseases affect lung compliance primarily, whereas chest wall compliance (C_W) is affected by obesity and by diseases of thoracic nerves, muscles, bones, and joints.

Determinants of lung compliance

Surface tension. Surface tension is a phenomenon at a liquid-gas interface. The property is the result of the attractive forces, or cohesion, between like molecules at the boundary of the liquid and to their specific orientation. The attractive forces between adjacent liquid molecules at the surface are greater than those between liquid and gas molecules. The result is a net force exerted in the plane of the boundary that acts to preserve the integrity of the surface of separation and to resist rupture of the surface film of the liquid. This net force of attraction, or surface tension, tends to contract an exposed liquid surface such as a drop (one surface) or bubble (two surfaces) to the smallest possible area, minimizing the surface area/volume ratio. Surface tension is expressed in dynes/cm or ergs/cm^2.

Laplace's law. The surface tension of a soap bubble on the end of a tube tends to collapse the bubble, compressing the gas inside with a certain pressure if collapse is resisted. Laplace's law states that the pressure within a spherical liquid drop or bubble is directly proportional to the surface tension and inversely proportional to the radius; the equation that describes this relationship for a drop (one surface) is as follows:

$$P = \frac{2T}{r} \qquad (2)$$

where P is pressure in dynes/cm^2, T is surface tension in dynes/cm, and r is radius in cm. For a bubble (two surfaces) the relationship is as follows:

$$P = \frac{4T}{r} \qquad (3)$$

As surface tension increases or as the radius decreases, the pressure required to maintain the volume of a bubble increases. If we interconnect two bubbles with the same surface tension but different radii, that with the smaller radius (r_1) will empty into that with the larger radius (r_2) because P_1 is greater than P_2 (Fig. 6-4). The minimum radius and therefore maximum pressure are reached when the diameter of the bubble equals the diameter of the supporting tube. Since the volume of a spherical bubble is proportional to the cube of its radius, volume is a nonlinear function of the internal pressure. Fig. 6-5 shows this relationship for a bubble at the end of a tube. The Laplace relationship for a drop (one surface) is relevant for respiratory physiology because the liquid lining the pulmonary alveoli has one gas-liquid boundary.

Compliance, an important biophysical characteristic of the lungs and chest, is a measure of the elasticity of the connective tissue of airways, lungs, and blood vessels and the surface tension of the alveolar gas-liquid interface. We can isolate the effect of elasticity by removing the gas-liquid interface and thus the surface tension component. An excised de-aerated lung, suspended in saline to cancel the weight of the filling liquid, inflates with saline much more easily than the same lung suspended in air can be inflated with air. Fig. 6-6 compares the pressure-volume relationship for an excised lung during inflation with air to that during saline inflation. Since saline inflation abolishes the gas-liquid interface without changing elastic recoil, the curve on the left is compliance resulting from elasticity alone and that on the right is compliance resulting from both elasticity and surface tension.

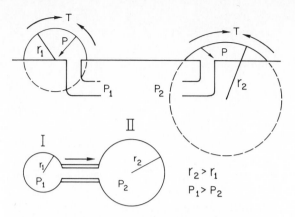

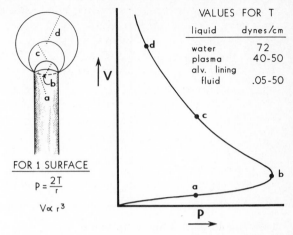

Fig. 6-4. Pressure-radius relationship for two bubbles of different size but having equal surface tension. Bubble I, with smaller radius (*r*), has a higher pressure (P_1) and will empty into bubble II when they are interconnected.

Fig. 6-5. Pressure-volume relationship of a bubble of radius *b* on the end of a tube. Surface tension is constant.

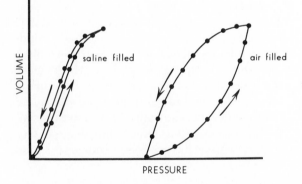

Fig. 6-6. Static pressure-volume curves of saline-filled and air-filled excised lungs, demonstrating the effects of elastic forces (left) and elastic plus surface tension forces (right) on static compliance of the lung.

Measuring lung compliance

Transpulmonary pressure, the difference between intrapleural pressure and alveolar pressure, is used to calculate lung compliance. As already stated, alveolar pressure is the same as mouth pressure when no air is flowing (Fig. 6-1). Under these conditions, intrapleural pressure is the same as transpul-

monary pressure, so C_L can be calculated by measuring the change in $P_{p\ell}$ at two levels of lung volume. $P_{p\ell}$ can be measured through a needle inserted between the ribs into the intrapleural space, but *changes* in $P_{p\ell}$ can be estimated on the basis of changes in esophageal pressure. The procedure for measuring esophageal pressure produces less discomfort, al-

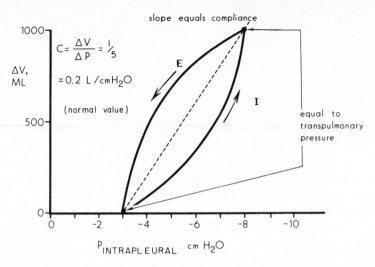

Fig. 6-7. Pressure-volume curve for the lung. Dynamic compliance of the lung is calculated from such a curve.

though some subjects disagree while the nasal tube with a small balloon is being positioned in the esophagus. After being positioned in the lower third of the esophagus, the balloon is inflated slightly to measure intraesophageal pressure.

Dynamic lung compliance is calculated by dividing the lung volume change during a tidal breath by the simultaneous change of intrapleural pressure (measured as the change in esophageal pressure) from the end of expiration to the end of inspiration. Fig. 6-7 shows an idealized compliance curve with normal values. A 1-L lung volume change is accompanied by a transpulmonary pressure change of 5 cm H_2O (the difference between -3 cm H_2O and -8 cm H_2O). Hence, lung compliance (C_L) is 1.0 L (BTPS) divided by 5.0 cm H_2O, or 0.2 L (BTPS)/cm H_2O. A continuous plot of changing lung volume versus changing intrapleural pressure during the course of a single breath creates a *hysteresis loop* because alveolar pressure reverses from inspiration (when it is "negative") to expiration (when it is positive).

TIME CONSTANTS FOR LUNG ELASTICITY

Although the lung is customarily discussed as if it were a perfectly elastic body or as if its elasticity were measured under static conditions, the compliance of the lung, in conjunction with the airway resistance (which affects the *rate* of air movement into or out of the lung), defines a *time constant* for the lung. Actually, different time constants can exist for different regions of the lung, depending on their regional compliance and the regional resistance to airflow.

The time constant is the product of the compliance and the resistance. It can be defined as the time (in seconds) required for inflation to 63% of the final volume, which would be achieved if the filling pressure were to remain constant indefinitely.

The time constant is represented by the equation shown at the top of p. 75.

Areas of the lung that have increased resistance or increased compliance will have longer time constants. They will accordingly require a longer time to be inflated to 63% of their po-

$$\text{Time constant (sec)} = \underset{\substack{\textbf{(Resistance} \\ \textbf{factor)}}}{\frac{\Delta P \text{ (cm } H_2O)}{\dot{V} \text{ (L/sec)}}} \times \underset{\substack{\textbf{(Compliance} \\ \textbf{factor)}}}{\frac{\Delta V \text{ (L)}}{\Delta P \text{ (cm } H_2O)}} = \frac{\text{cm } H_2O \times L}{L/\text{sec} \times \text{cm } H_2O} \qquad (4)$$

tential volume at any constant filling pressure. If the time for filling is limited, only the portions of the lung with short time constants will inflate to their expected capacity. If there is an inspiratory pause at the end of such an inspiration, there will be a regional adjustment, or redistribution, of the tidal volume, assuming that all the time constants are exceeded by the inspiratory pause. Those with shorter time constants will have received *proportionately* more air than those with longer time constants and will therefore contribute some of their air to those with longer time constants that were "underfilled" in the time available. If resistance *increases*, the value for pressure (cm H_2O) in the numerator will increase. If compliance *decreases*, the value for volume (L) in the numerator will decrease, so simultaneous opposite changes in resistance and compliance can result in no change occurring in the time constant. For example, if two regions of the lung have the same time constants, increasing the pressure at the mouth will produce the same pattern of volume change in both units; both will achieve 63% of their capacity in the same period of time (their time constant). If the resistance to one region is doubled without producing a change in compliance, the time constant will double, so it will require twice as long for that region of the lung to reach 63% of its volume.

Let us now reduce compliance by half in the same region. With the compliance reduced by half, the capacity for increasing the volume at a given pressure change will also be halved. The time for that region to fill to 63% of its *new* capacity will be halved, bringing it back to the original time constant. In this new condition, with both regions again having the same time constants, although the distribution of air is altered, the rates of pressure buildup within the alveoli are the same in both regions, so no redistribution will occur between the two regions at the end of an inspiration.

FREQUENCY DEPENDENCE OF DYNAMIC COMPLIANCE

From the discussion in the preceding section, it should be obvious that if the time constants of different regions of the lung are equal, the buildup of pressure in the alveoli will follow the *same time course*, independent of the volume change. Therefore, the distribution of inspired air within these regions will be independent of the pattern of breathing (frequency and tidal volume). There will be no redistribution of air within the lung at the end of an inspiration, and the measurement of dynamic compliance will not be affected by the breathing frequency. These conditions will not be met if the time constants are different in different regions of the lungs; this forms the basis for a sensitive test for early lung disease. Obstruction of small airways (less than 2 mm in diameter) will affect regional time constants for lung filling, so calculated dynamic compliance (C_{dyn}) will be reduced at higher breathing frequencies because of the reduced volume change within the time allowed in those regions with small, narrowed airways. Thus, a C_{dyn} at 60 to 80 breaths/min, which is less than 75% of the C_{dyn} measured at 20 breaths/min, is indicative of obstruction of small airways.

Obstruction of large airways affects the time constants of large regions of the lung but does not induce variable time constants within those regions. Therefore, one would not expect obstruction of large airways to produce a frequency dependence of C_{dyn}. The test is difficult to perform, but it is useful for early identification of small-airway disease. Of course, if there is a *regional* change of compliance without a change of regional resistance, one would see an effect on the total lung time constant. This would ordinarily affect C_{dyn} at low breathing frequencies and would not require the observation at high breathing frequencies.

Elastance

Elastance is the transpulmonary pressure change (ΔP) required to produce a unit change of lung volume (ΔV); it is thus the reciprocal of compliance, so lungs with a larger compliance (greater ease of filling) have a lower elastance (smaller pressure change required to produce a given lung volume change). Since a transpulmonary pressure change of 5 cm H_2O normally produces a 1-L volume change, lung elastance is 5 cm H_2O divided by 1 L, or 5 cm H_2O/L (BTPS). Elastance, or the measure of the "vigor" with which the lung resists volume change, is in a sense analogous to resistance to flow in a mechanical system. Disregarding the difference caused by a time derivative (airway resistance is a measure of the vigor with which the lung resists volume change *per unit time*), the two terms can be handled in similar ways. That is, they can be summed algebraically to provide a meaningful measurement for the entire system. As indicated in Chapter 2, the resistance of the total pulmonary system is the sum of the individual resistances:

$$R_{tot} = R_n + R_{aw} + R_{lar} \qquad (5)$$

Similarly, the total elastance of the lung-chest system is the sum of the individual elastances:

$$El_T = El_L + El_W \qquad (6)$$

Lung elastance and chest wall elastance are normally about equal; the total elastance of the lung-chest system is about twice that of the lung alone:

$$El_T = 5 \text{ cm } H_2O/L + 5 \text{ cm } H_2O/L = \qquad (7)$$
$$10 \text{ cm } H_2O/L \text{ (BTPS)}$$

COMPLIANCE IN LUNG DISEASE

Diseases that change the elastic properties of the lung or the surface tension of the gas-liquid interface within the lung affect lung compliance. Certain diseases decrease lung compliance (the lungs become stiff), whereas other diseases increase compliance (loss of normal lung elasticity).

At first glance an increase of lung compliance might appear advantageous because such a lung can be inflated with less effort. On the contrary, increased lung compliance is a serious problem. Increased compliance reduces transpulmonary pressure, the force that holds small airways open. Reduced airway caliber increases airway resistance, disturbing the distribution of inspired gas within the lung and severely limiting expiratory flow rate. Pulmonary emphysema increases compliance; this disease of the lung parenchyma destroys the fine network of alveolar capillaries and alveolar septa and diminishes lung elasticity.

The patient with increased lung compliance breathes with his lungs more fully inflated. The thorax enlarges ("barrel-chest"), and the hemidiaphragms descend, tending to flatten. FRC increases and the RV/TLC ratio may increase to 0.6 or 0.7, more than twice the normal value of 0.2 to 0.3. Increasing compliance causes increasing lung overinflation and decreasing transpulmonary pressure; a plot of the measured values inscribes the characteristic sigmoid compliance curve of emphysema. However, this is a self-limiting process; increasing compliance ultimately causes lung failure.

Decreased lung compliance is also a serious problem. In this case there is difficulty with inspiration. As compliance decreases, a greater transpulmonary pressure change is required to produce a given lung volume change. The greater inspiratory effort needed to produce this change means that the work of breathing increases as compliance decreases. Pulmonary interstitial fibrosis, a relatively irreversible condition caused by a variety of diseases that affect the lung parenchyma, decreases lung compliance. Pulmonary edema and vascular congestion also decrease compliance but are often reversible. Reduction of the amount of lung tissue available for expansion, a condition resulting from neoplasm or surgical excision of lung tissue, reduces compliance despite the fact that elasticity of the remaining lung and *specific compliance* (C_L/V_A) are unchanged. Surfactant deficiency also reduces lung compliance.

Regardless of cause, as compliance decreases, breathing becomes rapid and shallow, increasing dead space ventilation. Total pulmonary ventilation rate then increases sharply, providing adequate alveolar ventilation despite the low tidal volume. The work of breathing thus increases even more. Progressively decreasing lung compliance quickly compromises breathing efficiency.

The condition of progressive small-airway disease, which causes a frequency dependence of compliance, has already been described. Although there is an increase in C_{dyn} when it is measured at an elevated breathing frequency, it is actually caused by a change in the time constants in the lung and not by a change in lung compliance. When C_{dyn} is measured at a slow breathing frequency, the value is ordinarily within the limits of normal. Thus, changes in C_{dyn} measured at high breathing frequencies are not usually indicative of abnormal compliance of the lung.

Alveolar pressure-volume relationship

Fluid lines the alveoli, and the surface tension at the gas-liquid interface affects alveolar filling. This was presented earlier in a discussion of Laplace's law. To progress further in understanding the *actual* alveolar pressure-volume relationship, it is necessary to recognize that elastance of the alveoli and the surrounding tissue also affects the relationship. This complex relationship is shown in Figs. 6-8 and 6-9. Surface tension forces predominate when

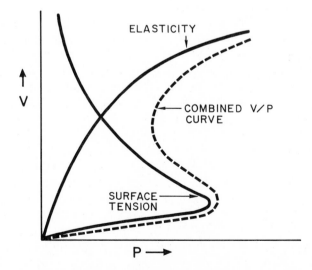

Fig. 6-8. Theoretic pressure-volume curve for an alveolus that has unchanging surface tension. The combined curve is the sum of the elasticity curve and the surface tension curve.

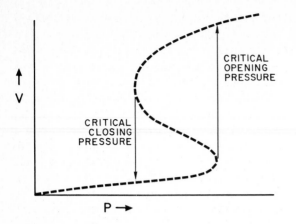

Fig. 6-9. Pressure-volume curve for an alveolus that has unchanging surface tension, showing the "critical opening pressure" and the "critical closing pressure."

alveoli are small, and elastic forces predominate when alveoli are inflated. In the process of opening a collapsed alveolus, pressure increases steadily, overcoming alveolar surface tension until the alveolar radius equals that of the alveolar duct; any further pressure increase will snap the alveolus open. The pressure necessary to reach this point, termed *critical opening pressure*, is determined primarily by alveolar surface tension and by the diameter of the alveolar duct. Beyond this pressure, elasticity is the chief determinant of the pressure-volume curve.

In the process of closing an open alveolus, the pressure-volume relationship initially reflects alveolar elasticity, but as volume continues to decrease, surface tension becomes the more important factor. The point at which further pressure decrease allows the alveolus to collapse is called *critical closing pressure*. Fig. 6-9 shows these two critical points.

The pressure-volume relationship during alveolar inflation differs from that during deflation. Thus, at a given pressure, inspiratory alveolar volume differs from expiratory alveolar volume. The lung reflects its recent history

with respect to volume change; this characteristic is termed *hysteresis*.

Pulmonary surfactant

All open alveoli are exposed to the same airway pressure on the inside and to the opposing intrapleural pressure on the outside. The difference, or transpulmonary pressure, is thus essentially the same for all open alveoli regardless of their size. Laplace's law, as well as other pressure-volume considerations, suggests that as transpulmonary pressure increases, large alveoli should get larger, small alveoli should get smaller, and collapsed alveoli should never open; indeed, small alveoli should empty into larger alveoli and tend to collapse. How does the lung inflate evenly if the only factors involved are alveolar elasticity and a fixed surface tension? The relatively even distribution of ventilation within the lung implies that some other factor is operating. The identification and solution of this problem is one of the most fascinating chapters in the history of respiratory physiology.

A chemical substance in the alveolar lining fluid varies surface tension as alveolar volume changes and is called *pulmonary surfactant.** Strictly speaking, the plural, pulmonary *surfactants*, is preferable because there is a family of phospholipid surfactants; for simplicity we will call them pulmonary surfactant.

The early work of von Neergard more than 50 years ago highlighted the importance of surface tension in lung compliance, and he indicated that surface tension in the lung must be inexplicably lower than predicted. Pattle in England studied the stability of lung foam (generated by lethal gas in gas warfare experiments) and concluded that the surface tension must be near 0 because of a material secreted in the lungs. Clements in the United States showed

---

*Detergents also decrease surface tension; however, they differ from surfactants in that they are entirely soluble in the liquid phase and thus do not change the surface tension as surface area changes.

the dependence of surface tension on surface area and contributed much to our understanding of the structure of surfactant. Avery and coworkers demonstrated that infants with hyaline membrane disease (respiratory distress syndrome of the newborn) had a deficit in surface-tension–lowering activity and related it to surfactant deficiency or inactivation. Many other investigators have contributed to our current understanding of the characteristics of surface tension in the lung and the dependence of these characteristics on surfactant.

Pulmonary surfactant is probably produced in the type II pneumonocytes in the lung. It is formed by the synthesis of fatty acids, which are incorporated into phospholipids, such as dipalmitoyl lecithin. Lecithin, which is present in the highest concentration and is thus the most important surfactant, must contain two saturated fatty acid residues to exhibit surfactant properties.

The surface-active lecithin has a relatively short half-life of 14 hours. The fate of the phospholipids is unknown, although there is evidence that macrophages play a role in their removal from the lining. It is likely that the entire metabolic cycle, from synthesis to removal, occurs within the lung.

The surfactant molecule has a *hydrophobic end* (water insoluble) and a *hydrophilic end* (water soluble). It thus remains at the gas-liquid interface oriented so that the polar (hydrophilic) portion of the molecule is in the liquid phase and the nonpolar (hydrophobic) portion is in the gas phase. The interruption of the surface by surfactant molecules decreases surface tension. The surface tension of the alveolar lining fluid, which might otherwise be about 72 dynes/cm (the surface tension of water), is reduced to a *mean* tension of 20 to 25 dynes/cm. As the boundary area containing pulmonary surfactant contracts, surface tension falls; as it expands, surface tension increases. Decreased surface area increases the number of surfactant molecules per unit area, decreasing surface tension; increased surface area decreases sur-

factant concentration, increasing surface tension. This effect promotes alveolar stability. The resistance of the boundary to compression is related to the surface density (number of molecules per unit area) of surfactant; as the boundary contracts, it offers progressively greater resistance to further compression. This effect also promotes alveolar stability.

The surfactant effect of lung washings or lung extracts can be demonstrated with a Wilhelmi balance (Fig. 6-10). In this apparatus surface tension is continuously measured as a slowly moving barrier changes the area containing surfactant. Fig. 6-11 shows an idealized curve for the area-surface tension relationship of an alveolar extract. As area is first decreased and then increased, a hysteresis loop is recorded, presumably because of a change in the orientation of surfactant molecules as their concentration changes. However, the significance of this hysteresis is not fully understood.

Since alveolar surface tension decreases more rapidly than alveolar radius, small alveoli enlarge with even less pressure than large alveoli; since transpulmonary pressure is essentially equal for all lung units, pulmonary surfactant increases lung compliance and favors even distribution of inspired gas. Surfactant has significance for alveolar liquid balance. If alveolar surface tension were as high as that of serum, approximately 55 dynes/cm, the alveoli would fill with plasma transudate. A high surface tension favors movement of liquid from pulmonary capillaries and interstices into alveolar spaces and may cause alveolar collapse. The low surface tension of healthy lungs, an essential element in the balance of forces, including colloid osmotic pressure and capillary hydrostatic pressure, favors alveolar dryness. The movement and spread of surfactant molecules and the concomitant movement of the hypophase may also have significance for alveolar clearance and alveolar configuration.

Note that the factors affecting the alveolar pressure-volume relationship are very complex. Fortuitously, the lung acts like an elastic

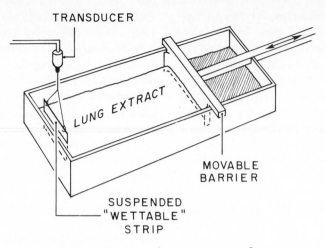

Fig. 6-10. Wilhelmi balance for measuring surface tension.

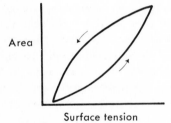

Fig. 6-11. Idealized curve for the area versus surface tension relationship of normal lung extract, which contains surfactant.

body that obeys Hooke's law in that most of the "elastance" is determined by surface tension phenomena. Without surfactant, the lung could not function as an efficient system for gas exchange between the environment and arterial blood.

SURFACTANT DEFICIENCY

Pulmonary surfactant deficiency increases the surface tension of the alveolar lining fluid but, more importantly, it reduces the amplitude of the alveolar surface tension fluctuations that normally occur with each breath. As a re-

sult, compliance decreases, the work of breathing increases, alveolar hypoventilation develops, ventilation-perfusion mismatching increases, and lung diffusion-perfusion relationships become grossly abnormal. This impairment of lung function produces arterial hypoxemia and respiratory acidosis. If extreme, the hypoxemia tends to produce metabolic acidosis as well.

By interfering with normal production of surfactant, removing it, or inactivating it, various conditions cause surfactant deficiency. These include:

1. Hypoxia.
2. Acidosis.
3. Abnormalities of pulmonary circulation, such as embolism and vascular congestion.
4. Atelectasis.
5. Pulmonary edema and transudation (the accumulation of fluid in interstitial and alveolar spaces).
6. Extracorporeal circulation (cardiopulmonary bypass).
7. Hyperoxia. In the usual clinical setting O_2 is administered in relatively low concentration with frequent interruption

necessitated by patient activity and nursing care. However, long-term administration of O_2 in excessive concentration can aggravate the ventilation-perfusion distribution and diffusion problems of patients with bronchopulmonary disease. Surfactant deficiency may be involved in these adverse effects.

8. Pulmonary lavage.
9. Aspiration of various foreign materials, including hydrocarbons.
10. Drowning.
11. Respiratory distress syndrome of the newborn infant or the adult.
12. Asphyxia.

Clinical problems associated with surfactant deficiency

The conditions just listed impair lung function by depleting alveolar surfactant. Surfactant depletion occurs more often than is clinically recognized, especially after abdominal surgery. This clinical catastrophe, adult respiratory distress syndrome, complicates a variety of medical conditions and surgical procedures.

In a typical case, gas exchange deteriorates within 24 to 36 hours after surgery. Arterial hypoxemia is the first clinically observable indication. Oxygen administration relieves this hypoxemia only temporarily. Pulmonary deterioration progresses from decreased compliance to frank alveolar hypoventilation, serious ventilation-perfusion abnormalities, and respiratory acidosis. Assisted ventilation is then effective, but only briefly; inflation pressure must be increased continually to maintain adequate alveolar ventilation. Despite apparently adequate pulmonary ventilation, patchy atelectasis produces regions of shuntlike (venous admixture–like) effect, aggravating arterial hypoxemia. Drastic measures are needed. These include assisted ventilation with 35% O_2 in nitrogen, positive end-expiratory pressure, diuretics, and glucocorticosteroids. Arterial blood gases and pH should be closely monitored.

Factors conducive to development of the adult respiratory distress syndrome, such as hypoxia, atelectasis, acidosis, pulmonary edema, or excessive hyperoxia during the immediate postoperative period, should be detected early and treated effectively as they arise. Clinical problems related to surfactant deficiency in the newborn are discussed in the section on respiratory distress syndrome of the newborn in Chapter 15.

RESISTANCE TO BREATHING

Poiseuille's law relates the factors that determine laminar gas flow through a smooth unbranched tube of fixed dimensions:

$$\dot{V} = \frac{\pi r^4 \Delta P}{8L\eta} \tag{8}$$

where $\dot{V}$ is volumetric flow rate, r is tube radius, ΔP is driving pressure (pressure difference between two arbitrary points in the tube), L is tube length, and η is gas viscosity.

All these factors are variables except for $\pi/8$, which is constant. $\dot{V}$ is a function of r^4; tube radius profoundly affects flow rate. If all other factors remain constant, doubling tube radius increases gas flow by a factor of 16. A slight decrease of airway caliber caused by secretions, edema, or bronchoconstriction increases airway resistance greatly; to maintain the same flow rate requires a correspondingly great increase in driving pressure. Poiseuille's equation also shows that flow rate is inversely related both to tube length (L) and to the viscosity (η) of the gas. Other factors remaining constant, volumetric flow rate is a linear function of, and proportional to, driving pressure; Poiseuille's law for a laminar flow regime (character) may then be simplified:

$$\Delta P = K_1 \times \dot{V} \tag{9}$$

The constant K_1 incorporates dynamic gas viscosity as well as tube length and radius. A Reynolds' number (N_R) (Chapter 2 and Appendix, Respiratory calculations) greater than 2,000 generally indicates turbulent flow. The equation that relates driving pressure to volumetric flow rate during turbulence is as follows:

$$\Delta P = \frac{f \times L}{4\pi^2 r^5} \times \dot{V}^2 \tag{10}$$

where f is a friction factor that incorporates the roughness of the tube surface as well as Reynolds' number. As N_R increases, (1) f becomes less dependent on it and (2) density becomes increasingly important, whereas viscosity becomes less so. Reynolds' numbers of 10,000 occur in the trachea during exercise. The other symbols in this equation have the same meaning as those in Poiseuille's equation. If all other conditions remain constant, the relationship between driving pressure and the resultant volumetric flow rate for a turbulent flow regime is as follows:

$$\Delta P = K_2 \times \dot{V}^2 \tag{11}$$

The constant K_2 incorporates f (a function of density relative to viscosity—the reciprocal of kinematic viscosity) as well as tube length and radius.

During expiration, increased linear flow velocity changes the flow regime from a laminar pattern in the bronchioles to turbulent flow in the large airways. A mixed flow regime occurs during quiet spontaneous breathing. The following equation, combining the separate equations for laminar and turbulent flow, relates driving pressure to resultant volumetric flow rate:

$$\Delta P = K_1 \times \dot{V} + K_2 \times \dot{V}^2 \tag{12}$$

The first term of the right-hand member of the equation is for laminar flow and the second term is for turbulent flow. Note that laminar flow relates to dynamic viscosity, whereas turbulent flow relates to kinematic viscosity.

Physiologic aspects of airway resistance

Details of the physical aspects of airflow and airway resistance (R_{aw}) are presented in Chapter 2. The *physiology* of R_{aw} is presented here

in context with the mechanics of breathing. *Compliance,* as just discussed, is concerned with the *elastic* component that resists lung volume change. *Resistance* is concerned with the *nonelastic* component that resists change of the volume of gas in the lungs.

R_{aw} is the ratio of driving pressure to the resultant volumetric flow rate; its units are cm $H_2O \times L^{-1} \times sec^{-1}$. For a healthy adult, R_{aw} values range from 2 to 3 cm $H_2O \times L^{-1} \times sec^{-1}$ measured at an arbitrary flow rate of 0.5 L/sec; this is a flow rate usually achieved in quiet breathing during both inspiration and expiration. If R_{aw} were measured at a higher arbitrary flow rate of, for example, 1.0 L/sec, normal values would be higher.

The reason for dependence of R_{aw} on flow rate is that the relationship between ΔP and $\dot{V}$ is different for laminar as opposed to turbulent flow, and the flow pattern (for example, the proportion of flow that is turbulent) depends on the flow velocity in a given conduit. (Refer to Rohrer's equation and the discussion of flow patterns in Chapter 2 for a review of the physical determinants of R_{aw}.)

In addition to the effect of the gas characteristics on R_{aw}, the size and shape of the airways also affect the measured R_{aw}. For example, R_{aw} decreases with increasing lung volume. This relates to radial traction on the airways as the lung expands. The increased airway caliber reduces resistance to laminar flow according to Poiseuille's law. Furthermore, the larger airway radius implies a lesser velocity for the same airflow rate, and this tends to make flow more laminar (less turbulent) for any given flow rate. All this decreases R_{aw}.

At a given lung volume, R_{aw} is less during inspiration than during expiration. This is because intrapleural pressure decreases during inspiration. The reduced (more "negative") intrapleural pressure is distributed throughout the lung tissue (modified by the hydrostatic effect of the weight of the lung), whereas intraluminal pressure varies from the "negative" value of alveolar pressure to atmospheric pressure at the nose or mouth; hence, transmural pressure is, on the average, greater during inspiration and smaller during expiration at a given lung volume. Thus, although *transpulmonary* pressure (pressure across the alveoli) is not different, airflow dynamics produce a kinetic pressure difference within the airway, which adds to or subtracts from the transpulmonary pressure, to determine the transmural pressure (pressure difference between the intrapleural space and the lumen of the airways). This results in greater dilation of the airways at any given lung volume and the *same flow rate* during inspiration and expiration.

Airways lengthen during inspiration and shorten during expiration; however, inspiratory airway lengthening cancels only a small fraction of the resistance decrease associated with increasing airway caliber. Similarly, during expiration airway shortening affects resistance only slightly.

Factors that decrease airway caliber increase R_{aw}, sometimes greatly. These factors include bronchial secretion, edema, vascular congestion of the mucosa, and constriction of bronchial smooth muscle (bronchoconstriction) from chemical (for example, histamine) or parasympathetic (vagal) stimulation.

A less obvious cause of increased R_{aw} is loss of lung elasticity. Increased lung compliance decreases transpulmonary (distending) pressure; intrapleural pressure more closely approximates intrapulmonary (alveolar) pressure. The diameter of small airways decreases, increasing R_{aw}.

Factors that limit expiratory flow rate

Expiratory flow rate is limited by airway resistance, transpulmonary pressure, and intrapulmonary pressure (Fig. 6-12). As gas flows through an airway, the pressure diminishes steadily along the stream. During *forced* expi-

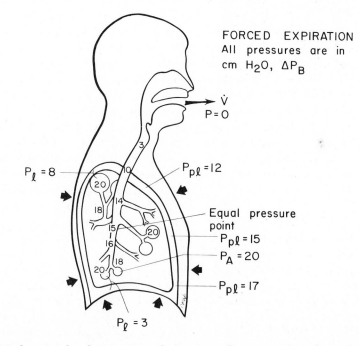

Fig. 6-12. Mechanism that limits maximal expiratory flow rate. Forced expiration increases intrapleural pressure, reversing transpulmonary pressure relationship. This reversal collapses nonrigid airways to produce an expiratory "check-valve."

ration, the expiratory flow rate at which intrapleural pressure becomes "positive" depends on transpulmonary pressure (a function of lung compliance) and the airway resistance. Compliance and airway resistance thus interact to determine the point of reversal of transmural pressure. If this pressure reversal occurs in peripheral airways, these airways, unsupported by cartilage, tend to collapse. If the resistance of small, peripheral airways increases, the pressure drop is greater along these less well-supported airways and they tend to collapse at a modest expiratory flow rate. This flow-limiting ("check-valve") mechanism produces the characteristic plateaus in the isovolume pressure-flow curves of healthy subjects. In pulmonary emphysema this effect is exaggerated by loss of lung elasticity and by airway collapsibility, so that air enters the lung with relative ease but is trapped during expiration behind a segment of bronchial collapse.

WORK OF BREATHING

Breathing involves muscular work. During inspiration, as muscles increase the volume of the thorax, elastic tissue is stretched and deformed and surface tension is overcome, creating a subatmospheric intrapulmonary pressure so that air flows into the lungs. Work is necessary to overcome the factors that resist lung inflation. This work of breathing is generally expressed in two ways: mechanical work and metabolic work.

Mechanical work of breathing

Physical work is defined as force times distance. The work of inspiration is expressed in terms of pressure change (ΔP) times volume change (ΔV) in units of cm H_2O × liters rather than kilograms × meters. In Fig. 6-13 the total work of quiet inspiration (sum of all shaded areas) is divided into the work required to overcome elasticity (approximately 65%) and the nonelastic work required to overcome friction (about 35%). About 80% of the nonelastic

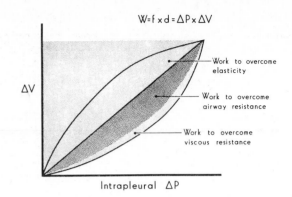

$$W = f \times d = \Delta P \times \Delta V$$

ΔV

Work to overcome elasticity

Work to overcome airway resistance

Work to overcome viscous resistance

Intrapleural ΔP

Fig. 6-13. Work of inspiration (total shaded area) consists of the work to overcome elasticity plus airway resistance plus viscous resistance. As work is done to overcome elasticity during inspiration, energy for the succeeding passive expiration is stored in the system.

work is used to overcome airway resistance, whereas 20% is used to overcome the viscous resistance of the lung. Quiet spontaneous expiration is passive, and the work required is recovered from energy stored in the lung-chest system during the preceding inspiration. The rest of the stored energy is transformed into heat and thus wasted. When expiration is active, more work is done per breath.

As compliance decreases or as resistance increases, the work of breathing increases. Fig. 6-14 illustrates the work of breathing in health, in restrictive lung disease (with decreased compliance), and in obstructive lung disease (with increased resistance).

Metabolic work of breathing

The work of breathing appears more meaningful to a physiologist when expressed in metabolic terms. It is calculated as the *additional* O_2 consumption required for breathing multiplied by the mechanical equivalent for O_2 consumption, expressed in units of ml (STPD) of O_2/L (BTPS) of ventilation. The metabolic cost is low during quiet breathing but increases

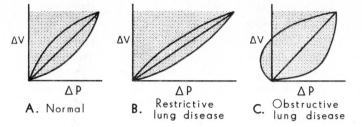

Fig. 6-14. Analysis of the work of breathing (shaded areas) for **A,** a healthy subject; **B,** a patient with restrictive ventilatory impairment; and **C,** a patient with chronic diffuse obstructive bronchopulmonary disease.

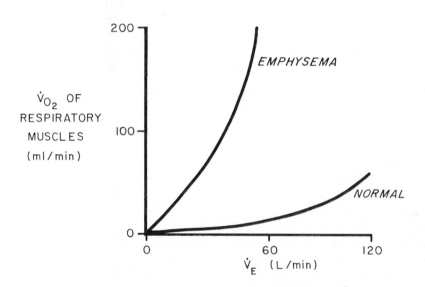

Fig. 6-15. Relationship of oxygen cost of breathing to expiratory minute volume for a healthy subject and for a patient with bronchitis-emphysema syndrome. (After Campbell, E. J. M., Westlake, E. K., and Cherniack, R. M.: J. Appl. Physiol. **11:**303, 1957.)

steadily as ventilation increases. Fig. 6-15 shows this relationship.

Energy cost of breathing

Obstructive lung disease increases the cost of breathing. In severe cases the O_2 cost of increased ventilation exceeds the additional O_2 provided by the increased effort. Thus, a patient with advanced emphysema may actually supply less O_2 to his metabolizing tissues as a result of increasing pulmonary ventilation, aggravating hypoxemia. Furthermore, such increased work of breathing may produce extra CO_2 at a rate in excess of the patient's ability to eliminate it, aggravating hypercapnic acidosis.

We cannot measure the O_2 consumption of the respiratory muscles directly. We estimate the O_2 cost of breathing by measuring total O_2 consumption at several different levels of pulmonary ventilation. Assuming that the O_2 consumption increments represent the metabolic cost of additional ventilation at each level, the O_2 cost of breathing at rest is estimated by extrapolation of the curve to the O_2 consumption axis (control ventilation). By this method the O_2 cost of resting breathing is usually found to be 0.5 to 1.0 ml (STPD) of O_2/L (BTPS) of ventilation. The efficiency of breathing is calculated in percent as 100 times the work output per metabolic cost or as 100 times the mechanical work per metabolic work. The mechanical efficiency of breathing is approximately 10% and is thus similar to that of other mechanical work done by the body.

CHAPTER 7

DIFFUSION OF GASES IN THE LUNG

The continuous exchange of O_2 and CO_2 between blood and the atmosphere is accomplished by the simultaneous processes of pulmonary ventilation, pulmonary perfusion, and alveocapillary diffusion.

Inspired air and alveolar gas mix to varying degrees in the airways. However, most of that mixing is *convective* because of bulk movement of air within the airways; *diffusion* of gases in those airways is not important for mixing. However, diffusion contributes to mixing and air movement in the *terminal* airways, where distances are short, airway caliber is narrow, and airway volume changes may not occur.

Most references to gas diffusion as a factor in the process of gas exchange consider the movement of *dissolved* gases in extracellular water, through membranes, and within cells. The diffusion pathway for O_2 in the lung is from the alveolus through the alveolar lining liquid, the alveolocapillary membrane, the plasma, and into the erythrocyte, where it combines with hemoglobin. For CO_2 the diffusion pathway in the lung is considered to be from inside the erythrocyte (where CO_2 is released from buffers and hemoglobin), into and through the plasma, through the alveolocapillary membrane and lining fluid, and into the alveoli.

Sixty to seventy years ago there was a vigorous debate as to whether CO_2 and O_2 moved only by diffusion or whether an active process was involved in hastening equilibration. It was concluded to the satisfaction of most physiologists, until recently, that the kinetics of O_2 and CO_2 transfer can be explained completely in terms of the action of catalysts, such as carbonic anhydrase and the rapid coupling and uncoupling of respiratory gases with hemoglobin. However, recent evidence suggests that the diffusion of O_2 and CO across the mammalian alveolocapillary and placental membranes is facilitated by cytochrome P-450. This cytochrome, a hemoprotein attached to the endoplasmic reticulum within the cells, is also involved in certain biologic oxidation and hydroxylation reactions. Cytochrome P-450 may facilitate diffusion by acting as a fixed-site (bucket-brigade) O_2 and CO carrier. It is estimated that facilitated diffusion accounts for a large fraction of the O_2 that moves across the placental membrane and about 10% to 15% of the O_2 that moves across the alveolocapillary membrane. A variety of drugs and gases combine with cytochrome P-450, blocking this gas transfer mechanism.

DETERMINANTS OF GAS DIFFUSION

In healthy subjects, the process of diffusion rapidly equalizes the pressure of gases in the alveoli with gas pressures inside the erythrocytes. Part of the time required for pressure equilibration is required for diffusion through the fluid spaces, and part is used for the chemical reactions of O_2 and CO_2 with hemoglobin and CO_2 with blood buffer systems.

Largely because of differences in solubility between the two gases, CO_2 diffuses more than 20 times as fast as O_2. However, the rate of the chemical reactions of CO_2 with the bicarbonate buffer system is much slower than the rate of reaction of O_2 with hemoglobin. Thus, there is less difference in the time required for *total* equilibration of O_2 and CO_2 pressures during pulmonary gas exchange than appears at first glance. Despite the equilibration times for *diffusion* being markedly different and factors affecting the diffusion of gases across the alveolocapillary membrane having minimal effect on CO_2 equilibration, other factors, such as carbonic anhydrase inhibitors, can interfere with CO_2 transfer in the lungs and result in CO_2 retention because of incomplete equilibration.

At rest, blood traverses the alveolocapillary bed in about 0.75 second (mean transit time). However, greatly increased cardiac output, as during exercise, can sharply reduce transit time. At rest, blood gases ordinarily equilibrate within 0.3 to 0.4 second, and CO_2 has been reported to require even less time to reach equilibrium. Thus, incomplete equilibration of gas pressures as a result of reduced *time* for diffusion occurs during high cardiac output states and can contribute to widening the alveolar-arterial P_{O_2} difference during strenuous exercise.

Increased P_{O_2} difference between alveolar gas and mixed venous blood requires a larger volume of O_2 transfer per volume of blood to achieve equilibrium. For example, during vigorous exercise O_2 extraction increases, reducing mixed venous blood O_2 content and P_{O_2}. Assuming adequate $\dot{V}_A$, alveolar P_{O_2} will be normal, and more O_2 will be transferred before equalization of O_2 pressure in the alveoli and pulmonary capillaries. If transit time decreases, for example, during vigorous exercise, the increased alveolar-arterial P_{O_2} difference may be contributed to by the larger P_{O_2} difference between alveolar gas and mixed venous blood.

If gas diffusion across the alveolocapillary membrane is impaired, the mean driving pressure would have to increase for an equal volume of O_2 to be transferred by diffusion. Thus, the *rate* of transfer per unit of driving pressure is reduced when the capacity of the lung for diffusion is reduced.

The volume of gas transfer *per unit time* depends on three factors: (1) the physiochemical characteristics of the gas to be transferred, (2) the driving pressure across the alveolocapillary membrane (between the alveolar gas and the inside of the erythrocyte), and (3) the characteristics of the lung with respect to membrane area and thickness through which the gases must diffuse.

Gas characteristics

Molecular weight. At a given temperature the product mv^2 is constant; thus, larger gas molecules move more slowly. Since the rate of diffusion of a gas is directly proportional to the velocity of its molecules, larger gas molecules diffuse more slowly whether in gas or liquid. Since the mass of a molecule m is reciprocally related to v^2, the relative rates of diffusion of two gases are inversely proportional to the square roots of their molecular weights, or densities (Graham's law). Thus, on the basis of molecular weight only, O_2 diffuses slightly faster than CO_2:

$$\frac{\sqrt{44}}{\sqrt{32}} = \frac{6.63}{5.66} = 1.17 \qquad (1)$$

Gas temperature. Just as smaller molecules diffuse more rapidly at any given temperature (mv^2 is a constant), a given molecule diffuses more rapidly as temperature increases. Increasing temperature increases kinetic energy (mv^2). Since mass remains constant, the velocity of molecular movement increases. Because kinetic energy is a function of v^2, the rate of diffusion of a gas, in mixture with another gas or in a liquid, is directly proportional to the square root of the absolute temperature.

In healthy persons, lung temperature remains approximately 37° C (310° K) and hence is not usually considered by the physiologist as a variable affecting the rate of diffusion of gases within the lung or the rate of gas transfer across the alveolocapillary membrane. However, in metabolically active tissues, for example in skeletal muscles during exercise, temperature can increase by several degrees Celsius. The elevated temperature increases the gas diffusion rate and facilitates the transfer of O_2 and CO_2 in those areas where larger volumes of gas must be transferred per unit time.

Solubility coefficient. The rate of transfer of a gas across a biologic membrane depends on the solubility coefficient (C_s) of that gas in the aqueous phase of the membrane. At 38° C, CO_2 is approximately 21 times as soluble as O_2 in the aqueous fluids of the body and diffuses much faster than O_2 across the alveolocapillary membrane. Impaired diffusion interferes with O_2 transfer long before CO_2 transfer is affected; indeed, outward diffusion of CO_2 is never a clinical problem except in patients whose diffusion is so severely impaired that life can be maintained only by administration of high P_{O_2} mixtures.

However, in body fluids the relative diffusion rates of O_2 and CO_2 depend on solubility *and* molecular weight. Thus, although somewhat heavier, the much more soluble CO_2 diffuses about 20 times faster than O_2 per unit driving pressure across the water-containing alveolocapillary membrane.

The driving pressure for O_2 at the arterial end of the pulmonary capillary is ordinarily 40 to 50 torr (from an alveolar P_{O_2} of 95 to 100 to a mixed venous P_{O_2} of perhaps 50 torr), whereas the driving pressure for CO_2 is about 6 torr (mixed venous P_{CO_2} of 46; $P_{A_{CO_2}}$ about 40). Thus, there is an approximately eightfold difference between the driving pressures for O_2 and CO_2 in favor of O_2. This reduces the difference in absolute diffusion rates (the result of solubility differences) to a factor of about $2^1/_2$ in favor of CO_2. If the reaction rate for HCO_3^- to CO_2 is a limiting factor, the driving pressure for CO_2 may not be at the theoretic level and the difference between diffusion rates for CO_2 and

O_2 might be even less than that suggested on the basis of solubility differences alone.

Transmembrane pressure difference

The volume of a gas that diffuses across the alveolocapillary membrane per unit time is directly related to the mean gas pressure difference between alveolus and pulmonary capillary. The greater the mean gas pressure difference, the larger will be the volume of gas that diffuses across the alveolocapillary membrane. Three factors maintain the pressure differences that promote the transfer of O_2 and CO_2 across the alveolocapillary membrane.

Alveolar ventilation. As alveolar ventilation increases, the composition of alveolar gas approaches that of inspired air. Normal alveolar ventilation maintains a P_{O_2} of approximately 100 torr and a P_{CO_2} of 40 torr, creating a *source* of O_2 and a *sink* for CO_2 as these gases diffuse across the alveolocapillary membrane.

Pulmonary capillary blood flow. There is an exponential rise in the P_{O_2} of venous blood as it flows through the capillaries in the lungs. Blood flow through the capillary keeps the P_{O_2} at the pulmonary arterial end more near the mixed venous level, and as blood flow increases, a greater portion of the blood has a lower P_{O_2}. Blood with a lower P_{O_2} serves as a more effective sink for O_2, keeping the blood P_{O_2} low and facilitating the transfer of O_2 across the membrane.

The reverse condition applies to CO_2 transfer. As pulmonary capillary blood flow increases, a larger volume of blood toward the pulmonary arterial end of the capillary has a P_{CO_2} closer to that of mixed venous blood. It thus serves as a larger source of CO_2, keeping the mean driving pressure higher so that more CO_2 is transferred from blood to alveoli.

Chemical reactions. Hemoglobin is a sink for the stream of O_2 molecules that moves from alveolar gas into the erythrocyte.

After combining with hemoglobin, O_2 is no longer in solution and exerts no back pressure, except that caused by the molecules remaining in solution, which are in equilibrium with the combined O_2. Thus, a large volume of O_2 can be transferred with only a slight buildup of P_{O_2}. The back pressure thus developed is inversely related to the affinity of hemoglobin for O_2. In this way large volumes of O_2 are transferred without eliminating the driving pressure required for the diffusion process.

The CO_2-buffering mechanism of blood, including carbaminohemoglobin, is a source of CO_2, favoring a CO_2 pressure difference, despite the stream of CO_2 molecules across the alveolocapillary membrane. The kinetics of the CO_2 reactions in blood favor the maintenance of a normal pressure difference. The velocity of the chemical reactions is sufficiently great to remove O_2 from solution and to supply CO_2 for diffusion from the erythrocyte.

Lung characteristics

Membrane area. The total volume of gas that diffuses across the alveolocapillary membrane per unit time is limited by the area of membrane available for diffusion. Lung size as well as the distribution of alveolar ventilation and pulmonary capillary blood flow are important determinants of this gas-exchanging area. Thus, the rate of diffusion is directly related to the functioning area of the alveolocapillary membrane.

Diffusion distance. The rate of diffusion is inversely related to the length of the pathway between the alveolus and the hemoglobin molecule within the erythrocyte. The pathway involved in the diffusion process from alveolus to hemoglobin molecule can be divided into five steps: (1) the liquid alveolar lining layer; (2) the alveolocapillary membrane, where diffusion depends on the pressure gradient from alveolar gas to pulmonary capillary plasma, tissue thickness and characteristics, and gas-exchanging surface area; (3) diffusion in plasma until the gas molecule meets the erythrocyte membrane; (4) diffusion across the erythrocyte membrane; and (5) random movement until

contact and chemical combination with a hemoglobin molecule occur.

The diffusion pathway across the alveolocapillary membrane varies normally from 0.1 to 0.5 μm, but in disease it may increase greatly; appreciable reduction of alveolocapillary membrane thickness by any circumstances appears unlikely. The sum of the distances in steps 3, 4, and 5, from membrane to hemoglobin molecule, is sometimes called intracapillary distance.

Liquid viscosity. The rate of diffusion of a gas is inversely related to the viscosity of the liquid through which it diffuses. Viscosity is essentially constant for the alveolar lining liquid, for the aqueous phase of the alveolocapillary membrane, and for the blood plasma in the pulmonary capillary.

Summary equation. All factors that affect the rate of gas diffusion across the alveolocapillary membrane are represented in the following equation:

$$\dot{V} \propto \frac{C_s \times T \times A \times dP}{\sqrt{MW} \times L \times \eta} \qquad (2)$$

where $\dot{V}$ is the volumetric rate of gas transfer by diffusion, C_s is the solubility coefficient, T is the absolute temperature, A is the area of the gas-exchanging membrane, dP is the difference in gas pressure across the diffusion path, MW is the molecular weight of the gas, L is the length of diffusion pathway, and η is the viscosity of the liquid.

The pressure gradient, dP, in turn, is a function of alveolar ventilation, pulmonary capillary blood flow, and the velocity of the chemical reactions involved.

Pulmonary diffusing capacity

Pulmonary diffusing capacity (D_L), or lung transfer factor (T_L), is a measure of the lung *conductance* for a gas. This term expresses quantitatively the pulmonary transfer of a specific gas under standardized conditions of driving pressure across the diffusion pathway.

Gas transfer between alveoli and pulmonary

capillary blood obeys the fundamental law of diffusion:

$$\frac{dV}{dt} = D(P_1 - P_2) \tag{3}$$

where dV/dt is the rate of transfer of a given gas in milliliters per minute across a given membrane, D is the diffusion coefficient for that gas in the membrane being studied and is expressed as $ml \times min^{-1} \times torr^{-1}$, and $(P_1 - P_2)$ is the pressure difference in torr for that gas between the two sides of the membrane.

D is directly proportional to the solubility of that gas in the membrane under stated conditions and to the total membrane surface area available for diffusion, but D is inversely proportional to membrane thickness and to the square root of the molecular weight of the gas.

This definition of D is specific for the pulmonary system and, as such, D is written with a subscript. D_L is defined as the *pulmonary diffusing capacity* and calculated as the volume of a specific gas (STPD) that can be transferred per minute per torr of driving pressure. It is expressed as follows:

$$D_L = \frac{\dot{V}}{(P_A - P_{\bar{v}})} \tag{4}$$

Division of volume transferred per minute by the gas pressure difference normalizes pulmonary diffusing capacity and thus facilitates comparison of the transfer rates of different gases across the lung. Changes of pulmonary diffusing capacity thus reflect changes in the lung.

D_L is a measure of the conductance across the lung, since it increases as the ease of gas transfer increases. The reciprocal of D_L is "resistance" to gas transfer. In the case of O_2, with which pulmonary diffusing capacity is most concerned, the resistance to gas transfer by diffusion consists of three series resistances: that in the alveoli $(1/D_A)$, that across the membrane $(1/D_M)$, and the resistance to gas diffusion associated with the rate limitation of O_2 removal by hemoglobin $(1/D_b)$. The resistance to O_2

transfer contributed by blood reactions is, more specifically, inversely related to the reaction rate of O_2 with hemoglobin and to the volume of blood (hemoglobin) in the capillary. These are expressed as:

$$\frac{1}{D_b} = \frac{1}{\theta V_c} \tag{5}$$

where θ is a term for the reaction rate of O_2 with hemoglobin and V_c is capillary blood volume. (It is not clear why the term is not Q_c, since blood volume is conventionally abbreviated Q; however, the term is well entrenched and changing it might create more difficulty than continuing to use an inconsistent designation.)

Thus, the three series resistances are additive, providing a measure of the total resistance to O_2 transfer in the lung:

$$\frac{1}{D_L} = \frac{1}{D_A} + \frac{1}{D_M} + \frac{1}{\theta V_c} \tag{6}$$

D_A refers only to the component of diffusion from the center of the alveolus to its wall and is probably negligible because of the short distance for diffusion within the alveolus.

This process should not be confused with the diffusion of gases within terminal airways, an aspect of delivery of inspired gas to the alveoli. Diffusion within airways is not included in the definition of D_L and is not measured by the diffusing capacity test, since the method considers only the driving pressure in the alveoli, P_A.

Diffusing capacity of the membrane, D_M, and the factor related to blood reactions, θV_c, account about equally for the major resistance to O_2 transfer across the lung. The two factors can be separated by measuring the D_L for CO at a low and a high level of O_2, thus measuring the effect of changing the blood reaction rates on total $D_{L_{CO}}$. Note that $D_{L_{CO}}$ is affected by all the factors that affect $D_{L_{O_2}}$, including blood reaction rates, since both CO and O_2 react similarly with hemoglobin despite having strikingly different affinities.

Measurement of pulmonary diffusing capacity

The D_L of a gas is defined as the volume in milliliters (STPD) that diffuses across the alveolocapillary membrane per minute per torr of mean pressure difference. In general, D_L is calculated as follows:

$$D_L = \frac{\text{Rate of gas transfer}}{\substack{\text{Mean alveolar} - \text{Mean pulmonary} \\ \text{gas tension} \quad \text{capillary gas tension}}} \quad (7)$$

D_L limits the transfer of any gas that undergoes large volume transfer before decrease of transmembrane pressure difference. Because of specific chemical reactions that occur in the blood, this condition applies to three gases: CO_2, O_2, and CO. As indicated earlier, the higher membrane diffusing capacity for CO_2, as compared with O_2 (a result of their respective water solubilities), implies that diffusion impairment must produce hypoxemia before it produces CO_2 retention and hypercapnic acidosis.

A gas suitable for the measurement of D_L must be much more soluble in blood than it is in the alveolocapillary membrane to maintain an effective driving pressure. To be suitable for this test, a gas must also be readily and accurately analyzable. Finally, the factors affecting the diffusing capacity must be related to the factors that affect the diffusing capacity for O_2, which is the gas of physiologic importance. Carbon monoxide is a test gas that meets these criteria and is used for the measurement of D_L.

The diffusing capacities for O_2 and CO are affected by some of the same factors, since both gases combine with hemoglobin. Hemoglobin removes CO from solution very effectively, forming carboxyhemoglobin. The affinity of hemoglobin for CO is from 200 to 300 times as great as that for O_2 (Haldane number). At equilibrium at sea level a P_{CO} of 1.46 torr, or 0.065%, produces the same percent saturation of hemoglobin as does a P_{O_2} of 100 torr, or

14.0% O_2. Thus, P_{CO} back pressure is nearly 0 when blood CO concentration is low.

The dynamics of CO uptake differ from that of O_2 uptake in the lungs because mixed venous blood has appreciable O_2 content and tension as it enters the pulmonary capillaries; the rate of diffusion of O_2, but not CO, depends on a diminishing pressure gradient as blood traverses the pulmonary capillary. Thus, CO transfer is not limited by the rate of pulmonary capillary blood flow; it is limited by the rate of diffusion across the alveolocapillary membrane, by diffusion across the erythrocyte membrane, and by the rate of the subsequent chemical combination of CO with hemoglobin (θ).

$D_{L_{CO}}$ can be calculated from measurements of the transfer rate and the mean alveolar P_{CO} during the time of measurement, assuming mean pulmonary capillary P_{CO} (back pressure) to be 0. It is difficult to calculate $D_{L_{O_2}}$ because *mean* pulmonary capillary P_{O_2} cannot be measured. Subjects who smoke cigarettes or have otherwise been exposed to CO may have appreciable carboxyhemoglobin levels in the blood, invalidating the test results.

Two methods are commonly used to determine pulmonary diffusing capacity for carbon monoxide ($D_{L_{CO}}$): the breath-holding method and the steady-state method. The breath-holding method is now used more widely; the subject inspires a gas mixture containing 0.4% CO and an inert insoluble gas, such as helium or neon, in air and holds a single breath in the lungs for 10 seconds. The volume of CO removed by the blood is calculated from the alveolar volume and the change in P_{CO} in the alveolar gas during the breath-holding period. In this method mean pulmonary capillary P_{CO} is neglected. $D_{L_{CO}}$ is then calculated as follows:

$$D_{L_{CO}} \text{ (ml} \times \text{min}^{-1} \times \text{torr}^{-1}) = \quad (8)$$
$$\frac{60 \times V_A}{t(P_B - 47)} \ln \left[\frac{F_{Init_{CO}}}{F_{Final_{CO}}} \right]$$

where V_A is alveolar volume, t is breath-holding time in seconds, $F_{Init_{CO}}$ is fractional concentration of CO in alveolar gas at the beginning of the breath-holding period, and $F_{Final_{CO}}$ is fractional concentration of CO in alveolar gas at the end of the breath-holding period. A disadvantage of this method is that very ill or dyspneic patients, or subjects who are exercising may have difficulty in holding their breath for the required 10 seconds.

In such cases the steady-state measurement can usually be made. This consists of breathing from a gas mixture containing 0.25% CO for a measured interval of time, during which mixed expired gas is collected and an alveolar gas sample is taken. The rate of CO uptake per minute is calculated, and the mean alveolar CO pressure is determined by analysis of the alveolar gas sample. For the most accurate measurement, blood samples should also be obtained for determination of P_{CO} to estimate the CO back pressure.

The combination of differing solubility and molecular weight explains why $D_{L_{O_2}}$ is 1.23 times greater than $D_{L_{CO}}$:

$$\frac{D_{O_2}}{D_{CO}} = \frac{O_2 \text{ solubility}}{CO \text{ solubility}} \times \frac{\sqrt{MW\ CO}}{\sqrt{MW\ O_2}} = \quad (9)$$

$$\frac{0.024}{0.018} \times \frac{\sqrt{28}}{\sqrt{32}} = 1.23$$

where solubility is in $vol \times vol^{-1} \times (760\ torr)^{-1}$ at 35° C. Thus, pulmonary diffusing capacity for CO is converted to that for O_2 by multiplying $D_{L_{CO}}$ by the factor 1.23. A similar calculation for CO_2 in relation to O_2 indicates that it must diffuse at about 20 times the rate of O_2 through an aqueous medium:

$$\frac{D_{CO_2}}{D_{O_2}} = \frac{C_{S_{CO_2}}}{C_{S_{O_2}}} \times \frac{\sqrt{MW\ O_2}}{\sqrt{MW\ CO_2}} = \quad (10)$$

$$\frac{0.592}{0.024} \times \frac{\sqrt{32}}{\sqrt{44}} = 24.7 \times 0.853 = 21.0$$

Despite the great difference in solubility, *total* $D_{L_{CO_2}}$ is not much greater than that for O_2. This is because CO_2 reacts more slowly with hemoglobin and blood buffers. When diffusing capacity is reduced, there is little impairment of CO_2 transfer, from which we conclude that $D_{L_{CO_2}}$ is high. Factors that impair D_L do not interfere with CO_2 transfer, but other factors, such as decreased transit time (reduced time for equilibration in the lung) and carbonic anhydrase inhibitors (that reduce the $HCO_3^- \leftrightarrows CO_2$ equilibration rate), cause arterial-alveolar P_{CO_2} differences. Although $D_{M_{CO_2}}$ is high, $D_{b_{CO_2}}$ is much less than that for O_2, so the sums of the transfer and equilibration rates are similar.

Factors that affect pulmonary diffusing capacity

Body position. D_L is greater in the recumbent position by 15% to 20% over that measured with the subject upright. Two factors are probably responsible for this finding: (1) pulmonary blood volume increases when a subject is recumbent, and (2) pulmonary blood flow is distributed more evenly when a subject is recumbent, tending to match more closely the distribution of ventilation within the lung, thus providing a larger effective area for diffusion.

Body size. D_L increases with body size. Thus, D_L for men is, on the average, larger than the D_L for women. After adjusting for differences of body size, the mean differences for men and women of the same age disappear. D_L increases during growth, although the increase is not proportionately so large as the weight increase. This probably means that the effective area for diffusion is *proportionately* larger in children than it is in adults.

Physical exercise. The D_L of healthy subjects increases by 25% to 35% during muscular exercise; most of the increase is achieved with moderate levels of physical activity. The increase probably results from several factors:

1. Increased ventilation of certain lung areas.
2. Increased lung perfusion, with improved distribution of $\dot{V}_A/\dot{Q}_c$ ratios, bringing the mean P_{CO} nearer to 0 in the capillary

blood. Furthermore, pulmonary capillary blood volume increases, which in itself increases D_L.

3. During exercise hemoglobin concentration increases as a result of sympathoadrenal discharge, probably also as a result of splenic contraction (not of great importance in man), and perhaps as a result of slightly decreased plasma volume from osmotic shift of water during prolonged exercise. Increased hemoglobin increases D_b slightly, partly because of the reduction of CO back pressure at any given rate of CO uptake.

4. During heavy exercise decreased mixed venous P_{O_2} may decrease competition for hemoglobin and thereby decrease the back pressure of CO (usually considered negligible, but it is, in fact, not quite 0).

Pulmonary disease. Diseases that decrease D_L do so by reducing effective surface area and/or by increasing diffusion distance.

1. Reduced effective surface area.
   a. Loss of lung tissue by excision or destruction of lung decreases both alveolar gas volume and capillary blood volume.
   b. Alveolar closure or regional airway obstruction decreases alveolar volume.
   c. Capillary obstruction, pulmonary embolism, or regional vasoconstriction reduces capillary volume.
   d. Mismatching of ventilation with perfusion reduces the effective, or functioning, membrane area for gas transfer.

2. Increased diffusion distance (increased length of diffusion pathway, or alveolocapillary diffusion block).
   a. Thickened alveolocapillary membrane (for example, fibrosis) increases diffusion distance and decreases D_L. Such conditions probably also decrease D_L by producing regions of decreased compliance, impairing the distribution of ventilation, and thus reducing the effective membrane area for diffusion.
   b. Accumulation of fluid in the lung decreases D_L. Fluid may accumulate within the alveolocapillary membrane itself (interstitial edema) or on the alveolar surface (intraalveolar edema) because of increased permeability, increased intracapillary pressure, or increased surface tension as a result of surfactant deficiency.
   c. Increased intracapillary diffusion distance also affects D_L. Low hemoglobin concentration (anemia) increases the effective intracapillary diffusion distance. It also diminishes the sink for CO and favors the development of CO back pressure.

The clinical syndrome of *alveolocapillary diffusion block* includes a variety of bronchopulmonary diseases that have in common the feature of increased alveolocapillary diffusion pathway. It is now recognized that increased diffusion pathway is less important than the effect on ventilation-perfusion matching. Regional compliance changes that result from these conditions greatly change the distribution of ventilation, disturbing $\dot{V}_A/\dot{Q}_c$ ratios and in turn decreasing the area available for gas transfer. The diseases that produce this pathophysiologic condition include pulmonary berylliosis, asbestosis, sarcoidosis, interstitial lung disease, adenomatosis, alveolar proteinosis, pulmonary edema, and to some extent, mitral stenosis.

The clinical picture includes hypoxemia and cyanosis, which are aggravated by exercise, alveolar hyperventilation, decreased arterial blood P_{CO_2}, and often essentially normal ventilatory capacity.

Tests of D_L cannot distinguish between lengthened diffusion pathway on the one hand and decreased surface area on the other; furthermore, D_L may decrease by a combination of the two. Attempts to relate pulmonary diffusing capacity to alveolar volume (D_L/V_A) can be misleading, since V_A does not reliably reflect *effective* area, although if V_A is reduced, D_L is predictably low. If $\dot{V}_A/\dot{Q}_c$ ratios (Chapter 9) are uniform throughout the lung, D_L/V_A helps to differentiate the cause of decreased D_L; however, $\dot{V}_A/\dot{Q}_c$ ratios are often also abnormal in patients who have reduced D_L.

GAS POCKETS

The absorption of gas from pockets within the body involves solubility, diffusion, and perfusion. Gas pockets in the body gradually decrease in size and disappear or, if the walls are rigid, develop a "negative" pressure. The rate of disappearance of a gas depends on its composition and the metabolic rate and circulation of the adjacent tissues, both of which may be affected by physical activity. There are two characteristics of a gas that affect the rate at which it is absorbed from a pocket: *solubility* and *diffusivity*. Solubility determines the amount of gas that can dissolve in the surrounding tissue per torr of pressure. The greater the solubility, the more rapid a gas is absorbed. The diffusivity of a gas is the rate at which it diffuses from a point of higher pressure to a point of lower pressure. It applies to dissolved gases as well as to gases in mixture. According to Graham's law the rate is inversely proportional to the square root of the molecular weight of the gas. Thus, both solubility and diffusivity are factors that affect the rate at which a gas leaves a closed pocket.

Immediately after creation of a closed gas pocket, all gases in the area begin to equilibrate between the pocket and the surrounding tissue. The gas in the pocket soon reaches a composition reflecting the initial composition, as modified by the inward movement of gases having a higher pressure in the tissues than in the pocket and by the outward movement of gases having a higher pressure in the pocket than in the tissues. Those gases with the highest solubility, greatest diffusivity, and largest pressure differences move most rapidly in the equilibration process. For example, CO_2 moves rapidly into a pocket of air. Oxygen moves out of the pocket simultaneously because of a large O_2 pressure difference, from about 145 torr in the pocket to perhaps 50 torr in the surrounding tissue. Either the volume (if the pocket is collapsible) or the pressure (if the pocket is rigid, as in the middle ear) changes in response to the early adjustment of gas composition. After the composition is adjusted according to the individual gas pressures, the volume decreases progressively as gas is absorbed from the pocket.

Why is gas absorbed from a collapsible gas pocket until the pocket disappears? Gas pockets disappear because they are ultimately subject to the atmosphere and its pressure; the blood supply in their walls is essentially venous, and venous blood is incompletely saturated. Blood, in its passage through metabolizing tissues, may lose 60 torr of P_{O_2} but gain only 5 torr of P_{CO_2}. This uneven exchange leaves venous blood with a 55 torr deficit in total gas pressure; however, the partial pressures of the various gases comprising a pocket add up to a value that is close to atmospheric pressure. After the rapid initial composition changes, during which any large gradients are minimized, there is for each gas a pressure gradient from the gas pocket to the blood leaving the vicinity of the pocket. Each gas present diffuses along this pressure gradient into the blood, and the pocket is graduallly absorbed. Although CO_2 is much more soluble than N_2 in body fluids, a pocket contains both as long as it lasts; complete loss of CO_2, which is not possible, would leave a reverse CO_2 tension gradient. The pace of CO_2 loss is set by the gas that diffuses from the pocket most slowly. The presence of N_2 in a gas pocket retards absorption greatly; it is clear that atmospheric nitrogen delays atelectasis of occluded alveoli and is thus of value for air-breathing animals.

Gas pockets occur within the body as a result of trauma, disease, obstruction of spaces such as the middle ear or paranasal sinuses, rapid decompression with aerobullosis,* or experimental production. Two such gas pockets in particular are well studied—pneumothorax and pneumoperitoneum. If the pocket is in the middle ear, where volume is fixed by bone structure, the gas loss is often replaced by a fluid transudate.

It is impossible to completely eliminate dissolved N_2 from body fluids by pure O_2 breathing as long as the skin is exposed to air; even though relatively insoluble, N_2 trickles across the skin barrier into the body. It was suggested in Chapter 1 that O_2 uptake by dry skin occurs but is not very important. However, skin has a layer of cornified epithelium, the removal of which may decrease the diffusion barrier to gases. It may be that scrubbed, wet skin permits passage of more O_2 than is commonly supposed and is even more permeable to CO_2. Scholander found that the nitrogen/argon ratio in the swim bladder of deep-sea fish is similar to the ratio of these two gases in air, and he concluded that the swim-bladder N_2 of those fish is not derived from metabolism but rather from gases dissolved in the water.

APNEIC OXYGENATION

If an animal breathes pure O_2 long enough to eliminate almost all the N_2 from its body and is then anesthetized so deeply that breathing is arrested, this animal can consume O_2 and survive for an hour or more with no breathing movements. This phenomenon was first called "diffusion respiration," but the later term *apneic oxygenation* is preferable because O_2

---

*See Glossary, hypobarogenous aerobullosis.

moves down the trachea not by diffusion, but by convection.

The respiratory exchange ratio (R_E) of such an animal is less than 1 during the experiment. Carbon dioxide entering the lung does not keep pace with the O_2 leaving the lung for the pulmonary circulation. If the animal's lung volume remains constant at FRC and if the airway is open, a pressure gradient forces O_2 from the outside down through the airway and into the lung. As the experiment goes on, only a fraction of the CO_2 produced reaches the lungs.

When alveolar P_{CO_2} reaches the level of venous blood, no more CO_2 diffuses into the lung. Most of the CO_2 is stored in the tissues, where the buffering capacity for CO_2 is high. The P_{CO_2} of the returning mixed venous blood increases (as does alveolar P_{CO_2}), but most of the gas movement across the lung is O_2 uptake, and the respiratory exchange ratio remains very low.

The remaining CO_2 increases the level of CO_2 stores all over the body. Oxygen uptake occurs almost entirely in the lungs, and the respiratory exchange ratio is low. The resulting uneven gas exchange with the pulmonary circulation creates an intrapulmonary pressure deficit, drawing a column of O_2 from the outside down the airways.

With a constant flow of gas into the lungs, there is no way of disposing of CO_2 (except through the skin). P_{CO_2} increases gradually to very high levels. The profound respiratory acidosis eventually produces a H^+ concentration of about 10 times normal, and the animal dies. Tromethamine (THAM buffer) infusion can keep the pH at normal levels and prolong survival of the experimental animal.

CHAPTER 8

PULMONARY CIRCULATION

The cardiovascular system consists of the heart, which functions as a variable output pump, and the blood vessels, which also react adaptively to changing physiologic conditions. The primary function of the cardiovascular system is to circulate the blood—distributing it according to regional needs, transporting O_2 and nutrients to metabolizing body tissues, and removing CO_2 and other products of metabolism. In addition, the circulation is involved in the regulation of body temperature, delivers leukocytes and antibodies for defense and immune processes, and plays an important role in the transport of various chemical mediators, or hormones. For all of these functions; the continuous, efficient, and adaptive performance of the heart is essential.

The cardiac output, or volume of blood that passes through the heart in 1 minute during rest, is nearly equal to the total blood volume. In response to physical activity, fever, or certain emotions, cardiac output increases. This is accomplished by some combination of increased cardiac rate and increased stroke output, the product of which is cardiac output.

The circulatory system consists of two rather different segments—the *pulmonary* circulation and the *systemic* circulation—which are connected in series. The systemic circuit is a high-resistance circuit with a large pressure difference between its arteries and veins, whereas the pulmonary circuit, which accommodates the same blood flow, normally offers only slight resistance. The pulmonary blood flow is dis-

tributed to a *single* organ, whereas the systemic circuit supplies *numerous* organs that have various functions; pulmonary blood volume is considerably less than systemic blood volume. Because the pulmonary circulation is a low-pressure, low-resistance vascular system in series with the systemic circulation, the flow through one system is identical with the flow through the other over any appreciable period of time, unless there are abnormal vascular communications (shunts) in the heart or lungs.

During diastole the venous blood flows from the right atrium through the tricuspid valve to fill the right ventricle, a process that is facilitated by atrial contraction. During systole, pressure increases within the right ventricular cavity, the tricuspid valve closes, and blood is ejected through the pulmonic valve into the main pulmonary artery. The variable volume of blood that remains in the ventricle after systole is termed its *residual volume*.

The pulmonary circulation is anatomically and functionally unique. It is more elaborate than that of any other organ, and the pulmonary blood vessels are well adapted to maintain the critical distribution of pressure and flow that optimizes respiratory gas exchange. The pulmonary circulation serves several important functions: (1) respiratory gas exchange (arterializing venous blood); (2) transport of fluid and solutes across the walls of the pulmonary exchange vessels; (3) transport of biologically important substances, such as hormones and chemical mediators, including serotonin, norepinephrine, certain prostaglandins, angiotensin I, and bradykinin, to and from the lung; (4) filtration of particulates; and (5) acting as a variable capacity blood reservoir.

The pulmonary vascular system filters all the blood that flows from right ventricle to left atrium. It removes most microthrombi, although some bypass the pulmonary capillaries through the varying arteriovenous shunts. The pulmonary circulation supplies nutrients and substrates for the metabolic activity of the lung parenchyma, including surfactant synthesis. By contrast, the source of substrates for the production of mucus is the bronchial (systemic) circulation.

The pulmonary circulation, primarily the venous side, serves as a reservoir of blood for the left ventricle. The volume of this reservoir is a factor in the regulation of total blood volume, via the Gauer-Henry volume receptors located in the large pulmonary veins and left atrium.

The main pulmonary artery divides into right and left branches, and each of these divides further, closely paralleling the arborization of the airway. Anatomically, the pulmonary vasculature does not normally contain the muscular type of arteriole that is the stopcock of the systemic circulation. The terminal branches of the pulmonary artery enter directly into dense alveolocapillary networks. In the alveoli, pulmonary capillary blood is separated from alveolar gas by a remarkably thin, continuous, submicroscopic layer of tissue, termed the *alveolocapillary membrane*. The existence of this membrane was first demonstrated by electron microscopy.

Mixed venous blood enters the pulmonary capillaries and, prior to exit, is fully arterialized by diffusion of CO_2 and O_2 across the alveolocapillary membrane. Oxygenated arterial blood then flows into the pulmonary venous system, which in turn empties into the left atrium via the four pulmonary veins. Paradoxically, the pulmonary artery contains mixed venous blood, whereas the pulmonary veins contain arterial blood.

Technics for study of the human pulmonary circulation have developed rapidly since 1929, when Forssmann performed the first right heart catheterization (on himself). This technic was subsequently developed and applied by Cournand for the study of pulmonary hemodynamics of human subjects in health and disease. Much basic physiologic information has been gained in this way, and excellent technics for diagnosis of cardiopulmonary diseases are now available.

PULMONARY BLOOD VOLUME

The total blood volume constitutes slightly less than 10% of the body weight. The pulmonary vascular bed normally contains about 10% of the circulating blood volume; thus, pulmonary blood volume is estimated to be about 500 ml but varies considerably in response to changing physiologic conditions. The capacity of the pulmonary capillary bed is estimated to be about 100 ml. When the output of the right ventricle and the input to the left atrium are equal, pulmonary blood volume remains constant. However, small differences between input and output can result in large changes of pulmonary blood volume if these differences continue for many heartbeats. The mechanism that regulates pulmonary blood volume is probably described by Starling's law of the heart, which relates the force of contraction and emptying of the ventricle to diastolic volume, a quantity that in turn is related to filling pressure. Left ventricular filling pressure probably regulates the output of the left ventricle. Hence, outflow from the pulmonary vascular bed matches the input from the right ventricle. The regulation of pulmonary blood volume probably involves more than simple passive reliance on the balance between right and left ventricular outputs.

The apparently simple series configuration of the pulmonary and systemic segments of the circulation is not entirely as it seems. The bronchial arterial circulation returns some venous blood to the pulmonary veins and left ventricle. There are precapillary anastomoses between bronchial and pulmonary arteries that under certain circumstances can increase left ventricular output without a parallel increase of right ventricular output. The thebesian circulation also increases left ventricular output, returning some coronary venous blood to the left atrium rather than through the coronary sinus to the right atrium. These channels vary from individual to individual and from health to disease. However, pulmonary blood flow is not passively affected by such changes in the balance between right and left ventricular outputs.

Other factors also affect pulmonary blood volume. It fluctuates during each cardiac cycle, the volume increasing during systole as pulmonary arterial and venous pressures increase. The magnitude of the volume change is related to the compliance of the pulmonary blood vessels. Pulmonary blood volume also fluctuates during each breathing cycle. During inspiration, more "negative" intrathoracic pressure reduces vena caval blood pressure, which in turn increases right ventricular output and pulmonary blood volume. By contrast, each expiration increases intrathoracic pressure relative to systemic arterial pressure, tending to decrease the *net* systolic pressure (in reference to diastolic pressure, which increases during expiration). This effect tends to cause a slight increase of left ventricular output. Thus, breathing produces an oscillating effect on the heart, with right ventricular output exceeding left ventricular output during inspiration, whereas left exceeds right during expiration.

Body position has an important effect on pulmonary blood volume. In the upright (standing) position, blood pools in the dependent parts of the systemic circulation (abdomen and legs). This reduces venous return, causing an approximately 25% reduction of pulmonary blood volume and cardiac output as compared with that in the supine position. Positive end-expiratory pressure (PEEP) ventilation, which is used to prevent or treat lung collapse in cer-

tain clinical conditions, also decreases pulmonary blood volume and cardiac output by impeding venous return.

PULMONARY BLOOD FLOW

The anatomy and physiology of pulmonary blood flow and lung perfusion are important for the field of circulation as well as the field of respiration. It is essential to understand the factors that determine pulmonary vascular pressures, vascular resistance, and the *distribution* of pulmonary blood flow within the lung as a background for understanding respiratory physiology.

Measurement of pulmonary blood flow

Pulmonary blood flow can be measured by any of several methods. The direct Fick method was the first to be developed and remains the reference standard for other methods. The Fick principle can be applied to any flowing stream of fluid that an indicator either enters or leaves, provided the *rate of entry or exit* of the indicator together with its *concentrations* on both sides of the site of entry or exit can all be measured. The fluid flow rate during any given period of time equals the quantity of indicator entering or leaving the stream during that same period of time, divided by the difference between the indicator concentration before and after the site of entry or exit. A basic requirement of the Fick principle is that the indicator must be thoroughly mixed with the flowing stream at each of the two sampling sites.* Therefore, in measuring pulmonary blood flow, blood samples for analysis must be obtained downstream from each ventricle, which in the absence of circulatory shunts serve as mixing chambers for the entire

---

*Oxygen is a suitable indicator for the direct Fick method because the pulmonary rate of O_2 uptake and blood O_2 concentrations are readily measurable. Furthermore, O_2 uptake is a relatively stable ongoing process that is not unduly sensitive to various slight, moment-to-moment cardiopulmonary fluctuations as, for example, is the process of CO_2 output.

bloodstream. This requires a right heart catheterization.

After right heart catheterization is accomplished, the catheter tip is placed in the pulmonary artery for withdrawal of the mixed venous blood sample. An indwelling arterial needle is inserted into a systemic artery, such as the brachial, radial, or femoral artery. A steady state of rest of the circulation and respiration is approached as closely as possible. Mixed expired gas is collected over a precisely timed interval. Samples of systemic arterial and mixed venous blood are slowly and simultaneously drawn at a constant rate from the two sources, midway during the expired gas collection. Because blood O_2 content fluctuates constantly, and during exercise or hyperventilation may do so greatly, blood samples must be withdrawn slowly and at a constant rate over a period of 10 seconds, or preferably longer, so that a *time* average sample is obtained.

The Fick principle states that the volume of O_2 taken up by the blood flowing through the lungs per minute ($\dot{V}_{O_2}$) equals the product of total pulmonary blood flow in milliliters per minute ($\dot{Q}$) and the arteriovenous blood O_2 content difference in milliliters of O_2/100 ml of blood:

$$\dot{V}_{O_2} = \dot{Q} \times (C_{a_{O_2}} - C_{\bar{v}_{O_2}}) \qquad (1)$$

The units most frequently used in this equation are ml (STPD) of O_2/min = (ml of blood flow/min) $\times$ ml (STPD) of O_2/100 ml of blood. Solving the equation for $\dot{Q}$:

$$\dot{Q} = \frac{\dot{V}_{O_2}}{(C_{a_{O_2}} - C_{\bar{v}_{O_2}})} \qquad (2)$$

Although the direct Fick method is the standard, it has three disadvantages: (1) it requires right heart catheterization, (2) it is valid only during a steady state of the subject, and (3) it requires careful analysis of arterial and mixed venous blood samples for O_2 content and mixed expired gas samples for O_2 uptake.

The most widely used method for measuring

pulmonary blood flow (cardiac output) is the *indicator-dilution method.* A single bolus of an indicator (for example, indocyanine green dye, cool saline, or radioiodinated serum albumin) is injected into a peripheral vein, and its concentration is measured continuously at a downstream site in the systemic arterial system. If a technic is used (usually graphic or mathematical) to eliminate the effect of recirculating indicator, the mean concentration of indicator per unit of time can be calculated. This result, together with the *known* amount of indicator injected, permits calculation of pulmonary blood flow:

$$\text{Mean indicator concentration} = \qquad (3)$$
$$\frac{\text{Amount of indicator injected}}{\text{Time interval} \times \text{Blood flow rate}}$$

$$\text{Blood flow rate} = \qquad (4)$$
$$\frac{\text{Amount of indicator injected}}{\text{Time interval} \times \text{Mean indicator concentration}}$$

The mean indicator concentration is determined by integrating the area under the concentration curve recorded from the arterial site and dividing by the integration time interval. Thus, the denominator on the right side of equation (4) is the area obtained by integration of the recorded curve, expressed in terms of indicator concentration multiplied by seconds.

The most widely used indicator for clinical measurement of pulmonary blood flow and cardiac output is cool saline (thermal indicator). Indicator "concentration" is in terms of °C difference between arterial blood temperature and saline (room) temperature. A thermistor thermometer of suitable sensitivity and response time is used to measure temperature in the systemic artery.

Another method of calculating pulmonary blood flow involves measuring the uptake of a chemically inert soluble gas. The most frequently used example of this method involves measurement of the rate of uptake of N_2O and the mean alveolar P_{N_2O} during a breath-holding period. The applicable equation is as follows:

$$\dot{Q} = \dot{V}_{N_2O} \times (P_{N_2O} \times C_S) \qquad (5)$$

where $\dot{Q}$ is blood flow, $\dot{V}_{N_2O}$ is the uptake rate of nitrous oxide, and C_S is the solubility coefficient of the gas in blood.

This method came into wider use after it was adapted to the body plethysmograph. The inert gas uptake method measures only pulmonary capillary blood flow because shunt blood flow does not take up the inert gas. Some of the very soluble N_2O dissolves in the tissues that line the airways, giving values for pulmonary blood flow that are somewhat higher than those measured by other methods unless a correction is made for that error.

Distribution of pulmonary blood flow

Because the pulmonary circulation is a low pressure system (mean pulmonary arterial blood pressure is 12 torr) that operates in our 1-g gravity field, the distribution of pulmonary blood flow is uneven and affected most in the upright standing position. The effect of gravity on the distribution of pulmonary blood flow has led to the concept of four *lung zones*, in which different hemodynamic conditions govern blood flow.

Zone 1. Because of low vascular resistance, pulmonary arterial pressure is low. In fact, when we are sitting or standing quietly, it is too low to cause blood to rise to the lung apices. Hence, the pulmonary capillaries are collapsed and unperfused even though the alveoli are ventilated. This lung zone includes all ventilated regions where alveolar pressure is equal to or greater than the pulmonary arterial pressure.

Zone 2. In this middle region of the lung, arterial pressure exceeds alveolar pressure and the capillaries are perfused. However, alveolar pressure exceeds pulmonary venous pressure and determines the effective perfusion pressure. Because alveolar pressure is essentially the same at all lung levels and arterial pressure increases at progressively lower lung levels as a result of hydrostatic effect, the effective per-fusion pressure (inflow pressure minus outflow pressure) increases at lower lung levels. Thus, from the level at which arterial pressure equals alveolar pressure (where perfusion begins) down to the level at which venous pressure equals alveolar pressure (below which the hydrostatic pressure difference across the alveolar capillary region does not change), blood flow increases progressively down the vertical dimension of the lung. The effect of venous pressure is not reflected in the effective perfusion pressure, and the resistance to blood flow is determined by the difference between arterial and alveolar pressure at each level.

Zone 3. In this middle-to-lower region of the upright lung venous pressure reflects the hydrostatic effect of the column of blood on the venous side of the pulmonary circulation and exceeds alveolar pressure. Vascular resistance is affected by the *difference* between arterial and venous pressure at each level, which remains constant throughout the vertical dimension of this zone. However, the vascular "distending pressure" increases because of increasing hydrostatic pressure in both arteries and veins, and the mean diameters of the vessels increase at lower levels in the zone. From Poiseuille's law, it is clear, even with the same driving pressure (arterial minus venous), that flow must increase in vessels of larger diameter; hence, there is reduced vascular resistance and a gradient of flow down zone 3, as well as down zone 2.

Zone 4. In this lowest lung zone the pressure relationships in the alveolar region are the same as in zone 3. However, extra-alveolar vessels affect the vascular resistance, changing the flow at different levels in this zone. These extra-alveolar vessels are exposed to pressures other than alveolar, resulting in different transmural pressure. They are slightly larger than alveolar vessels, about 100 μm in diameter, and are affected more by pleural pressure than by alveolar pressure. In this zone, therefore, blood flow *decreases* at lower levels because of the compressing effects of increasing interstitial pressure, which is related to, but not identical with, intrapleural pressure.

This effect on vascular resistance is important because the transmission of alveolar pressure to the small vessels affects regional, and sometimes total, vascular resistance and thus pressure-flow patterns throughout the lung.

A change of the degree of lung inflation affects the calculated pulmonary vascular resistance. Resistance is minimal when transpulmonary pressure (inflation pressure) is about 7 cm H_2O. Resistance increases as transpulmonary pressure increases and the lung inflates. An explanation, not accepted by all physiologists, is that lung inflation stretches the alveolar blood vessels, tending to narrow them as the lung expands.

As lung volume decreases from functional residual capacity (mean transpulmonary pressure approximately 7 cm H_2O), vascular resistance again increases. When the lung is collapsed, total vascular resistance is nearly twice the minimum value. (This compares with approximately 4 times the minimum at maximal lung inflation.) The cause of this increase is not completely understood, but it is probably related to compression and kinking of extra-alveolar vessels. Blood continues to flow through collapsed lung at a somewhat reduced flow rate, a reduction that results from the increased vascular resistance.

PULMONARY ARTERIAL PRESSURE

Confusion often arises because of failure to distinguish clearly among the different pressure measurements that can be made in a stream of fluid flowing through a tube. It is necessary to distinguish *driving* pressure, *lateral* pressure, *end* pressures (coming and going), and *transmural* pressure.

Hemodynamic analysis of the pulmonary circulation is complicated by the same factors that complicate study of the systemic circulation:

1. Blood vessels are not rigid tubes.

2. Blood vessels are not of uniform caliber.
3. Blood vessels are not perfectly straight.
4. Blood vessels branch irregularly.
5. Blood flow is pulsatile, not steady.
6. Blood is a nonhomogeneous, nonnewtonian liquid.

The pulmonary circulation lies within the thoracic cavity, where it is subject to the intrathoracic pressure, which it reflects immediately and with great fidelity. The intrathoracic pressure changes that occur during breathing, cough, and Valsalva and Müller maneuvers are readily detected by pressure-sensing devices placed within the pulmonary artery or veins. Such pressure increases are uniformly applied and thus tend to support the pulmonary vessels, rather than causing disruptive stress. Vagal receptors in the pulmonary conus sense increased transmural pressure and reflexly decrease blood pressure and heart rate.

The mean pulmonary arterial pressure at rest is about one eighth of the systemic arterial pressure. The pulmonary vascular bed is relatively distensible and readily accommodates increased blood flow and volume. Exercise increases pulmonary arterial pressure slightly because flow increases relatively more than resistance decreases. Following unilateral pulmonary artery ligation, pulmonary arterial pressure increases transiently but returns to a normal level after a short time. A comparison of typical hemodynamic values for the pulmonary as opposed to systemic circulation is given in Table 4.

Pulmonary arterial hypertension can result from four different pathophysiologic conditions: (1) increased pulmonary arterial blood flow and volume, as in left-to-right circulatory shunts; (2) increased resistance of the pulmonary vasculature or of the venous side of the pulmonary circulation, as in rheumatic mitral valvular disease; (3) hypoxia, with or without acidosis, as at altitude; and (4) massive loss or obstruction of the pulmonary vascular bed, as in thromboembolic disease.

Table 4. Typical hemodynamic values for the pulmonary as opposed to systemic circulation

	Pulmonary circulation	Systemic circulation
Arterial pressure (torr)		
Systolic	25	125
Diastolic	8	80
Mean	12	95
Capillary pressure (torr)	6-9	25
Blood flow (L $\times$ min^{-1} $\times$ M^{-2})	3.1	3.1
Calculated total vascular resistance index (dynes $\times$ sec $\times$ cm^{-5} $\times$ M^{-2})	100-200	1,800
Blood volume (ml)	500	5,000

PULMONARY VASCULAR RESISTANCE

Resistance is a *calculated* quantity that actually consists of several separate components. The concept includes all factors that cause a pressure loss along the intravascular course of the flowing bloodstream. The chief components of total calculated resistance at a given flow rate are viscosity and density of the blood, and length and cross-sectional area of the vascular segment under study.

Resistance may also be defined as the impedance to blood flow through a given segment of the circulation; this may be a total circuit, such as the systemic or pulmonary circuit, a region such as the hand, or an organ, such as the brain. Resistance is generally expressed in terms of pressure loss per unit of blood flow.

In contrast to airflow resistance in the bronchopulmonary system, which increases as flow increases (largely because of increased turbulence), vascular resistance tends to decrease as flow increases because the greater pressure that increases blood flow dilates the compliant vascular bed. About 60% of the resistance in the pulmonary vascular system resides in its capillary bed. By contrast only 25% of the total resistance of the systemic vascular system resides in its capillaries. Thus, the pulmonary capillaries play an important role in regulating both pulmonary vascular resistance and the distribution of pulmonary blood flow. Despite the many factors just discussed that complicate

hemodynamic analysis of the pulmonary circulation, it is common to calculate and express pulmonary vascular resistance as if the blood vessels were rigid, the blood were a newtonian fluid, and Poiseuille's law applied. If these were the conditions, resistance could be calculated accurately by analogy with Ohm's law:

$$\text{Resistance} = \frac{\text{Arterial mean pressure gradient (torr)}}{\text{Blood flow (ml/sec)}} \quad (6)$$

Aperia's formula treats the hemodynamic data so as to give the result in CGS values:

$$R \text{ (dynes} \times \text{sec} \times \text{cm}^{-5}) = \frac{(P_1 - P_2) \times 1,330}{\text{Blood flow}} \quad (7)$$

where R is resistance, $(P_1 - P_2)$ is pressure loss across the resistance bed in torr, and blood flow is blood flow through the resistance bed in milliliters per second. The pressure drop across the resistance to be calculated must be determined. Usually, both entrance and exit pressures are measured. The exit pressure for the systemic circuit is so unrelated to the entering pressure that in practice it is often disregarded. However, in the pulmonary vascular bed this is certainly not the case, and the actual pressure gradient must therefore be measured.

The transmural pressure across the alveolar wall (alveolar intrapulmonary pressure minus intrapleural pressure) can become great enough under certain conditions to interfere significantly with pulmonary capillary flow. When this happens, should equation 7 be calculated as shown, or should the pressure drop be taken as pulmonary arterial pressure minus alveolar transmural pressure? Permutt concluded that in calculating the resistance to flow of a river containing a waterfall, it is meaningless to calculate from the river source to the bottom of the waterfall. When high alveolar transmural pressure is the cause of increased resistance to flow in the pulmonary capillaries, the flow downstream from the alveoli to the pulmonary vein is a waterfall. In this situation the equation should read as follows:

$$\text{Pulmonary vascular resistance} = \tag{12}$$

$$\frac{\begin{array}{c}\text{Pulmonary arterial} \\ \text{mean pressure}\end{array} - \begin{array}{c}\text{Alveolar} \\ \text{transmural pressure}\end{array}}{\text{Cardiac output}}$$

Resistance is calculated from measurements of arterial blood flow and blood pressure (driving pressure); since these are subject to considerable error, the calculated resistance will be correspondingly in error. Small changes in resistance may therefore be of no significance. Changes in calculated resistance cannot be interpreted without consideration of arterial pressure changes and, in the pulmonary circuit, alterations of pulmonary venous or alveolar pressure as well. Changes in resistance may result from the distending effect of the inflow or exit pressure, or conversely, a change in the state of the vascular bed may be masked by alteration in the distending pressure. Other hemodynamic factors remaining equal and unchanged in a given subject, changes in calculated resistance are presumed to reflect changes in vascular cross-sectional area. However, a decrease in calculated resistance may be caused by either increased vascular distention by higher entering pressure or actual vasodilation. Another problem that arises in interpreting resistance values is the variable effect of body size. As in the case of cardiac output, the validity of using body surface area (BSA) to "take out" body size as a variable is subject to discussion.

Total pulmonary vascular resistance index (TPVRI) is a calculation of the vascular resistance from the pulmonary artery to the left atrium, whereas pulmonary arteriolar resistance index (PARI) is a calculation of the vascular resistance from the pulmonary artery to a pulmonary vein. The word *arteriolar* is used here loosely because (1) vessels comparable to the thick-walled, heavily muscled systemic ar-

Total pulmonary vascular resistance, TPVR (dynes $\times$ sec $\times$ cm^{-5}) = $\tag{8}$

$$\frac{[\text{Pulmonary arterial mean pressure (torr)}] \times 60 \times 1,330*}{\text{Cardiac output (ml/min)}}$$

Total pulmonary vascular resistance index, TPVRI (dynes $\times$ sec $\times$ cm^{-5} $\times$ M^{-2}) = TPVR/BSA (M^2) $\tag{9}$

Pulmonary arteriolar resistance, PAR (dynes $\times$ sec $\times$ cm^{-5}) = $\tag{10}$

$$\frac{\left[\begin{array}{c}\text{Pulmonary arterial mean} \\ \text{pressure (torr)}\end{array} - \begin{array}{c}\text{Pulmonary artery mean} \\ \text{wedge pressure (torr)}\end{array}\right] \times 60 \times 1,330*}{\text{Cardiac output (ml/min)}}$$

Pulmonary arteriolar resistance index, PARI (dynes $\times$ sec $\times$ cm^{-5} $\times$ M^{-2}) = PAR/BSA (M^2) $\tag{11}$

---

*1330 (mercury density $\times$ acceleration caused by gravity) is used in this formula to convert pressure from units of torr to CGS units of dynes/cm². This value varies slightly with temperature (mercury density varies with temperature), altitude, and latitude (acceleration caused by gravity, g, varies both with altitude and latitude).

terioles are not found in healthy lung* and (2) the vascular segment involved comprises pre-capillary, capillary, and postcapillary blood vessels. Furthermore, as already indicated, the capillaries contribute more than half the total pulmonary vascular resistance, so pulmonary arteriolar resistance (PAR) should probably be considered to be primarily pulmonary capillary resistance (PCR). Table 5 shows calculation of typical normal values for pulmonary vascular resistance.

To make meaningful calculations, it is necessary to measure the blood flows correctly and, when shunts are present, to use the *appropriate* flows in the resistance formula.

The important comparison of TPVRI with PARI is facilitated by calculation of percent of predicted for each as shown in equation 13.

$$\text{Percent of predicted} = \qquad (13)$$

$$\frac{\substack{\text{Value obtained from cardiac} \\ \text{catheterization data (found)}}}{\substack{\text{Typical normal mean value} \\ \text{(predicted)}}} \times 100$$

---

*However, such vessels often develop after prolonged, severe pulmonary arterial hypertension.

Clinically, the comparison of PARI with TPVRI provides important information as to *where* the circulatory resistance is located. Calculations of PARI both *before* and *after* exercise, O_2 breathing, and injection of certain drugs provide important information on whether pulmonary vascular resistance is fixed or reversible.

In clinical practice, chronic obstruction of the pulmonary circulation results from either diffuse constriction or obliteration of small pulmonary blood vessels or, in the left atrium, from thrombus, tumor, or mitral valvular disease. A third situation is the intense pulmonary vascular constriction that intervenes secondarily when pulmonary capillary pressure rises to edema-threatening levels. This occurs in mitral stenosis or high-flow, left-to-right shunts; in the latter case the pressure rise is termed an *Eisenmenger reaction*.

Also of clinical interest is the fact that development of increased peripheral vascular resistance and consequent arterial hypertension can mask a pressure gradient across a pulmonic or aortic cardiac valve, so that both diagnostic pressure gradient and cardiac murmur disappear. The value of this hemodynamic fact is apparent.

Table 5. Calculation of typical normal values* for pulmonary vascular resistance

	High normal	Low normal
Cardiac index ($\text{ml} \times \text{min}^{-1} \times \text{M}^{-2}$)	3,100	3,100
Pulmonary arterial mean pressure (torr)	15†	12†
Pulmonary artery mean wedge pressure (torr)	9	6
TPVRI		
Range: 309-386	$\dfrac{15 \times 1{,}330 \times 60}{3{,}100} =$	$\dfrac{12 \times 1{,}330 \times 60}{3{,}100} =$
Mean: 348	386 dynes $\times$ sec $\times$ cm^{-5} $\times$ M^{-2}	309 dynes $\times$ sec $\times$ cm^{-5} $\times$ M^{-2}
PARI		
Range: 77-232	$\dfrac{(15\text{-}6) \times 1{,}330 \times 60}{3{,}100} =$	$\dfrac{(12\text{-}9) \times 1{,}330 \times 60}{3{,}100} =$
Mean: 154	232 dynes $\times$ sec $\times$ cm^{-5} $\times$ M^{-2}	77 dynes $\times$ sec $\times$ cm^{-5} $\times$ M^{-2}

*Assume typical normal values for healthy man at supine rest.
†Pulmonary arterial mean pressure increases with altitude.

Lung inflation and pulmonary perfusion

As already noted, pulmonary arterial pressure is not sufficient in the normal, resting, erect, sea-level dweller to perfuse the upper portions of the lungs. However, it appears that perfusion of these areas is assisted by lung inflation. Riley has devised an analogy to explain this assistance. Groups of alveoli, or lobules, are clustered together to form a small globular mass. Each such mass touches other similar masses; however, there are spaces between these masses just as there are spaces between Ping-Pong balls stored in a basket. These spaces are occupied, in part, by pulmonary blood vessels of various intermediate sizes. Each globe increases in size during inspiration but retains its globular shape. When this occurs, the spaces between the masses increase in volume, increasing the space between adjacent globes. The pressure in the blood vessels within these spaces decreases, sucking up pulmonary arterial blood from more dependent areas. Quiet breathing is generally not of sufficient volume to promote perfusion of the lung apices in the erect person; however, deep breathing, such as the hyperpnea of exercise is sufficient. In addition, according to Permutt, the small vessels that cause resistance to blood flow are closely surrounded by alveolar pressure.

PULMONARY VASCULAR REACTIVITY

Although pulmonary blood vessels have a rich autonomic nerve supply, they are relatively unresponsive to it. The effects of changes in O_2 and CO_2 pressures on pulmonary vessels are *opposite* to the effects of these gases on systemic vessels. Alveolar hypoxia is a potent constrictor of pulmonary blood vessels (*hypoxic pulmonary vasoconstriction*), increasing pulmonary vascular resistance and pulmonary arterial pressure, whereas increased P_{O_2} dilates these vessels. Despite years of research the mechanism of hypoxic pulmonary vasoconstriction remains unknown. The reactivity of pul-

monary blood vessels to changing respiratory gas tensions is an important homeostatic factor in maintaing optimal ventilation-perfusion relationships in the lung. The tone of the pulmonary vessels is modulated by action of the sympathetic nervous system, histamine, and prostaglandins. Pulmonary vessels are relatively unresponsive to various drugs that exert powerful effects on systemic blood vessels.

Clinically, the effect of hypoxia on the pulmonary vasculature may result in serious elevation of pulmonary arterial pressure, with consequent increase of right ventricular work. The mechanism is of importance in patients with chronic mountain sickness, as well as in those with pulmonary insufficiency and cor pulmonale. High-altitude disease of cattle ("brisket disease") involves the same mechanism. Hypoxia and acidosis exert a synergistic vasoconstrictor effect on the pulmonary vasculature. The following equation describes this combined action:

$$P = K + aH + bS + \omega HS \qquad (14)$$

where P is pulmonary arterial mean pressure in torr, K, a, b, and ω are coefficients, S is arterial oxyhemoglobin unsaturation in percent, and H is H^+ concentration in $m\mu Eq/L$. In view of this synergism it is difficult to evaluate the degree to which increased calculated pulmonary vascular resistance depends on structural changes and the degree to which it depends on potentially reversible factors. Acute O_2 administration, although relieving hypoxia, simultaneously decreases alveolar ventilation, thereby increasing acidosis and tending to maintain pulmonary vasoconstriction.

A great deal of research has yielded relatively few drugs that have potent effects on the pulmonary circulation. Silove, holding blood flow rate constant in the isolated lobe of newborn calf lung, found that isoproterenol consistently produces pulmonary vasodilation, whereas norepinephrine has a variable vasoconstrictor effect that depends on the initial conditions of P_{O_2} and pH. Serotonin (5-hydroxytryptamine) constricts both the bronchi and the pulmonary vasculature, increasing pulmonary arterial pressure. Intravenous nicotine administered to anesthetized, intact dogs causes a significant rise in pulmonary arterial pressure. Experimental evidence has implicated the adrenal medulla in the response. The isolated perfused lung is refractory to nicotine, as is the intact lung after adrenalectomy. Nicotine causes pulmonary hypertension only when the adrenal glands are intact. Other conditions that cause pulmonary hypertension, such as elevated intracranial pressure and Cushing's syndrome, also have an important adrenal medullary component. Other agents believed to have a direct pulmonary vascular effect should be reexamined to determine whether they act directly on the pulmonary vasculature or exert their effects primarily through the release of epinephrine from the adrenal medulla.

Intravascular injection of small volumes of autologous hemolyzed blood produces a prompt, marked increase of pulmonary arterial pressure in experimental animals. Injection of small doses of adenosine diphosphate (ADP) causes a similar reaction, together with decreased platelet count and formation of platelet and fibrin thrombi.

The pressor response to hypoxia of normal subjects is abolished by an infusion of acetyl-

choline. Tolazoline (Priscoline), like acetylcholine, decreases pulmonary arterial pressure in many patients in whom it is initially elevated. Table 6 lists factors that are known to affect pulmonary vascular tone.

The uncommon clinical entity *primary pulmonary hypertension* is a disease of children and young, usually female, adults characterized by abnormally high pulmonary arterial pressure, sometimes exceeding systemic arterial blood pressure. The initial symptoms are usually exertional syncope and dependent edema resulting from right heart failure. The primary pathophysiologic disorder is increased resistance to blood flow in small pulmonary arteries and precapillary vessels. The disease is usually fatal within several years of the onset of symptoms. No specific therapy is known.

DETECTION OF VENOUS-TO-ARTERIAL CIRCULATORY SHUNTS

Central shunts can be defined as abnormal communications between the two sides of the circulation. Advances in thoracic surgery have made the accurate preoperative diagnosis of circulatory shunts a matter of practical concern. Shunt detection and estimation are important aspects of the diagnosis of cardiopulmonary diseases. Shunts are of three types with respect to direction of shunt flow: (1) right-to-left, or venous-to-arterial, (2) left-to-right, and (3) bidirectional. Shunt detection is basically detection of flow, and all methods of detection or semiquantitation involve either simultaneous withdrawal and analysis of blood samples for O_2 content from various parts of the circulation, or the injection or inhalation of various indicator substances.

Venous-to-arterial shunts produce arterial hypoxemia because a certain fraction of the mixed venous blood bypasses the alveolar gas. Pulmonary arteriovenous fistula is an example of such a vascular abnormality. In bronchiectasis, large abnormal shunts develop between the bronchial and pulmonary arteries. The O_2

Table 6. Factors that affect pulmonary vascular tone

Dilators	Constrictors
Beta adrenergic agonists	Hypoxia
Acetylcholine	Hypercapnia
Histamine H_2-receptors	Sympathetic nerves
Bradykinin	Alpha adrenergic agonists
Prostaglandins I_2, E_1	Histamine H_1-receptors
Theophylline	Serotonin
	Angiotensin II
	Prostaglandin $F_{2\alpha}$

method for detection of venous-to-arterial circulatory shunts is described in Chapter 17.

If Xe^{133}, an inert radioactive gas,* is dissolved in saline or blood and injected intravenously, the proportion of the injected dose that appears in the systemic arterial blood is a measure of pulmonary venous-to-arterial shunting. This relatively insoluble, foreign, radioactive gas is almost completely cleared from the blood during a single passage through the pulmonary capillaries of *ventilated* alveoli, so that radioactivity appearing in the systemic circulation must have come from shunted blood. Xe^{133} injection has been combined with a conventional indicator-dilution curve by dissolving the gas in solutions of indocyanine green dye. After making certain assumptions, the proportion of the cardiac output shunted from right to left can be calculated. This calculation give values for ve-

nous-to-arterial *pulmonary* shunt and does not include shunts of other types. It is the most specific method available.

Hydrogen is also used to detect right-to-left shunts. Hydrogen-saturated saline or blood is injected through a cardiac catheter placed in the right heart. The hydrogen is detected by a platinum electrode placed in a systemic artery. Another method involves the injection of indocyanine green dye into the right side of the circulation and sampling from the left side via a systemic artery. A densitometer system, such as is commonly used for cardiac output, records the concentration of indicator in the arterial blood and also measures the appearance time of injections made at various locations within the right heart. Angiocardiography can also be used to detect and localize shunts. Radiopaque contrast medium is injected in the right heart and observed roentgenographically as it appears in the left side of the heart.

---

*Xe^{133} is a radioactive isotope of xenon that has a half-life of 5.27 days.

CHAPTER 9

DISTRIBUTION OF INSPIRED AIR, DISTRIBUTION OF PULMONARY BLOOD FLOW, AND VENTILATION-PERFUSION RATIO

Even under physiologic conditions inspired gas and pulmonary blood flow are unevenly distributed. Diffuse bronchopulmonary diseases often exaggerate this nonuniform distribution of ventilation and perfusion. Indeed, ventilation-perfusion ratio inequality is the most common clinical cause of arterial hypoxemia.

NONUNIFORM DISTRIBUTION OF VENTILATION
Physiologic causes

1. During inspiration the shape of the thoracic cage and the movement of the ribs increase lung volume proportionately more at the base of the lung than at the apices. The volume of the upper part of the chest increases only two thirds as much per 100 gm of lung tissue as that of the lower chest because the upper ribs are less curved and the upper thoracic cage less mobile.

2. The descent of the hemidiaphragms expands the lower lobes of the lungs more than the upper lobes; downward movement of the lung above the hilum (upper lobes) must stretch the supporting trachea and is thus less than the downward movement of the lower lobes.

3. At any given level of the upright lung, inspiration expands the peripheral lung more than the deeper tissue. Thoracic expansion decreases intrapleural pressure; this expands the lung by "pulling" it out. The expansion of deeper lung tissue is also limited by its larger, stiffer supporting airways. Thus, in addition to the vertical maldistribution of ventilation, there is also an uneven distribution at any given level in the lung.

4. The distribution of a single inspiration within the lung is sequentially uneven. In the upright lung the weight of lung tissue (lung density is 0.2 that of water) and blood results in a more positive (less "negative") intrapleural pressure at the bottom of the thorax. The intrapulmonic pressure is atmospheric throughout the lung when the airway is open and air is not moving. Hence, *transpulmonary* pressure is less in the dependent (lower) lung regions than in the upper regions. The lower lung regions are less inflated because the degree of stretch of the lung at any level is related to the transpulmonary pressure at that level (Fig. 9-1).

At the end of a maximal expiration (at residual volume [RV]), the intrapleural pressure at the bottom of the lung is normally *positive* because of the weight of the lung above it. This

109

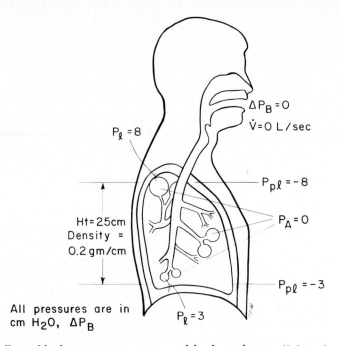

$\Delta P_B = 0$

$\dot{V} = 0$ L/sec

$P_\ell = 8$

$P_{p\ell} = -8$

$P_A = 0$

Ht = 25cm
Density =
0.2 gm/cm

$P_{p\ell} = -3$

All pressures are in
cm H_2O, ΔP_B

$P_\ell = 3$

Fig. 9-1. The effect of hydrostatic pressure caused by lung density (0.2 gm/cm vertical distance) on intrapleural pressure at different levels of lung height. Note that alveoli exposed to more "negative" pressure (toward the top) have greater transpulmonary pressure and are more expanded than those toward the bottom, where intrapleural pressure is less "negative."

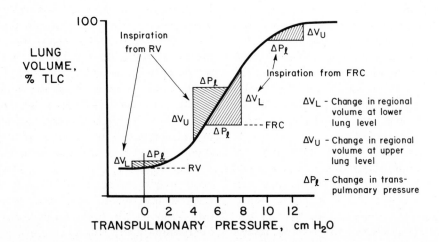

LUNG
VOLUME,
% TLC

Inspiration
from RV

ΔV_U

ΔP_ℓ

Inspiration from FRC

ΔP_ℓ

ΔV_L

ΔV_U

- - - - FRC

ΔP_ℓ

ΔV_L

ΔP_ℓ

- - - - RV

ΔV_L – Change in regional
volume at lower
lung level

ΔV_U – Change in regional
volume at upper
lung level

ΔP_ℓ – Change in transpulmonary pressure

0   2   4   6   8   10   12

TRANSPULMONARY   PRESSURE,   cm H_2O

Fig. 9-2. Effect of the lung volume at the beginning of inspiration on the vertical distribution of inspired air and relationship of volume to regional lung compliance.

dependent region is collapsed, and expansion of the entire lung must occur before intrapleural pressure becomes "negative" at the lung base and the dependent portion of the lung begins to fill. Because there is a pressure *difference* between apex and base (as long as the upright position is maintained), the upper part of the lung is on a steep portion of the sigmoid lung compliance curve, as shown on the left in Fig. 9-2. It therefore receives all the inspired air until the dependent regions open and begin to receive ventilation.

A strikingly different distribution of ventilation occurs if tidal breathing starts from functional residual capacity (FRC) instead of from RV. At this lung volume the lower region is usually open but has a smaller transpulmonary pressure than is present in the upper lobes. Therefore, as shown on the right in Fig. 9-2, the sigmoid compliance curve and the vertical gradient of transpulmonary pressure at FRC indicate that a normal inspiration goes preferentially to the lower lobes. The upper lung is already in the region where compliance decreases as volume increases and receives a progressively smaller portion of the inspired air as the inspired volume increases.

The lung presents an apparent paradox with respect to regional volume and ventilation. The dependent region contains a smaller volume of gas (per unit of resting lung volume) but receives a larger proportion of ventilation. The upper region contains a larger volume of gas at rest (is more expanded) but undergoes a smaller lung volume *change* during inspiration. This difference is the basis for the *closing volume test*, which measures the degree of lung expansion required to maintain a "negative" intrapleural pressure in the most dependent regions so that all the lung shares in ventilation.

West and co-workers demonstrated that the effect of gravity and lung weight on the distribution of compliance accounts for most of the vertical nonuniformity of distribution of ventilation. Of course, the anatomic causes of uneven distribution remain operative in the grav-

ity-free state, but they do not cause regional lung collapse and permit a more even distribution of compliance in the lung at any given lung volume.

Pathologic causes

Physiologic factors produce a certain degree of uneven distribution of inspired gas; pathologic changes of lung or airway exaggerate this uneven distribution of ventilation. Regional elasticity changes, such as pulmonary fibrosis, affect lung compliance, and less compliant lung regions inflate less for a given transpulmonary pressure difference. Regional obstruction of airways, such as a check-valve mechanism in pulmonary disease or masses that compress the airways, increases resistance to air flow, and some lung regions are ventilated inadequately. Intrathoracic fluid accumulation may limit regional expansion, change compliance, and produce nonuniform distribution of inspired gas.

NONUNIFORM DISTRIBUTION OF PERFUSION
Physiologic causes

1. The weight of the column of blood in the pulmonary circulation produces a vertical hydrostatic pressure gradient in the pulmonary blood vessels. Thus, although the arteriovenous pressure difference may be the same in all pulmonary vessels because these pressures are measured at the level of the heart, hydrostatic pressure is greater in the dependent small vessels, dilating them. Poiseuille's law indicates the powerful effect of blood vessel diameter on blood flow, in which a twofold increase of radius, for example, causes a sixteenfold increase of blood flow, other factors remaining unchanged. As a result, pulmonary capillary blood flow is much greater in the dependent lung regions and decreases almost linearly from the bottom of the healthy upright human lung to the apex, where it reaches low values.

The caliber of the entire pulmonary vascular

bed depends on the magnitude of the pulmonary arterial pressure. The lung level below which capillaries remain open and perfused depends on the arterial pressure, but the vertical arterial pressure gradient is independent of the absolute pressure. As long as the heart is pumping a column of blood into the pulmonary arterial system, there is nonuniform distribution of blood flow within the lung.

The uneven distribution of blood flow, resulting from the hydrostatic pressure gradient within the pulmonary blood vessels, impairs pulmonary gas exchange to some extent. Hence, arterial blood P_{O_2} decreases slightly when a healthy subject arises from a supine to a sitting or standing position. When a healthy subject is accelerated in a centrifuge, maldistribution of blood flow increases and may become severe. Conversely, in the weightless state, such as during orbital space flight, the distribution of pulmonary blood flow is more uniform and, because the distribution of ventilation is also more uniform, lung efficiency for gas exchange is optimal.

2. Because of the acute angle at which the right pulmonary artery branches from the main pulmonary artery, momentum carries relatively more blood into the left pulmonary artery. This difference increases as blood flow velocity increases, as, for example, when cardiac output increases or the pulmonary artery constricts. Thus, there is also a nonuniform distribution of blood flow at any given level within the lung. However, the pattern and cause of this distribution differ from that of the uneven distribution of ventilation related to lung height (vertical maldistribution).

Pathologic causes

Any alteration in the pulmonary circulation that produces a regional change in resistance to blood flow aggravates the uneven distribution of pulmonary perfusion. Kinking or compression of blood vessels caused by intrathoracic masses or embolic obstruction of pulmonary vessels contributes greatly to nonuniform distribution of pulmonary blood flow. A regional vasoconstriction, whether by direct action on blood vessels or mediated through the autonomic nervous system, also contributes to nonuniform pulmonary perfusion.

DISTRIBUTION OF VENTILATION-PERFUSION RATIOS

The gas-exchanging function of the lungs is achieved through interaction of the ventilatory gas stream with the blood perfusing the gas-exchange regions; hence, the ventilation-perfusion relationship, abbreviated $\dot{V}_A/\dot{Q}_c$ ratio, has great physiologic inportance. Various terms have been used to describe the abnormalities related to the distribution of the $\dot{V}_A/\dot{Q}_c$ ratio; these include inequality, nonuniformity, unevenness, and inhomogeneity. Concern for the $\dot{V}_A/\dot{Q}_c$ ratio is directed toward its distribution within the lung. The overall (mean) ratio reflects the average resting alveolar ventilation (about 4 L [BTPS]/min) and the average normal pulmonary capillary blood flow (about 5 L/min). The overall (or mean) calculated $\dot{V}_A/\dot{Q}_c$ ratio is thus 0.8. However, ventilation and perfusion must be distributed to the same areas to accomplish gas exchange.

The importance of matching the distribution of ventilation with the distribution of perfusion is illustrated in the following *reductio ad absurdum*. Assume that total pulmonary ventilation and total pulmonary capillary blood flow are both normal so that the overall mean $\dot{V}_A/\dot{Q}_c$ ratio is 0.8. However, assume also that the entire ventilation goes to the right lung, whereas the entire perfusion goes to the left lung. The $\dot{V}_A/\dot{Q}_c$ ratio for the right lung is therefore infinity, whereas the $\dot{V}_A/\dot{Q}_c$ ratio for the left lung is 0. No gas exchange would occur in either lung, and the condition is obviously incompatible with life.

Fatal mismatching of ventilation with perfusion occurred in emphysema patients after unilateral lung transplantation; blood flow went preferentially to the new lung because of high vascular resistance in the old one, and inspired gas went primarily to the old, abnormally compliant lung.

There is normally a nonuniform distribution of both ventilation and perfusion in the lung. Furthermore, there is a greater proportionate ventilation and a greater proportionate perfusion in the lower, or dependent, regions of the lung. However, the patterns of unevenness for ventilation do not precisely match those for perfusion, resulting in $\dot{V}_A/\dot{Q}_c$ variations throughout the lung.

As shown in Fig. 9-3, ventilation per unit of resting lung volume increases progressively from lung apex to base in a healthy subject in the upright position. The mechanics of thoracic volume change account for some of this maldistribution, but much of it results from the effect of gravity and lung weight on regional lung volume at FRC. There is also a progressive in-

crease of perfusion per unit of resting lung volume from lung apex to base in the upright position. This also results primarily from the effect of gravity, which produces a greater hydrostatic blood pressure at the lung base, dilating small pulmonary vessels.

The effect of gravity on the vertical gradient for perfusion is greater than that on the vertical gradient for ventilation (Fig. 9-3). Note the steeper slope for perfusion increase than for ventilation increase at low lung levels. This results in a nonuniform $\dot{V}_A/\dot{Q}_c$ ratio that is greater at the apex and smaller in the lower lobes. Note that it is the ratio of two changing flow rates, and that when the denominator increases more rapidly than the numerator, the ratio decreases. This is what occurs in the healthy upright human subject, producing an approximately fivefold increase in the $\dot{V}_A/\dot{Q}_c$ ratio from the bottom to the top of the lung.

MEASURING THE DISTRIBUTION OF $\dot{V}_A/\dot{Q}_c$ RATIOS

The degree of nonuniform distribution of inspired gas is commonly studied by means of the single-breath nitrogen test. This test has the virtue of being simple, rapid, and harmless. After a single deep inhalation of pure O_2, the subject expires steadily at a measured rate to RV level while the N_2 concentration in the expired gas stream is recorded with a nitrogen analyzer. Analysis of the record of N_2 concentration versus volume of gas expired yields information regarding the uniformity of distribution of inspired gas.

A better analysis of the distribution of ventilation involves measuring the distribution of an inhaled radioactive gas during a brief period of ventilation. A mixture containing a low concentration of Xe^{133} in air is inhaled, and the distribution of a single breath is recorded. The subject then continues to breathe the air-Xe^{133} mixture spontaneously for a few minutes, while scintillation counters display the pattern of radioactivity that develops in the lungs. The re-

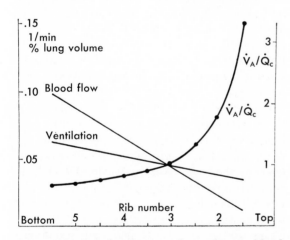

Fig. 9-3. Vertical distribution of ventilation, blood flow, and ventilation/perfusion ratio in the healthy upright human lung. Because blood flow decreases more rapidly than ventilation from the bottom to the top of the lung, ventilation/perfusion ratio rises slowly at first, then rapidly. (From West, J. B.: Ventilation/blood flow and gas exchange, ed. 2, Oxford and Edinburgh, 1970, Blackwell Scientific Publications, p. 33).

gional distribution of Xe^{133} during the initial breath indicates the distribution of inspired air, whereas the distribution of radioactivity after a few minutes of spontaneous breathing indicates regional lung *volume*, permitting calculation of regional ventilation per unit of lung volume. Radiation exposure is minimized during this test by using Xe^{133}, an isotope that has a short half-life (about 5.3 days) and is eliminated quickly by ventilation after completion of the test, and by using modern scintillation counters that register very low levels of radiation.

A test for gross disturbance of the distribution of pulmonary blood flow involves the breathing of pure O_2 for 15 minutes, after which a sample of arterial blood is drawn and analyzed for O_2 pressure. Failure to achieve an arterial P_{O_2} above about 550 torr (at sea level) indicates venous-to-arterial shunting, which may be thought of as a lung region having a $\dot{V}_A/\dot{Q}_c$ of 0 because there is perfusion without ventilation.

Another procedure for evaluating the distribution of pulmonary blood flow involves intravenous injection of macroaggregated serum albumin labeled with technetium-99m (Tc^{99m}), a radioactive isotope that has a half-life of about 6.3 hours. The injected aggregates lodge in pulmonary capillaries where blood is flowing. The perfused areas of the lung are then mapped by external scanning to produce a *lung scan*.

A recently developed method that provides quantitative data on the distribution of pulmonary blood flow also involves the use of Xe^{133}. The gas is dissolved in saline and injected into a peripheral vein. Scintillation counters placed on the chest wall display the distribution of radioactivity during a brief period of breath-holding after injection of the dissolved gas in the same way that the distribution of ventilation is displayed using Xe^{133}. The radioactive gas is distributed within the lung according to the pattern of blood flow. As Xe^{133} passes through the gas-exchanging vessels, it diffuses out of the capillaries and into the alveoli. During the breath-holding period it remains in the alveoli, where its distribution is recorded. Regions having more perfusion accumulate more radioactivity, a relationship that is reflected in the pattern of Xe^{133} distribution. The distribution of $\dot{V}_A$ can now be related to the distribution of $\dot{Q}_c$, and both can be expressed in terms of flow units per unit of regional lung volume at rest.

Other radioactive gases can also be used to study the distribution of $\dot{V}_A/\dot{Q}_c$ ratios in health and disease. Yet another method involves measuring the relative uptake rates of inert gases that have different solubilities.

CONSEQUENCES OF NONUNIFORM $\dot{V}_A/\dot{Q}_c$ RATIO DISTRIBUTION

Corrected to milliliters of ventilation per 100 gm of lung tissue, the upper lobes are ventilated approximately 65% but are perfused only about 10% as much as the lower lobes; blood flow is more disproportionate than ventilation between upper and lower lobes. The $\dot{V}_A/\dot{Q}_c$ ratio is much higher in the upper lobes (3.3) than in the lower lobes (0.66). There is thus a fivefold difference in the $\dot{V}_A/\dot{Q}_c$ ratio between upper and lower lobes. Because much of the ventilation and most of the blood flow go to the lower lobes, their $\dot{V}_A/\dot{Q}_c$ ratio is closer to the overall mean value of 0.8.

Alveolar gas composition differs from region to region of the lung because ventilation and perfusion, which determine O_2 and CO_2 exchange, are nonuniformly distributed and imperfectly matched. Only if $\dot{V}_A/\dot{Q}_c$ ratios were evenly distributed throughout both lungs would a sample of expired gas reflect the true mean gas pressures to which the pulmonary capillary blood was exposed.

There is a sequential emptying pattern of the lung that is related to the lung volume at which the gas is expired. The composition of a sample of alveolar gas reflects this pattern of emptying. Hence, an alveolar sample would represent the mean alveolar pressures for O_2 and CO_2 at any given instant only if all the alveolar gas were included. This consideration is important for the calculation of anatomic dead space, which depends on accurate measurement of the mean alveolar P_{CO_2}.

PHYSIOLOGIC ADJUSTMENTS TO NONUNIFORM $\dot{V}_A/\dot{Q}_c$ RATIO DISTRIBUTION

Regional lung responses improve the distribution of $\dot{V}_A/\dot{Q}_c$ ratios, restoring a more even pattern after alteration by such factors as postural change or bronchopulmonary disease. Hyperperfused regions remove more O_2 from alveolar gas, decreasing alveolar P_{O_2}; this regional hypoxemia causes regional vasoconstric-

tion, diverting blood to other lung regions. Even slight regional vasoconstriction strongly affects the distribution of perfusion; blood flow decreases in the region of vasoconstriction, and because total blood flow remains unchanged, perfusion of other regions increases.

In regions of relative hyperventilation and high $\dot{V}_A/\dot{Q}_c$ ratio, alveolar P_{CO_2} is low because of CO_2 washout. Regional hypocapnia produces local bronchoconstriction, decreasing the $\dot{V}_A/\dot{Q}_c$ ratio in that region where it was high and redistributing ventilation to regions where $\dot{V}_A/\dot{Q}_c$ was low, while *total* $\dot{V}_A$ remains unchanged.

The regional responses affecting the distri-

Table 7. Regional responses affecting distribution of $\dot{V}_A/\dot{Q}_c$ ratios within the lung

Regional abnormality	Effect	Reflex response	Result
Decreased $\dot{Q}$ or increased $\dot{V}$ (high $\dot{V}_A/\dot{Q}_c$ ratio)	Regional hypocapnia	Bronchoconstriction	Decreased regional $\dot{V}$ (reduced $\dot{V}_A/\dot{Q}_c$ ratio)
Decreased $\dot{V}$ or increased $\dot{Q}$ (low $\dot{V}_A/\dot{Q}_c$ ratio)	Regional hypoxemia	Vasoconstriction	Decreased regional $\dot{Q}$ (increased $\dot{V}_A/\dot{Q}_c$ ratio)

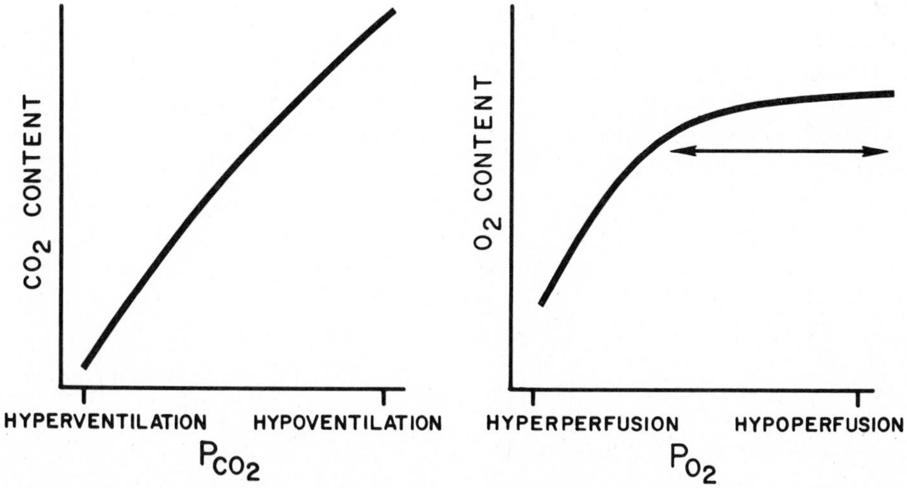

Fig. 9-4. Importance of CO_2-dissociation curve (left) and oxyhemoglobin dissociation curve (right) for gas exchange in areas of high or low $\dot{V}_A/\dot{Q}_c$.

bution of $\dot{V}_A/\dot{Q}_c$ ratios within the lung are summarized in Table 7. These responses constitute a local homeostatic mechanism, favoring equalization of $\dot{V}_A/\dot{Q}_c$ ratio distribution.

Despite the surprising degree of nonuniformity of distribution and mismatching of ventilation and perfusion, the *efficiency* of gas exchange is 97% to 98% of the theoretic maximum value for both O_2 and CO_2. This calculation takes 100% as the maximum amount of each gas that would exchange if the normal total ventilation and total perfusion were perfectly distributed and matched throughout both lungs. The high efficiency of gas exchange, despite striking variations of $\dot{V}_A/\dot{Q}_c$ ratio distribution, is a result of the shapes of the dissociation curves for CO_2 and O_2 (Fig. 9-4). The CO_2 dissociation curve (CO_2 content as a function of P_{CO_2}) is relatively steep and nearly linear in the physiologic range, facilitating efficient unloading of CO_2 in regions of hyperventilation (high $\dot{V}_A/\dot{Q}_c$) despite low $P_{a_{CO_2}}$. In contrast, the oxyhemoglobin dissociation curve is relatively flat in the physiologic range of lung P_{O_2}; thus, even in regions of hyperperfusion (relative hypoventilation and low P_{O_2}) O_2 content decreases little and blood loads O_2 efficiently, despite a low $\dot{V}_A/\dot{Q}_c$ ratio. As long as the overall mean $\dot{V}_A/\dot{Q}_c$ ratio is normal, the shapes of the dissociation curves for O_2 and CO_2 tend to maintain efficient gas exchange, despite regional variations in the distribution of ventilation and perfusion. If maldistribution of $\dot{V}_A/\dot{Q}_c$ is severe, hypoventilation and blood shunting through nonventi-

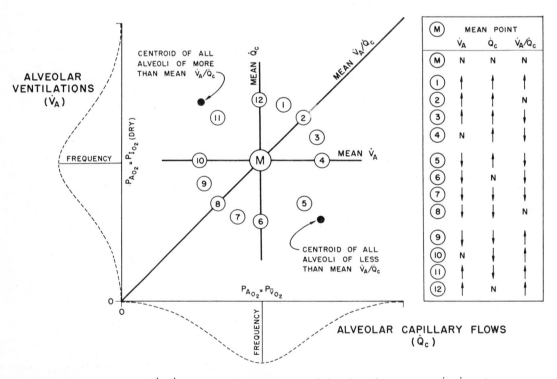

Fig. 9-5. Illustration of $\dot{V}_A/\dot{Q}_c$ ratios and classification of alveoli with respect to $\dot{V}_A/\dot{Q}_c$ relationships (schematic only; not based on actual data).

lated areas ($\dot{V}_A/\dot{Q}_c = 0$) are extreme and the physiologic mechanisms that maintain gas exchange cannot compensate.

CONSEQUENCES OF PATHOLOGICALLY NONUNIFORM $\dot{V}_A/\dot{Q}_c$ RATIO DISTRIBUTION

If the overall mean $\dot{V}_A/\dot{Q}_c$ ratio is normal, a pathologically nonuniform distribution of $\dot{V}_A/\dot{Q}_c$ ratios produces hypoxemia but not CO_2 retention. When ventilation and perfusion are very nonuniformly distributed and mismatched, regions of marked hyperventilation coexist in the lung with regions of marked hypoventilation. Regions of hyperventilation, high $\dot{V}_A/\dot{Q}_c$ ratio, and low blood CO_2 content compensate for regions of hypoventilation, low $\dot{V}_A/\dot{Q}_c$ ratio, and high blood CO_2 content. If overall alveolar ventilation is essentially normal, *average* arterial blood CO_2 content is also normal.

Regions of low $\dot{V}_A/\dot{Q}_c$ ratio produce hypoxemic blood. In regions of hyperventilation and high $\dot{V}_A/\dot{Q}_c$ ratio, blood O_2 content cannot increase because normal ventilation almost fully saturates hemoglobin. Thus, the mixture of blood from hyperventilating regions with that from hypoventilating regions is hypoxemic.

The population of hyperventilated alveoli, with greater than average $\dot{V}_A/\dot{Q}_c$ ratios (Fig. 9-5), having higher than average P_{O_2} values, contributes proportionately more O_2 to the expired gas. Because these same alveoli are hypoperfused, the O_2-rich blood that leaves them contributes proportionately less O_2 to the pulmonary venous blood. The population of alveoli with less than average $\dot{V}_A/\dot{Q}_c$ ratios has lower than average P_{O_2} values and undercontributes this low P_{O_2} to expired gas. Blood flowing through this population overcontributes its low P_{O_2} to pulmonary venous blood. Thus, even in the absence of an alveolar-arterial P_{O_2} gradient for any single alveolus, this mismatching of ventilation and perfusion gives rise to an overall alveolar-arterial P_{O_2} gradient.

The alveolar gas concentrations at all possible $\dot{V}_A/\dot{Q}_c$ ratios can be plotted on an O_2-CO_2 diagram (Fig. 9-6). The limits of the heavy line are the inspired gas point where $\dot{V}_A/\dot{Q}_c = \infty$ and the mixed venous blood point where $\dot{V}_A/\dot{Q}_c = 0$.

The consequences of large variations in the distribution of $\dot{V}_A/\dot{Q}_c$ ratios are complex and interesting. For example, in the healthy erect subject, because of relative hyperventilation of the upper lobes, much of the CO_2 is exchanged there. Because of the proportionately larger blood flow to the lower lobes, more of the O_2 is taken up there. Thus, the pattern of O_2 and CO_2 exchange differs from place to place within the lungs.

In chronic diffuse bronchopulmonary disease, maldistribution and mismatching of ventilation and perfusion commonly increase functional dead space and produce shuntlike effects, initially causing hypoxemia and finally CO_2 retention. Alveolar P_{O_2} may be normal or even increased as a result of compensatory hyperventilation. However, ventilation-perfusion problems must be distinguished from alveolar hypoventilation, which decreases alveolar P_{O_2} and increases alveolar P_{CO_2}.

THE O_2-CO_2 DIAGRAM

Our understanding of alveolar gas, its composition, its changes, and its physiologic significance is greatly facilitated by the O_2-CO_2 diagram. This diagram plots alveolar P_{CO_2} versus alveolar P_{O_2}, permitting simultaneous visual appreciation of the static and dynamic relationships of the two respiratory gases (Fig. 9-6). Oxygen pressure, or P_{O_2}, is plotted on the horizontal axis, and CO_2 pressure, or P_{CO_2}, on the vertical axis. In its simplest form the diagram shows the normal alveolar gas of healthy man at sea-level rest (alveolar $P_{O_2} = 100$ torr, alveolar $P_{CO_2} = 40$ torr), the saturated inspired air point (inspired $P_{O_2} = 150$ torr, inspired $P_{CO_2} = 0$), and a straight line joining these two points whose slope, R, is proportional to the respiratory exchange ratio.

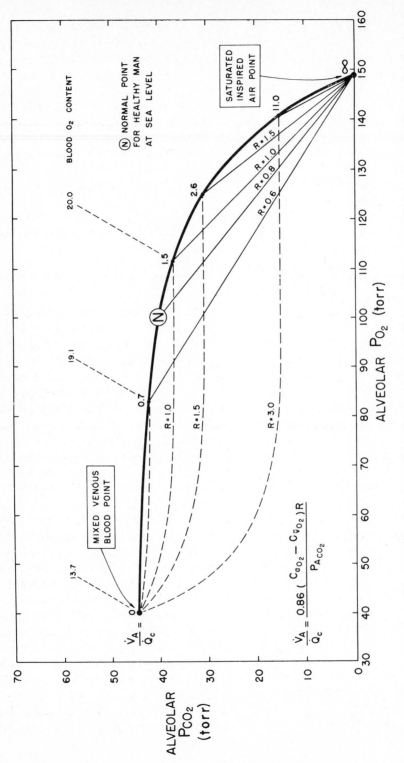

Fig. 9-6. O_2-CO_2 diagram. The heavy line indicates all possible combinations of O_2 and CO_2 tension that can theoretically exist in the alveoli and pulmonary capillary blood for the particular inspired gas, with mixed venous blood tensions indicated by the two heavy dots. Every point on this ventilation-perfusion line is determined by a particular $\dot{V}_A/\dot{Q}_c$ ratio. (From Rahn, H., and Fenn, W. O.: A graphical analysis of the respiratory gas exchange, Washington, D.C., 1955, The American Physiological Society.)

If pure O_2 is breathed, the R line slope on the O_2-CO_2 diagram is no longer proportional to the steady-state respiratory exchange ratio, R_s. Since no N_2 is present, the sums of P_{CO_2} and P_{O_2} must equal $P_B - 47$. A plot of this situation would show the inspired gas point (inspired $P_{O_2} = P_B - 47$, inspired $P_{CO_2} = 0$) and the alveolar gas point (alveolar $P_{O_2} = P_B - 47 - 40$, alveolar $P_{CO_2} = 40$). The R line slope is then -1; its slope is always -1 whenever pure O_2, or a mixture containing only O_2 and CO_2, is breathed, regardless of the metabolic respiratory quotient, R_s.

If a resting sea-level resident begins to hyperventilate with air, alveolar P_{O_2} is increased and alveolar P_{CO_2} is reduced (Fig. 16-3). Eventually, if a constant level of hyperventilation is maintained, the alveolar gas point comes to rest on the R line, the alveolar pathway during the intervening unsteady state having described a portion of a clockwise loop. Initially, alveolar P_{O_2} rises much more rapidly than alveolar P_{CO_2} drops.* With continued hyperventilation, however, alveolar P_{CO_2} gradually drops until the alveolar gas point reaches the R line and a steady state of hyperventilation is achieved—that is, there is no further change in the level of body CO_2 stores. Resumption of normal breathing is followed by alveolar gas value changes that complete the clockwise loop on the diagram; the alveolar gas values return to their original point on the R line. However, before this steady state is again achieved, alveolar P_{O_2} drops with more rapidity than alveolar P_{CO_2} rises, since it takes time to accumulate the metabolically produced CO_2 and augment the body stores.

The closed hyperventilation-and-recovery loop on the O_2-CO_2 diagram graphically por-

trays the impact of unsteady states on alveolar gas composition and respiratory exchange ratio. When CO_2 output equals CO_2 produced, a steady state exists; when CO_2 output equals current metabolic CO_2 production plus CO_2 from stores, R_A (alveolar R) is larger than R_s. When only a fraction of current metabolic CO_2 production is expired and the balance is being stored, R_A is less than R_s. Summarizing:

$$\frac{\dot{V}_{CO_2}}{\dot{V}_{O_2}} = R_s = R_A \text{ (steady state)}$$

$$\frac{\dot{V}_{CO_2} + CO_2 \text{ from stores}}{\dot{V}_{O_2}} = \text{High } R_A \text{ (unsteady state)}$$

$$\frac{\dot{V}_{CO_2} - CO_2 \text{ being stored}}{\dot{V}_{O_2}} = \text{Low } R_A \text{ (unsteady state)}$$

The R line slope on the O_2-CO_2 diagram is proportional to the respiratory exchange ratio, R_E, calculated from analysis of expired gas, except when pure O_2 is breathed. However, not one but many R lines can be drawn. When $\dot{V}_{CO_2} = \dot{V}_{O_2}$, R_E is 1 and the R line slope is -1; an R line slope steeper than -1 indicates an R_E greater than 1. Early in hyperventilation the slope of a line connecting the alveolar gas point with the inspired air point is steeper than 1, indicating an R_E greater than 1, or a CO_2 output that is in excess of O_2 uptake. During recovery from hyperventilation R_E is low, the R line slope on the O_2-CO_2 diagram is gradual, and much of the current metabolic CO_2 production is being stored rather than blown off.

Hypoventilation and recovery also produce a clockwise loop on the O_2-CO_2 diagram. An example of such a loop is seen during spontaneous breathing under general anesthesia. Initially, the drop in alveolar P_{O_2} far exceeds the rise in alveolar P_{CO_2}. As CO_2 stores increase, alveolar P_{CO_2} rises until a steady state for that level of ventilation is reached at the R line. Recovery from the anesthesia-induced ventilatory depression completes this clockwise loop but requires an extended period of many minutes,

---

*Large quantities of CO_2 are stored in the body, mostly as HCO_3^-. Substantial depletion of this stored CO_2 must occur before P_{CO_2} can fall appreciably. Since O_2 is not stored in appreciable quantities, alveolar P_{O_2} reacts more quickly to changes of pulmonary ventilation.

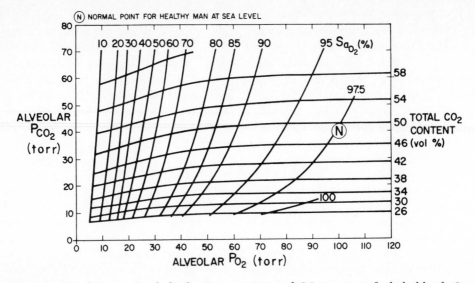

Fig. 9-7. O_2-CO_2 diagram. Isopleths for O_2 saturation and CO_2 content of whole blood. Oxyhemoglobin capacity is 20 vol%. Slope of $\dot{O}_2$ isopleths represents the Bohr effect, and slope of CO_2 isopleths represents the Haldane effect. (From Rahn, H., and Fenn, W. O.: A graphical analysis of the respiratory gas exchange, Washington, D.C., 1955, The American Physiological Society.)

during which the R line slope is greater while excess CO_2 stores are blown off in the expired gas.

Values for O_2 content and oxyhemoglobin saturation can be taken from a family of oxyhemoglobin dissociation curves plotted on an O_2-CO_2 diagram. Each curve is associated with a given P_{CO_2}—that is, a different Bohr effect. Such a plot is shown in Fig. 9-7.

The versatility of the O_2-CO_2 diagram is illustrated by Fig. 16-1, which shows the effects of departure from normal alveolar gas values. Hypoxia, CO_2 narcosis (not anesthesia at these P_{CO_2} values), hyperoxia, and hypocapnia surround the normal area. The rounded corners of these regions imply a synergism between adjacent effects.

CHAPTER 10

BLOOD-GAS TRANSPORT

HEMOGLOBIN

The transport of molecular O_2 within the circulatory systems of vertebrates is greatly facilitated by the hemoglobins—pigments that are remarkably adapted to their function. Hemoglobin increases blood O_2 content and capacity for any given loading pressure (P_{O_2}), whereas its intraerythrocytic location prevents the drastic colloid osmotic effect that would otherwise result if 15 gm/dL of protein were free in the plasma.

Ferrohemoglobin and ferrihemoglobin

Human erythrocytes are normally in the shape of biconcave discs; they consist of about one-third hemoglobin. Each of the four heme groups in the normal adult hemoglobin molecule (Hb A) has a polypeptide chain. These chains are of two types: alpha, which has 141 amino acid residues, and beta, which has 146 residues; each half-molecule of hemoglobin thus contains almost 300 amino acid residues.

Hemoglobin consists of a protein globin and a ferrous-protoporphyrin complex, ferroheme. Its iron content is 0.335% to 0.340%, and its molecular weight of about 67,000 corresponds to the presence of four hemes per molecule. Oxygen and carbon monoxide combine with ferrohemoglobin in the ratio of one gas molecule per ferroheme. The oxidation of ferroheme to ferriheme by the loss of one electron produces ferrihemoglobin, a derivative that combines with a number of anions but not with O_2 or CO. These reactions are reversible, the globin being unaffected in each case, and each of the compounds has a characteristic absorption spectrum. Ferrohemoglobin and ferrihemoglobin are also called hemoglobin and methemoglobin, respectively. The stable complex of the cyanide ion with methemoglobin, cyanmethemoglobin, finds use both as a standard in hemoglobinometry and in the treatment of cyanide poisoning. Since the various compounds of hemoglobin differ with respect to chemical and physical properties, erroneous results may be obtained from analysis of blood samples containing hemoglobin that is partially oxidized to ferrihemoglobin, denatured, or converted to another hemoglobin compound. Such changes may occur during the course of an analysis.

Methemoglobin is produced in nitrite poisoning and in toxic reactions to oxidant drugs.* Congenital methemoglobinemia is the result of a deficiency of diphosphopyridine nucleotide diaphorase; hereditary methemoglobinemia with and without mental retardation has been described. Hereditary methemoglobinemia is the result of an inherited defect in the enzyme-controlled reducing mechanism of the red blood cell, permitting accumulation of met-

---

*The aniline breakdown products of certain local anesthetics, such as the toluidine derivative prilocaine (Citanest), produce methemoglobin and, when administered in large doses, may even cause visible discoloration of the skin and mucous membranes. However, such methemoglobinemia is not clinically serious unless hypoxia or methemoglobinemia already exists; it is readily corrected by intravenous administration of methylene blue.

hemoglobin and resulting in heterogeneity with respect to the oxidation state of the heme iron after the hemoglobin molecule has been completely synthesized. A form of inherited methemoglobinemia has been described in which the globin moiety is apparently affected.

Carbon monoxide combines avidly with both hemoglobin and myoglobin, the respiratory pigment in "red" muscle cells. Its affinity for hemoglobin is about 210 times (Haldane number) as great as that for O_2. Carboxyhemoglobin, also called carbon monoxyhemoglobin, occurs in the blood of smokers and of individuals exposed to the exhaust fumes of internal combustion engines. The blood of firemen who have just attended a blaze may contain large amounts of carboxyhemoglobin. Carbon monoxide is very slowly oxidized in the body to CO_2. A small amount of CO is formed as a product of hemoglobin catabolism. Certain plants, for example, ocean kelp (*Nereocystis luetkeana*), produce CO in abundance.

Xe^{133} is a radioactive isotope with a half-life of 5.27 days and gamma emission of 81 kev that is used as an indicator for study of inspired gas and pulmonary blood flow distribution, as well as for determination of cardiac output. The gamma emission of Xe^{133} is readily detectable, yet sufficiently soft that relatively large doses produce little tissue damage. It is therefore of interest that xenon combines chemically with both hemoglobin and myoglobin, occupying a specific site in each molecule.

The biochemical structure and physiologic function of hemoglobin are intimately related. The enzymatic removal of a single histidine residue from the terminal end of the beta chain of globin (remote from heme) results in a pigment having a hyperbolic oxyhemoglobin dissociation curve, whereas removal from the alpha and beta chains of only five amino acid residues increases its affinity for O_2 50 times and eliminates the Bohr effect.

Fetal hemoglobin

Körber discovered in 1866 that the hemoglobin from human placental blood is more resistant to denaturation by aklali and by acid than the hemoglobin of adult blood. It is now known that this pigment is fetal hemoglobin (Hb F). Other species also have a fetal and an adult form of hemoglobin. The hemoglobin of a newborn infant is a mixture of fetal and adult forms. Hb F is present in the blood of normal infants for some months beyond the expected life span of the red cells in the peripheral circulation at birth. Replacement of Hb F by Hb A may be complete by the end of the first year of postnatal life; however, Hb F persists beyond infancy in some types of severe, chronic anemia. The structure of Hb F is an inherited characteristic, and its properties are characteristic for a given species. The control of its synthesis appears to differ from that of the normal and abnormal adult hemoglobins, since a patient may have Hb F in addition to two of the inherited adult forms. A small amount of Hb F may be present in all nonanemic adults, and elevated amounts are produced under the stress of acquired as well as congenital anemia; thus the production of this form is not restricted to the fetal period of life.

Abnormal hemoglobins

Considerable progress has been made in studying the genetics and biochemistry of Hb A synthesis. The discovery by Linus Pauling of the genetically determined biochemical abnormality of sickle cell hemoglobin (Hb S) opened up a new field in molecular biology. Hereditary variations of hemoglobin polypeptides are prototypes of abnormal protein synthesis. Within a relatively brief time, more than 30 abnormal hemoglobins have been described that differ from normal hemoglobin by a single amino acid residue in the alpha or beta chain. All but one can be explained on the basis of a single base change in the corresponding structural gene.

One abnormal hemoglobin, termed *Lepore,* is the result of an unequal crossover between beta and delta loci. Hemoglobins H and Barts are multimers of normal polypeptide chains, not hemoglobin variants. Unlike Hb F, the abnormal hemoglobins are very similar structurally and chemically to Hb A. An individual with two abnormal hemoglobin alleles, alike or unlike, has no Hb A in the red blood cells. Like Hb A, the abnormal hemoglobins are present in very low concentration at birth.

Before a hemoglobin is accepted as a new form and given a letter designation, characterization by electrophoresis with both the moving boundary and the zone technics at different pH's, chromatography, solubility, spectrophotometry with visible and ultraviolet light, and denaturation by alkali and cold are usually necessary.

Pauling demonstrated that Hb S is electrophoretically abnormal and that the hemoglobin in individuals with sickle cell trait, an asymptomatic condition, is a mixture of the abnormal form with normal Hb A. A single abnormal gene induces the synthesis of this abnormal hemoglobin. He originally suggested that sickling is caused by the chemically abnormal hemoglobin molecule, which on deoxygenation aggregates into rods and twists the erythrocyte out of shape. Deoxygenated Hb S is less soluble than deoxygenated normal hemoglobin or either type of oxyhemoglobin. The abnormality of Hb S is genetically determined; glutamic acid is replaced by valine at the sixth position in each of the two beta polypeptide chains. It has been suggested that this substitution creates a hydrophobic intramolecular bond that changes the configuration in such a way that molecular stacking occurs.

Reduced ferrohemoglobin is paramagnetic, whereas oxyhemoglobin and carboxyhemoglobin are diamagnetic. Normal human erythrocytes do not orient themselves in a magnetic field. However, deoxygenated sickled erythrocytes in a magnetic field of 3.5 kilogauss orient themselves with their long axes perpendicular to the magnetic lines of force, suggesting that Hb S molecules are linearly arranged.

OXYGEN TRANSPORT

Blood carries O_2 in two ways: (1) in physical solution as O_2 dissolved in the aqueous phase and (2) in a loose reversible chemical combination with hemoglobin, as oxyhemoglobin. In both cases the amount of O_2 held depends on the O_2 tension, or loading pressure, to which the blood is exposed.

Dissolved oxygen

Dissolved O_2, also termed O_2 in physical solution, comprises little more than 1% of the total blood O_2 content under ordinary physiologic conditions. The amount of O_2 dissolved in blood is directly proportional to the P_{O_2} to which it is exposed (Fig. 10-1). Henry's law implies that at constant temperature the amount of dissolved O_2 depends on the solubility coefficient (C_s) of O_2 in blood and is a linear function of P_{O_2}. Since the C_s for O_2 at 38° C is 0.003 vol%/torr, arterial blood that has a P_{O_2} of 95 torr contains about 0.29 vol% dissolved O_2. When a healthy subject breathes pure O_2 at sea level, alveolar P_{O_2} rises toward a theoretic maximum of 673 torr, arterial P_{O_2} exceeds 600 torr, and dissolved O_2 approaches 2 vol%. It is possible, but usually not of practical importance, to distinguish the fraction of dissolved O_2 that is in the blood plasma from the remainder that is dissolved in the aqueous phase within the blood cells.

Hyperbaric chambers increase total pressure to several times atmospheric pressure. During hyperbaric oxygenation, the concentration of dissolved O_2 increases proportionately in accordance with Henry's law and may then comprise a significant fraction of the total blood O_2 content. A subject breathing pure O_2 at 3-atm pressure has an alveolar P_{O_2} of approximately

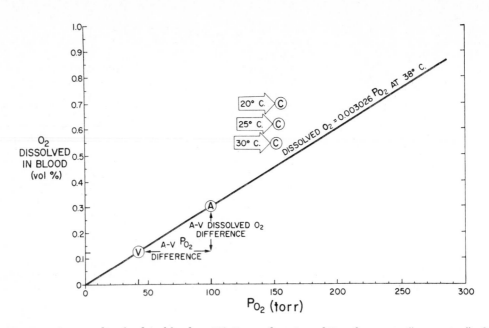

Fig. 10-1. Oxygen dissolved in blood at 38° C as a function of P_{O_2}; for use in "correction" of various blood samples for dissolved O_2 content in calculation of oxyhemoglobin saturation. Typical normal points are given for arterial, (A), mixed venous, (V), and air-equilibrated capacity, (C), blood samples at sea level.

2,000 torr, and the arterial blood contains about 6 vol% of dissolved O_2. This amount of dissolved O_2 would theoretically satisfy the O_2 requirements of a subject at rest. However, the toxicity of O_2 at high pressure limits the medical use of hyperbaric oxygenation to treatment of certain conditions by experts.

In homothermic animals temperature is not ordinarily a physiologically important variable affecting gases dissolved in blood, except during febrile or hypometabolic states such as hypothermia or hibernation. However, in certain poikilothermic species temperature is indeed an important variable, and for aquatic forms it may be a variable affecting the dissolved O_2 content of the aquatic environment as well as blood O_2 content. The effect of temperature on the dissolved O_2 content of whole blood is illustrated by the following data from Table 8. At a P_{O_2} of 760 torr, whole blood contains 2.32 vol

% of dissolved O_2 at 38° C, whereas it contains 3.29 vol% at 22° C.

In this regard the ice fish (*Chaenocephalus aceratus*) is an interesting example of vertebrate adaptation involving the relationship of dissolved O_2 to temperature. These fish attain a length of about 2 feet (60 cm) and are almost completely devoid of scales. They are truly anemic, virtually lacking both red blood cells and hemoglobin. The Antarctic Ocean water in which they live remains near 0° C throughout the year. The body temperature of this poikilothermic animal is approximately that of the surrounding frigid water, so that tissue metabolic demand for O_2 is low, whereas the low water temperature permits a good concentration of dissolved O_2.

It is interesting to compare the concentrations or pressures of various substances taken up and then released by the blood in arterial

Table 8. Dissolved oxygen in whole blood at various temperatures*

Temperature (° C)	Dissolved O_2 ml/100 ml blood P_{O_2} = 760 torr (vol%/atm)	Dissolved O_2 ml/100 ml blood/torr P_{O_2} (vol%/torr)
20	3.44	0.00453
22	3.29	0.00433
24	3.12	0.00411
26	3.00	0.00395
28	2.85	0.00375
30	2.73	0.00359
32	2.61	0.00343
34	2.52	0.00332
36	2.41	0.00317
38	2.32	0.00305
40	2.23	0.00293

*From Dittmer, D. S., and Grebe, R. M., editors: Handbook of respiration, Philadelphia, 1958, W. B. Saunders Co., p. 7.

blood samples with their concentrations or pressures in mixed venous blood samples. Such differences are termed *arteriovenous differences*. Given normal values for a healthy subject at rest, cardiac output equals 5.63 L/min, O_2 uptake equals 240 ml (STPD)/min, and arterial blood total O_2 content equals 18.97 vol %; the Fick equation relates these factors as follows:

$$\dot{Q} = \frac{\dot{V}_{O_2} \times 1/10}{C_{aO_2} - C_{\bar{v}O_2}}$$

$$5.63 = \frac{240 \times 1/10}{18.97 - 14.71} = \frac{24}{4.26}$$

Thus, in healthy man at rest the amount of O_2 extracted from the blood by the tissues (arteriovenous blood O_2 difference) is about 4 vol%; in contrast the arteriovenous difference for dissolved O_2 is about 0.18 vol%, or 4.5% of the total O_2 extracted.

Oxygen combined with hemoglobin

From the foregoing it is apparent that the amount of O_2 dissolved in blood or plasma is insufficient for tissue needs even at rest, and it certainly does not constitute the kind of reservoir required for intermittent physical activity, during which tissue O_2 demand may suddenly increase 15 to 20 times. In the resting subject more than 95% of the O_2 delivered to the tissues is transported in combination with hemoglobin, and during exercise this value may exceed 99%. The loading, transport, and unloading of O_2 are some of the physiologically significant functions of the remarkable pigment of vertebrate blood—hemoglobin.

Each molecule of hemoglobin contains four sites for combination with molecular O_2. Avogadro's law, defining the number of molecules per unit volume of gas, together with the molecular weight of hemoglobin, implies that 1 gm of hemoglobin can combine chemically with a maximum of about 1.36 ml (STPD) of O_2. One hundred milliliters of blood containing 15 gm of hemoglobin can combine with 15 × 1.36 = 20.4 ml (STPD) of O_2. The amount of O_2 actually combined with hemoglobin depends on blood P_{O_2}, since oxygenation is a reversible process that depends on the P_{O_2} to which the hemoglobin is exposed. Unlike dissolved O_2,

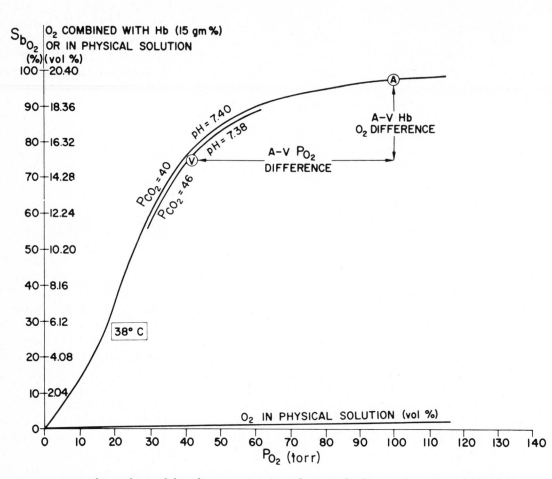

Fig. 10-2. The oxyhemoglobin dissociation curve, showing the basic relationship of blood O_2 transport. Its shape has great physiologic importance. The full curve above applies to the arterial blood of healthy man at rest, whereas the small section to its right applies to venous blood. Point Ⓐ represents normal values for arterial blood, and point Ⓥ, for venous blood. Changes in CO_2 pressure, pH, or temperature displace the oxyhemoglobin dissociation curve to the right or left. A physiologic shift from the venous to the arterial curve takes place as blood flows through the pulmonary capillaries, losing CO_2 and increasing in pH. The reverse shift occurs as blood flows through the systemic capillaries. Note that this effect, termed the Bohr shift, facilitates O_2 uptake in the lungs and O_2 dumping in the tissues. Note also the relatively small amount of O_2 carried by the blood in physical solution in the physiologic range of O_2 pressure.

the amount of O_2 combined with hemoglobin is *not* linearly related to P_{O_2} but is described by an S-shaped curve that slopes steeply between 10 and 50 torr P_{O_2} and has a nearly flat portion above 70 torr P_{O_2} (Fig. 10-2).

The unique shape of this oxyhemoglobin dissociation curve is an important example of physiologic adaptation. The relatively flat portion above 70 torr ensures the oxygenation of most hemoglobin despite wide variations in alveolar (and therefore arterial) P_{O_2}. On the other hand, the steep portion of the curve between 10 and 50 torr P_{O_2} assures unloading of large amounts of O_2 in the systemic capillaries in response to small tissue P_{O_2} decrements. The dissociation curves of various hemoglobins, including fetal hemoglobins and myoglobins, are beautiful examples of adaptation to environment.* As a result of the shape of the oxyhemoglobin dissociation curve, patients with initial hypoxemia from pulmonary insufficiency respond to altitude with relatively large decreases of arterial blood O_2 content and saturation.

Oxygen pressure versus oxygen content

The question is often asked concerning whether arterial blood O_2 *pressure* or *content* is more important for normal body function. The answer must be that they are *both* important. These two factors are inseparably related aspects of the same system, and each is related to a different aspect of O_2 supply. Oxygen pressure difference promotes diffusion of O_2 across membranes and into cells. Furthermore, tissue P_{O_2} provides an input to the homeostatic mechanism regulating O_2 delivery.

Gas pressure is one of the factors that determines the availability, or effective "local concentration," of gas molecules for physicochem-

ical reactions. The effects of any gas are thus a *direct* function of its *partial pressure*, not its concentration. The significance of P_{O_2}, as contrasted with O_2 content, depends further on the fact that this intensive factor can be detected by physiologic sensors anywhere within the system and that the information thus obtained can be used in a feedback control system.

Oxygen content, or concentration, determines how much O_2 can be transferred to the cells without producing a physiologically significant P_{O_2} decrease. At rest with a normal arteriovenous blood O_2 difference, mixed venous P_{O_2} remains above 30 to 40 torr. If arterial O_2 content is low, as in anemia or carbon monoxide poisoning, tissue P_{O_2} decreases to hypoxic levels when arteriovenous blood O_2 difference is only 4 vol%, even though arterial blood P_{O_2} is normal.

Blood O_2 *pressure*, or P_{O_2}, is measured directly by means of an O_2 electrode. Blood O_2 *content* is measured in several ways. The manometric method of Van Slyke and Neil measures total whole blood O_2 content (O_2 combined with hemoglobin plus dissolved O_2). Blood O_2 *capacity* is the O_2 content of a blood sample that has been exposed to a sufficiently high P_{O_2} so that all the hemoglobin is combined with O_2. Total O_2 content of the saturated capacity blood sample is then determined in the Van Slyke manometric apparatus. The dissolved O_2 content is subtracted from the total O_2 content of both content and capacity blood samples, giving the O_2 combined with hemoglobin for each. If the O_2 *actually* combined with hemoglobin is divided by the O_2 *capable* of combining with hemoglobin (content minus its dissolved O_2 divided by capacity minus its dissolved O_2), multiplication of this fraction by 100 gives oxyhemoglobin saturation in percent. Blood O_2 saturation (oxyhemoglobin saturation) is best calculated from analyses of O_2 content and capacity; however, it can be measured with oximeters of both spectrophotometric and re-

---

*The hemoglobin of the llama, an animal that is adapted to high altitude, has a dissociation curve considerably to the left of human adult hemoglobin; llama hemoglobin is 50% saturated at 19 torr P_{O_2}.

flectance type. These instruments are useful where rapid analysis of many blood samples is necessary, as during cardiac catheterization, but are less accurate than the chemical methods required to calibrate them. Reflectance oximeters in particular tend to give falsely high values for oxyhemoglobin saturation, the magnitude of the error depending on the O_2 pressure difference between blood sample and room air as well as the duration of blood sample exposure. Excessive familiarity with these instruments without concomitant thorough indoctrination in the proper anaerobic technic for handling blood samples can ruin laboratory personnel for careful work.

FACTORS AFFECTING OXYGEN TRANSPORT BY HEMOGLOBIN
Hemoglobin concentration

Because each gram of hemoglobin can combine with about 1.36 ml (STPD) of O_2, blood O_2 content depends not only on P_{O_2} but also on hemoglobin concentration. At any given P_{O_2}, increasing hemoglobin concentration increases blood O_2 content proportionately (Fig. 10-3).

Despite disagreement about the exact volume of O_2 that can combine with 1 gm of hemoglobin, the value 1.36 ml (STPD)/gm is widely used as a factor in calculations. Theoretically, 1 gm of hemoglobin can combine with 1.391 ml (STPD) of O_2, but this potential maximum is never actually achieved in vivo. The in vivo conditions that prevent achievement of the maximum saturation of hemoglobin with O_2 include the presence in circulating blood of small but variable amounts of carboxyhemoglobin and varying concentrations of inactive hemoglobins, such as the functionless pigment methemoglobin that increases in concentration as P_{O_2} increases. Because of these varying in vivo conditions, the value varies; hence, *calculation* of blood O_2 content and capacity using figures such as 1.36 (or 1.34 or 1.39) is almost certain to be less accurate than the actual laboratory measurement.

Blood pH

The affinity between O_2 and a given hemoglobin is represented by plotting oxyhemoglobin saturation (the percentage of hemoglobin combined with O_2) as a function of the P_{O_2} to which the blood is exposed. To eliminate hemoglobin concentration as a variable, we plot oxyhemoglobin saturation in percent rather than blood O_2 content as a function of P_{O_2}, simplifying the study of affinity. A curve presented in terms of oxyhemoglobin saturation reveals the effects of such factors as pH or temperature on the affinity of hemoglobin for O_2.

The relative position of an oxyhemoglobin dissociation curve is characterized by its P_{50} value, the P_{O_2} at which 50% of the given hemoglobin is saturated with O_2. The normal P_{50} for adult human blood is about 26 torr. P_{50} is affected by pH and thus also by P_{CO_2}. Decreasing pH, or increasing H^+ concentration, decreases the affinity between hemoglobin and O_2, shifting the oxyhemoglobin dissociation curve to the right (Figs. 10-2 and 10-4). Thus, to achieve a given level of oxyhemoglobin saturation, such as 50%, requires a higher P_{O_2} and, conversely, at a given P_{O_2} hemoglobin is less saturated with O_2. In body regions of high metabolic activity, such as exercising muscles that are producing CO_2 and metabolic acids, the pH-induced rightward shift of the oxyhemoglobin dissociation curve favors O_2 release.

Blood temperature

Increasing blood temperature decreases the affinity between hemoglobin and O_2, shifting the oxyhemoglobin dissociation curve to the right (Fig. 10-5). It is customary to consider the oxyhemoglobin dissociation curve for blood at physiologic temperature (38° C); at room temperature the curve is much to the left. In body regions of active metabolism where O_2 consumption rate is high, the elevated local temperature favors O_2 release at any given P_{O_2}, increasing the efficiency of O_2 transport.

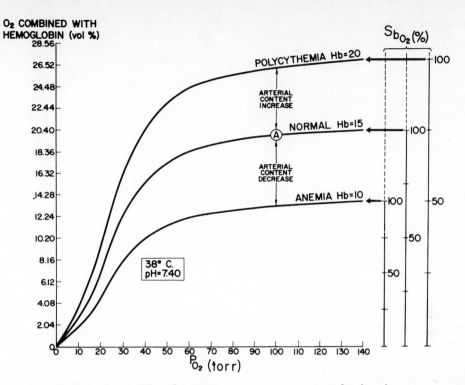

Fig. 10-3. Oxyhemoglobin dissociation curves in anemia and polycythemia.

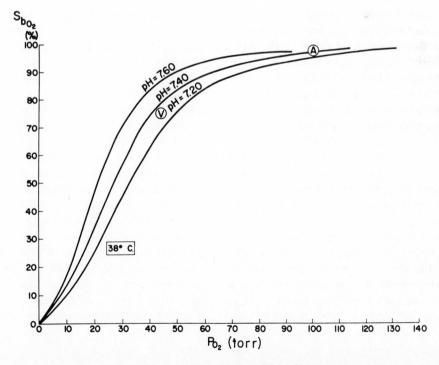

Fig. 10-4. Effect of pH on the oxyhemoglobin dissociation curve.

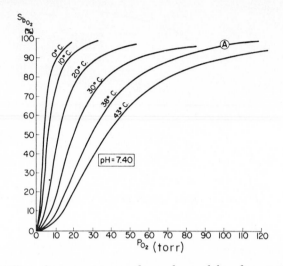

Fig. 10-5. Effect of temperature on the oxyhemoglobin dissociation curve.

2,3-Diphosphoglycerate (2,3-DPG)

The natural affinity of pure hemoglobin for O_2 is so great that it would not readily release O_2 at physiologic levels of tissue P_{O_2} without several ligands that enhance O_2 release: H^+, CO_2, and polyphosphate anions, such as the metabolic intermediary 2,3-DPG. These ligands favor O_2 release by stabilizing the deoxyconfiguration of the hemoglobin molecule (steric accommodation) and thus reducing its affinity for O_2. H^+ strengthen salt bridges within the hemoglobin molecule; CO_2 forms carbamino groups; and 2,3-DPG binds together subunits of the beta chains of the globin moiety of deoxyhemoglobin. Two of the four terminal valine residues of globin that bind CO_2 also bind 2,3-DPG. 2,3-DPG is only one of a variety of polyphosphate anions that combine with the basic groups of globin.

Erythrocytes have long been known to be rich in phosphate. Organic polyphosphate compounds within the erythrocyte, such as adenosine triphosphate (ATP) and in particular 2,3-DPG, play an important physiologic role in regulating the affinity between hemoglobin and O_2, and thus the position of the oxyhemoglobin dissociation curve of whole blood (Fig. 10-6). Erythrocytes contain the highest concentration of 2,3-DPG in the human body. The concentration of 2,3-DPG in the normal human erythrocyte is about 5 mM/L, many times higher than that of any other metabolic intermediate within the erythrocyte and on a molar basis is almost as great as hemoglobin concentration (molar ratio almost 1:1). Although ATP also affects the O_2 affinity of hemoglobin, its concentration is only about one fifth that of normal 2,3-DPG concentration; hence, its influence on O_2 affinity is small compared to that of 2,3-DPG.

Changes of 2,3-DPG concentration in the erythrocyte large enough to affect the affinity between hemoglobin and O_2 are measurable by chemical methods. As the anaerobic glycolytic process forms 2,3-DPG from 1,3-DPG, 2,3-DPG combines reversibly with deoxyhemoglobin (not oxyhemoglobin) in a 1:1 ratio, relieving the product inhibition of the enzyme 2,3-diphosphoglycerate mutase (2,3-DPG mutase) and thus facilitating further synthesis of 2,3-DPG. Free 2,3-DPG concentration is held con-

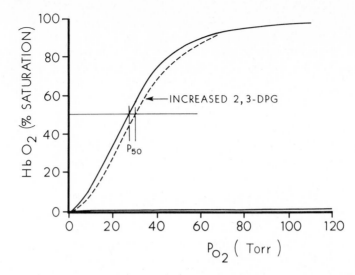

Fig. 10-6. Effect of 2,3-DPG on the oxyhemoglobin dissociation curve.

stant by a negative feedback mechanism. When oxyhemoglobin concentration increases, more 2,3-DPG is free, inhibiting synthesis and reducing glucose consumption rate within the erythrocyte. Thus, well-oxygenated erythrocytes metabolize glucose less rapidly.

When blood is removed from the circulation and stored in a blood bank, 2,3-DPG concentration falls, increasing O_2 affinity (left shift). 2,3-DPG concentration is only one-third normal in blood that has been stored for 1 week. How does transfusion of stored blood affect O_2 transport in the recipient?

As 2,3-DPG concentration increases within the erythrocyte, the affinity between O_2 and hemoglobin decreases and the oxyhemoglobin dissociation curve shifts to the right, an adaptive mechanism favoring O_2 release. Although pure Hb F has less affinity for O_2 than Hb A, fetal erythrocytes have greater affinity for O_2 than adult erythrocytes. For a given increase of 2,3-DPG concentration, the O_2 affinity of Hb A decreases more than that of Hb F. Because the oxyhemoglobin dissociation curve is essentially flat at alveolar O_2 pressures, oxyhemoglobin

saturation in the alveolar capillary is virtually unaffected by moderate 2,3-DPG increases. However, such increases decrease the affinity between hemoglobin and O_2 at the levels of P_{O_2} in metabolizing tissues, favoring O_2 release there, where it is needed. 2,3-DPG decreases O_2 affinity directly by binding to hemoglobin (right shift, ligand effect) and also indirectly by affecting intraerythrocytic pH. The erythrocyte membrane is very impermeable to the highly negative 2,3-DPG anion. 2,3-DPG synthesis alters the Donnan equilibrium, producing intraerythrocytic acidosis. If other factors remain constant at basal levels, doubling the normal erythrocyte 2,3-DPG to 30 μmoles/gm of hemoglobin increases P_{50} from 26.5 to 36.8 torr.

The average affinity between hemoglobin and O_2 in the blood of healthy human adults is normally less (P_{50} is higher) for women (P_{50} = 26.6 torr P_{O_2}) than for men (P_{50} = 25.1 torr P_{O_2}). This lower affinity probably results from a higher 2,3-DPG concentration in the erythrocyte. Although the cause of the higher 2,3-DPG concentration in women remains unknown, it may be associated with their lower hemoglobin concentration. The mean concentration of hemoglobin within the erythrocyte (MCHC) affects the interaction between 2,3-DPG and hemoglobin; as MCHC increases, P_{50} also increases.

Residence at high altitude, chronic hypoxia, chronic anemia, cyanotic congenital heart disease, and low-output cardiac insufficiency increase the concentration of organic phosphates within the erythrocyte, especially 2,3-DPG concentration, tending to maintain tissue oxygenation despite low blood O_2 content. Patients who have chronic diffuse bronchopulmonary disease in a stage of hypoxemia may also have high 2,3-DPG levels, apparently depending on whether or not the hematocrit is high. In dogs experimental anemia produced by plasma-for-blood exchange transfusion increases 2,3-DPG concentration within minutes.

Moderate hyperoxic hypobaria (258 torr, 100% O_2) decreases erythrocyte concentrations of both ATP (about 50%) and 2,3-DPG. Septic shock also decreases 2,3-DPG concentration.

In summary, during the course of a single circulation blood undergoes changes of P_{O_2}, pH, temperature, P_{CO_2}, and pressure. Physiologic shifts of the oxyhemoglobin dissociation curve favor O_2 release in regions of high metabolism where there is high O_2 consumption, high CO_2 production, and increased local temperature. Thus, each erythrocyte contains its own adaptive mechanisms that respond to hypoxia.

Interaction of 2,3-DPG and pH

Increasing H^+ concentration decreases O_2-Hb affinity, the H^+ acting as an *allosteric ligand* of hemoglobin. This effect is direct and immediate; the reaction proceeds as CO_2 enters the erythrocyte during its brief transit through the systemic capillaries (Bohr effect, right shift). Carbon dioxide also combines with hemoglobin at the same binding sites as 2,3-DPG. Hence, increasing P_{CO_2} displaces some 2,3-DPG molecules from hemoglobin, and sus-

tained hypercapnia decreases 2,3-DPG production. The time required for this 2,3-DPG response varies somewhat but is on the order of several hours. Because 2,3-DPG is also an important allosteric ligand of hemoglobin, and because decreasing 2,3-DPG concentration increases O_2-Hb affinity, after some hours of intraerythrocytic CO_2 acidosis, the oxyhemoglobin dissociation curve shifts back toward its original position. Thus, an acid-base disturbance that alters intraerythrocytic pH produces an immediate primary shift as a result of pH change, followed by a slower compensatory shift back toward the original position as 2,3-DPG concentration changes. Acidosis enhances O_2 release for only a few hours, whereas a primary increase of 2,3-DPG concentration has a sustained effect. A given change of 2,3-DPG has a greater effect if arterial P_{CO_2} and base concentration are low.

Metabolic acidosis and alkalosis produce significantly greater Bohr shifts in normal than in low DPG blood. By contrast, because of the effect of CO_2 on Hb-O_2 affinity, respiratory acidosis produces a greater Bohr effect in low DPG blood. The Bohr shift, especially in low DPG blood, thus differs appreciably depending on whether acid-base changes are metabolic or respiratory.

Carbon monoxide

This ubiquitous product of combustion combines avidly with hemoglobin to form carboxyhemoglobin (COHb), interfering with the oxygenation of hemoglobin. The affinity between carbon monoxide and hemoglobin is from 200 to 300 times greater than the affinity between O_2 and hemoglobin. Thus, small amounts of carbon monoxide can usurp a large proportion of the hemoglobin in blood, making it unavailable for O_2 transport. For example, at a P_{CO} of 0.12 torr, 50% of the hemoglobin is combined with carbon monoxide as COHb. Under these conditions both blood P_{O_2} and hemoglobin concentration can be normal, but O_2 content is

Table 9. Factors that shift the oxyhemoglobin dissociation curve

Right shift (Decreased affinity)	Left shift (Increased affinity)
Increased [H^+]	Decreased [H^+]
Increased P_{CO_2}	Decreased P_{CO}
Increased temperature	Decreased temperature
Increased 2,3-DPG	Decreased 2,3-DPG
	Carbon monoxide poisoning

greatly reduced. If the P_{CO} axis is compressed, the shape of the carbon monoxide–hemoglobin dissociation curve is almost identical to that of the oxyhemoglobin dissociation curve, suggesting that the process of combination of these two gases with hemoglobin is similar. Not only does carbon monoxide readily displace O_2 from hemoglobin, it also shifts the oxyhemoglobin dissociation curve to the left, further interfering with O_2 transport. At altitude the problem is even greater because more carbon monoxide forms during combustion and there is less ambient O_2 to compete with it. Thus, a patient with any hypoxemic condition who breathes carbon monoxide at altitude is at a special disadvantage.

Table 9 summarizes the important factors that shift the position of the oxyhemoglobin dissociation curve. A right shift means more O_2 unloading at a given P_{O_2} in the systemic capillaries.

Oxygen delivery rate

Oxygen delivery involves the processes of uptake and release of O_2 by hemoglobin in the erythrocyte and is influenced by many factors, such as P_{O_2} gradient, P_{CO_2}, pH, temperature, and concentrations of various electrolyte and nonelectrolyte substances, including 2,3-DPG. Oxygen delivery is studied by means of the polarographic method, which measures O_2 concentration in solution. When erythrocytes are near the dropping mercury electrode in the polarographic circuit, the electrode is a cathode on which all O_2 diffusing to its surface is instantly reduced and thus removed from solution. The dropping mercury electrode is thus comparable to an O_2-consuming living cell. The resulting polarographic diffusion current is directly proportional to the P_{O_2} of the solution. With blood, however, an *excess current* is observed, which is taken as a measure of the process

$$\text{Oxyhemoglobin} \rightarrow \text{Hemoglobin} + O_2$$

and considered to reflect the *oxygen delivery rate*. The diffusion current of blood divided by the diffusion current of a solution at the same P_{O_2} gives a ratio called *relative oxygen delivery rate*. Dissociation constants for oxyhemoglobin have been calculated using such measurements. Oxygen delivery rate increases as oxyhemoglobin saturation decreases. Blood from two individuals may differ significantly with respect to oxygen delivery rate.

Oxygen association in erythrocytes is a slower process than dissociation. Diffusion of O_2 through the erythrocyte membrane and the interior of the erythrocyte requires 10 times as long as does combination of dissolved hemoglobin with O_2. The increasing oxygen delivery rate of blood with decreasing oxyhemoglobin saturation is an intrinsic mechanism of blood itself that protects tissues against hypoxia. This intrinsic mechanism is in addition to other mechanisms, such as those regulating regional blood flow.

CARBON DIOXIDE TRANSPORT

Each minute the metabolizing cells of the human body consume about 250 ml of O_2 and produce about 200 ml of CO_2 for a metabolic respiratory quotient of about 0.8. The transport of this CO_2 by the blood from tissues to lungs is the subject of this section.

Atmospheric air contains only traces (0.03%) of CO_2. Unless CO_2 is added to inspired gas, the CO_2 present in venous blood, alveolar gas, and arterial blood originates in metabolizing body cells. Carbon dioxide diffuses from these tissue cells into the systemic capillary blood and is carried in the veins, both in chemical combination and in physical solution, to the lungs, where some of it diffuses into the alveolar gas to be eliminated in the exhalatory stream. The P_{CO_2} is greater in actively metabolizing cells than in blood flowing through the sytemic capillaries; carbon dioxide therefore diffuses from these cells into the plasma.

Carbon dioxide is carried in the blood as (1) dissolved CO_2, (2) carbonic acid, or H_2CO_3, (3) bicarbonate ions, or HCO_3^-, (4) carbamino-hemoglobin and other carbamino compounds, and (5) physiologically insignificant amounts of carbonate ion, or $CO_3^=$. When whole blood is chemically analyzed for total CO_2 content, all these molecular species are included. Since the CO_2 content of erythrocytes is considerably lower than that of plasma, it is essential to specify whether blood or plasma is being analyzed and to realize that the hematocrit is a variable affecting whole blood total CO_2 content.

Reactions, compounds, and consequences

In plasma. Of the CO_2 dissolved in plasma, a small amount reacts slowly with water to form carbonic acid; this H_2CO_3 dissociates into H^+ + HCO_3^-, and the resulting H^+ are buffered by plasma buffering systems.

Dissolved CO_2 in plasma also reacts with the free amino groups of various plasma proteins to form carbamino compounds. This rapid chemical reaction requires no catalyst:

$$R\text{---}NH_2 + CO_2 \rightleftharpoons R\text{---}NHCOO^- + H^+$$

In erythrocytes. However, most of the CO_2 that diffuses from tissue cells into the plasma enters the erythrocytes, where three events occur:

1. Some remains within the red blood cell as dissolved CO_2.

2. Some combines with hemoglobin to form carbamino compounds; the resulting H^+ are buffered by the hemoglobin molecule in a chemical process termed the *isohydric shift*. This process is facilitated by the simultaneous loss of O_2 from systemic capillary blood to the tissues because the conversion of oxyhemoglobin to reduced hemoglobin results in a weaker acid, which then takes up additional H^+ with little change of pH.

Carbon dioxide combines with hemoglobin (as well as other proteins) at the free amino ($-NH_2$) sites. In the hemoglobin molecule combination takes place in the globin moiety in close proximity to the heme portion. The presence of O_2 on the heme portion appears to interfere somewhat with carbamino compound formation. Carbon dioxide does not combine at $-NH_3^+$ sites, which, however, are in equilibrium with $-NH_2$:

$$
\begin{array}{ccc}
Hb\text{---}NH_2 & + CO_2 \rightleftharpoons & Hb\text{---}NHCOOH \\
\updownarrow & & \updownarrow \\
Hb\text{---}NH_3^+ & & Hb\text{---}NHCOO^- + H^+
\end{array}
$$

3. Some CO_2 combines with water to form H_2CO_3, which then dissociates to form H^+ and HCO_3^-. The conversion of CO_2 and H_2O into H_2CO_3 is very rapid because the enzyme, carbonic anhydrase, is concentrated within the erythrocyte. Carbonic anhydrase speeds the normally slow reaction but as a catalyst does not change its equilibrium. In blood the hydration of CO_2 is an important and rapid reaction only within the erythrocyte.

$$CO_2 + H_2O \overset{\overset{\text{Carbonic}}{\underset{\downarrow}{\text{anhydrase*}}}}{\rightleftharpoons} H_2CO_3 \rightleftharpoons HCO_3^- + H^+$$

This reaction also results in the formation of H^+, which are buffered by functional groups of the

---

*Actually, the enzyme carbonic anhydrase catalyzes the *hydroxylation* of CO_2 as follows: $CO_2 + OH^- \rightleftharpoons HCO_3^-$. However, the net effect is the same as that implied by the traditional equation given.

hemoglobin molecule with minimal change of pH. Again, the simultaneous conversion of some oxyhemoglobin to reduced hemoglobin facilitates the buffering (isohydric shift).

The preceding events result in an accumulation of HCO_3^- within the red blood cell. Some HCO_3^- diffuse out into the plasma to reestablish HCO_3^- concentration equilibrium between erythrocyte and plasma. If this diffusion of bicarbonate anions were accompanied by the diffusion of an equal number of cations, electric neutrality would be maintained within the erythrocyte. However, the erythrocyte membrane is not freely permeable to cations so that chloride anions from the plasma diffuse into the erythrocyte to preserve electric neutrality. This movement is termed the *chloride shift*. Simultaneously, some water moves into the erythrocyte to maintain osmotic equilibrium, resulting in a slight swelling of the erythrocytes in venous blood.

As O_2 uptake and CO_2 unloading proceed in the pulmonary capillaries, the reverse reactions occur.

Although plasma contains much more of the metabolically produced CO_2 than do the erythrocytes, and although plasma *transports* more than 60% of the CO_2 entering systemic capillary blood, chemical reactions within the erythrocyte account for almost all the additional HCO_3^- transported in the plasma. If carbonic anhydrase is inhibited, as by acetazolamide administration, the uncatalyzed reaction $CO_2 + H_2O \rightleftharpoons H_2CO_3$ proceeds slowly and will not be completed in the systemic capillaries or even in transit from veins to heart. The reverse reaction, $H_2CO_3 \rightleftharpoons CO_2 + H_2O$, which normally takes place in the fraction of a second that mixed venous blood is in the pulmonary capillaries, is also slow and continues long after the blood has left the pulmonary capillaries and entered the systemic circulation. Therefore, if carbonic anhydrase is inhibited, P_{CO_2} decreases gradually in venous blood until it reaches the pulmonary capillaries, where some CO_2 is

eliminated; however, P_{CO_2} rises as blood flows through the systemic arteries, and the unloading reaction slowly proceeds to completion; tissue P_{CO_2} rises as a result. An instantaneous method for measuring blood P_{CO_2} would be required to analyze the dynamics of this disturbance, but CO_2 retention under these conditions has been demonstrated.

Carbon dioxide dissociation curve

Just as the amount of O_2 in blood is a function of P_{O_2}, so the amount of CO_2 in blood is a function of P_{CO_2}. The solubility coefficient (C_s) for CO_2 in blood at 37° C is 0.063 vol%/torr. Chemical reactions that form HCO_3^- and the combination of CO_2 with hemoglobin account for most of the CO_2 content of blood. The CO_2 dissociation curve, or blood buffer curve, describes the formation of HCO_3^- from CO_2, or from dissociation or ionization of H_2CO_3, as a function of P_{CO_2} (Fig. 10-7). This curve is an experimentally determined curve resulting from the analysis of HCO_3^- in blood equilibrated with gas of various CO_2 pressures. The relationship between CO_2 pressure and CO_2 content is nearly linear in the physiologic range. The curvature, or departure from linearity, reflects the chemical reactions of CO_2 with water and blood buffers. The curve may be lowered by increasing the P_{O_2} of the equilibrating gas mixture, or it may be raised by lowering its O_2 pressure. This effect of changing the level of the CO_2 dissociation curve by varying the P_{O_2} is called the *Haldane effect*. Because of this effect, arterial blood has a somewhat lower dissociation curve than venous blood.

Carbon dioxide combines with the four terminal α-amino groups of the globin moiety to produce hemoglobin carbamates (carbaminohemoglobin). Deoxygenated hemoglobin combines with more CO_2 to form carbamates than does oxyhemoglobin; conversely, oxygenation of hemoglobin decreases its CO_2 capacity. This remarkable adaptation results from a change of the number of sites available for uptake of the

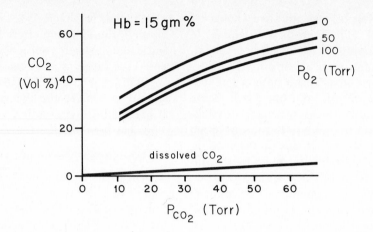

Fig. 10-7. CO_2-dissociation curves for whole blood with a hemoglobin concentration of 15 gm%. Dissolved CO_2 is shown at the bottom. The upper three curves show the effect of different P_{O_2} levels on the concentration of combined CO_2.

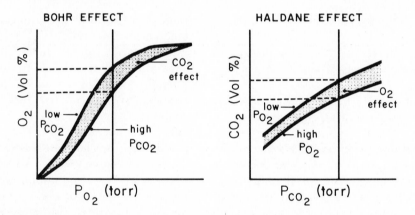

Fig. 10-8. Reciprocal interaction of O_2 and CO_2 on blood-gas transport. Increased P_{CO_2} decreases the affinity between hemoglobin and O_2 (Bohr effect), whereas decreased P_{O_2} increases CO_2 content (Haldane effect).

H^+ produced by carbamate formation. About 70% of the physiologic Haldane shift results from the changing affinity of hemoglobin for CO_2. In vitro the capacity of completely deoxygenated hemoglobin to form carbamino compounds is more than 3 times that of fully oxygenated hemoglobin. Hemoglobin carbamate formation is also a function of P_{CO_2}.

Interrelation of O_2 and CO_2 transport mechanisms

Oxygen unloading and CO_2 loading in systemic capillaries are mutually helpful processes. A reciprocal relationship exists so that increased P_{CO_2} aids in unloading O_2 and decreased P_{O_2} aids in loading CO_2 in the tissues. The reverse occurs in the lung, where decreas-

Table 10. Typical blood-gas and pH values for healthy man at rest*

	Inspired air	Alveolar gas	Arterial blood	Mixed venous blood	Arterio-venous difference
P_{H_2O} (torr)	Varies	47			
P_{O_2} (torr)	159†	104	100	42	58
S_{O_2} (%)			96	75	21
O_2 content (vol%)			18.97	14.71	4.26
O_2 combined with Hb (vol%)			18.67	14.59	4.08
O_2 in physical solution (vol%)			0.30	0.12	0.18
O_2 capacity of Hb (vol%)			19.45	19.45	0
P_{CO_2} (torr)	0.3†	40	40	46	6
Total CO_2 (vol%)			48.5	52.2	3.7
content‡ (mM/L)			21.8	23.5	1.7
Total CO_2 (vol%)			58.3	62.1	3.8
content§ (mM/L)			26.2	27.9	1.7
Combined CO_2§ (vol%)			55.6	59.0	3.4
CO_2 in physical solution§ (vol%)			2.78	3.13	0.35
Combined CO_2/Dissolved CO_2§			20.0/1	18.8/1	1.2/1
Plasma pH			7.40	7.376	0.024

*Sea level: P_B = 760 torr; assume Hb = 14.3 gm/dL.
†On basis of dry atmospheric air.
‡Whole blood.
§Plasma.

ing P_{CO_2} increases the affinity of hemoglobin for O_2 and increasing P_{O_2} reduces the affinity of hemoglobin for CO_2. These two effects, the *Haldane effect* on CO_2 loading and the *Bohr effect* on O_2 loading, result from the unique physicochemical properties of hemoglobin; they are contrasted in Fig. 10-8.

Since the oxyhemoglobin dissociation curve shifts to the right when P_{CO_2} increases, the affinity of hemoglobin for O_2 decreases; for a given P_{O_2} less hemoglobin is oxygenated. The O_2 released from hemoglobin as a result of increasing P_{CO_2} is available to the tissues.

Deoxygenation of hemoglobin increases its affinity for CO_2; thus at a given P_{CO_2} more CO_2 combines with hemoglobin, adding to that carried as HCO_3^- and as dissolved CO_2. Total blood CO_2 content increases.

These two mechanisms, both dependent on the characteristics of hemoglobin, facilitate the efficient exchange of respiratory gases in regions of high metabolic activity, where O_2 consumption and CO_2 production are increased. Table 10 shows typical blood-gas and pH values for healthy man at rest.

Body stores of carbon dioxide

Of the normal body gas stores, the CO_2 stores are the largest and the most complex. When pulmonary ventilation is eliminating CO_2 at precisely its production rate, CO_2 output equals metabolic CO_2 production and a steady state exists. However, any change in alveolar ventilation rate without a simultaneous precisely compensating change of CO_2 production produces an unsteady state, in turn changing the level of body CO_2 stores. If pulmonary ventilation rate without a simultaneous precisely compensating change of CO_2 production is greater than that required to rid the body of current CO_2 production, the rather large body reservoirs of stored CO_2 decrease. The body fluids, about 70% of body mass, normally hold 50 ml of CO_2 for each 100 ml of fluid (50 vol%); bone contains more than 100 vol% of CO_2. Thus, a 70-kgm man contains about 35 L of stored CO_2. This equals the resting metabolic CO_2 production for a period of about 140 minutes. When alveolar ventilation is subnormal, metabolic CO_2 is stored and the CO_2 reservoirs fill.

If CO_2 production remains constant, the re-

lationship between alveolar P_{CO_2} and alveolar ventilation is a rectangular hyperbola. If alveolar P_{CO_2} is halved; if ventilation is halved, P_{CO_2} is doubled. This relationship holds only after a new storage level is achieved and remains constant, that is, after a new steady state is achieved. Once attained, however, the alveolar ventilation rate must remain at the new level; if it changes, the level of CO_2 stores will follow it. The CO_2 stores of the body are readjusting almost continuously. The rate of adjustment of CO_2 stores during hyperventilation or hypoventilation with air is about one eighth as fast as that for O_2. Both processes are simple exponential functions of time.

CHAPTER 11

HYDROGEN ION REGULATION

Free hydrogen ions (H^+) are rare in most body fluids, but their concentration is very important. The activity of enzymes and the solubility of salts are dependent on H^+ concentration. At chemical neutrality there is only 1×10^{-7} (1/10,000,000) of a mole of H^+ per liter of solution. The concentration in arterial blood plasma is even less—about 4×10^{-8} (4/100,000,000) of a mole of H^+ per liter. However, gastric juice may contain 1 million times this concentration.

Chemically, any solution containing in excess of 1×10^{-7} mole of H^+ per liter is considered to be acidic, and any solution containing less than that concentration is alkaline, or basic. Note that the chemically neutral H^+ concentration of 1×10^{-7} mole per liter is acidic with respect to arterial blood plasma, which has a lower concentration.

What is an acid and what is a base?

Many years ago it was found that organic ash has an alkaline reaction. Since the most abundant cation in such ash is potassium (K^+), it was assumed that K^+ is a base. But K^+ in vitro does not reduce H^+ concentration. Organic ash is alkaline because of the anion associated with K^+ and not because of K^+ itself. Past literature refers to potassium and sodium as bases, but this usage is giving way to more descriptive and accurate terminology. An acid is any substance that increases H^+ concentration or that is a proton donor. Conversely, a base is any

substance that reduces H^+ concentration or that is a proton acceptor.

The hydrogen ion, or proton, does not exist free in aqueous solutions but rather is combined with a molecule of water as the hydrated hydronium ion, H_3O^+. Although it is more accurate to speak of hydronium ions, we may use the terms proton or hydrogen ion (H^+) for simplicity without introducing errors into these considerations.

Carbon dioxide combines with water to form carbonic acid, which then dissociates into H^+ and HCO_3^-. Since CO_2 increases H^+ concentration, it may be called an acid.* Since ammonia (NH_3) can accept a proton to form the ammonium ion (NH_4^+), ammonia is a base.

What is pH?

The concentration of hydrogen ions in a solution is expressed as gram-ionic weights per liter. At 25° C water has a H^+ concentration of 10^{-7} as well as a OH^- concentration of 10^{-7} moles per liter. Thus the pH of water at 25° C is 7. Greater accuracy is obtained if one substitutes the thermodynamic *activity* of the H^+ for its *concentration*.

It is obviously inconvenient to refer to H^+ concentrations such as 1/10,000,000 of a mole per liter. To avoid this inconvenience, acidity is usually expressed in terms of pH, which is defined as the logarithm of the reciprocal of the

---

*Actually, it is an acid *anhydride*.

H^+ concentration. In other words, the pH of a solution is the negative logarithm of its H^+ concentration. Accordingly, a solution at chemical neutrality with 1/10,000,000 (or 1×10^{-7}) mole of H^+ per liter has a pH of 7.

Note that as H^+ concentration increases, pH decreases. Note further that the concentration of H^+ in a solution at pH 6 is 10 times that in a solution at pH 7. Because of the logarithmic nature of the pH scale a decrease of 0.3 pH unit, although appearing small, actually represents a *doubling* of the H^+ concentration. The logarithmic nature of the pH scale must also be remembered when comparing pH differences and when making ratios involving pH.

pH homeostasis—concept and physiologic importance

Normal acidity within and around body cells is absolutely essential for maintenance of the dynamic, biochemical equilibrium that life processes involve. Cell metabolism and function require that acidity be kept within very narrow limits. Normal acidity is maintained within the body by a sensitive, well-integrated mechanism involving pH-sensitive receptors, kidneys, lungs, and several buffer systems.

Enzymes are biologic catalysts and, as such, speed the achievement of chemical equilibria. The physiologic importance of pH homeostasis becomes clear when we realize that a multitude of biochemical processes in any biologic system are catalyzed by specific enzymes and that each enzyme is optimally active at a specific pH. We may imagine then the biochemical chaos that results when appreciable shifts of pH occur, affecting the multitude of enzymes, each to a different degree and some actually in opposite directions. Accordingly, it is not surprising that the extreme range of plasma pH compatible with life in higher forms is from approximately 7.0 to 7.8. Hydrogen ion regulation is perhaps a better term than acid-base balance because it is indeed the maintenance of normal pH with which the homeostatic mechanisms are concerned.

The term *blood* pH always refers to *plasma* pH, which is higher than the intracellular pH of the erythrocyte. Note that *arterial* blood samples are required for clinical characterization of acid-base status and that blood temperature is an important variable.

BUFFER SYSTEMS AND THE HENDERSON-HASSELBALCH EQUATION

Strong acids, such as hydrochloric, sulfuric, and nitric acids, dissociate almost completely into H^+ and their associated anions. Because there is little attraction in solution of chloride, sulfate, or nitrate ions for H^+, these anions are very weak bases. However, weak acids are weak because they do not yield their H^+ readily. When they do, the anions formed remain rather avid for the H^+ they have lost and are therefore rather strong bases.

In low pH solutions where H^+ are relatively abundant, a H^+ lost from a weak organic acid is almost immediately replaced, so that at any instant most weak organic acid molecules are undissociated. As the pH increases, however, replacement of dissociated H^+ is slower, so that at any given instant a larger fraction of the organic acid molecules are dissociated. For any organic acid there is a pH at which only half of the organic acid molecules are undissociated; the other half are dissociated into H^+ and their anions, or bases. The pH at this point is termed the pK for that particular acid. *The pK is defined as the negative logarithm of the H^+ concentration at which half of the acid molecules are associated and half are dissociated.*

The relationships among pH, strength of a weak acid, or pK, and the base-to-acid concentration ratio for any buffer system are given by a modified form of the law of mass action called the Henderson-Hasselbalch equation:

$$pH = pK + \log_{10} \frac{[base]}{[acid]} \qquad (1)$$

where base is the anion (the acid molecule less its H^+). Some acids, such as carbonic, have 2 H^+, each of which may be lost. It is convenient, although not precisely accurate, to think of this as a step-by-step process. In such a case each H^+, or step, has its own pK. Under physiologic conditions the dissociation of only the first H^+ of carbonic acid is important, and we refer to this dissociation as the pK_1.

Phosphoric acid is an example of an acid with 3 H^+, each with its own pK. Physiologically, one is concerned primarily with the second of these (pK_2), which at normal body temperature is about 6.8. The Henderson-Hasselbalch equation for dissociation of this second H^+ of phosphoric acid is:

$$pH = 6.8 + \log_{10} \frac{[HPO_4^=]}{[H_2PO_4^-]} \qquad (2)$$

At pH 6.8, $HPO_4^=$ and $H_2PO_4^-$ are present in equal concentration. At pH 7.8 there is 10 times as much $HPO_4^=$ as $H_2PO_4^-$. At pH 5.8 there is 10 times as much $H_2PO_4^-$ as $HPO_4^=$. A phosphate buffer in which equal quantities of these ions are used resists large changes of pH. If acid is added, the free H^+ combine with $HPO_4^=$ to form $H_2PO_4^-$, with relatively little change in pH. If alkali is added to this pH 6.8 buffer, the pH reduction is minimized by release of H^+ from $H_2PO_4^-$ as it becomes $HPO_4^=$.

The *buffer capacity* of a solution is the amount of H^+ that can be added to or removed from a solution for a change of 1 pH unit. Buffer capacity depends on the concentration and nature of the buffer substances and on the pH in relation to the pK of the buffer. The slope of a buffer dissociation, or titration curve, is greatest at the pK of the buffer. It follows that buffers are most effective in the pH range that centers on their pK. Buffer capacity may also be defined as $d(V)/d(pH)$, or the slope of the acid-base titration curve. This definition, however, involving the ratio of a number to a logarithm, does not permit ready comparison of buffer slopes in different pH ranges. If H^+ concentration were used to express buffer capacity instead, direct comparison would be possible. *Effective buffer capacity* refers to the

in vivo capacity of organs to buffer perfusates and is more relevant to the physiologic behavior of intact living organisms.

Astrup suggested that the total surplus of acid or base in the *extracellular space* can be estimated by the following formula:

0.30 × Body weight (kgm) × Base excess or (3) deficit per liter of blood = Amount of $NaHCO_3$ or NH_4Cl required to restore standard plasma bicarbonate ion concentration to normal

However, more than half of the buffering capacity of the body is intracellular. It is therefore important to distinguish *blood* from *total body* acid-base balance. For example, after the experimental intravenous infusion of acid or base, acid-base changes in blood continue for hours, reflecting total body buffering capacity, metabolism, and compensating mechanisms.

The isohydric shift

In terms of buffer capacity, hemoglobin is the most important buffer in blood because blood contains about 15 gm of hemoglobin/100 ml and because the imidazole groups of globin histidine have a pK that is close to blood pH. Hemoglobin and oxyhemoglobin have different pK's, but each combines with H^+. Hemoglobin has a high pK, about 7.93; oxyhemoglobin has a much lower pK, about 6.68, and is the stronger acid. At an intracellular pH of 7.2 the ratio of Hb^-/HHb is about 1/5.4, whereas the ratio of $HbO_2^-/HHbO_2$ is 3.3/1. As some oxyhemoglobin molecules are losing O_2 to the tissues and becoming reduced hemoglobin, there is a rapid influx of H^+, many of which are taken up by hemoglobin with no change in pH. This buffer effect is known as the *isohydric shift*. At pH 7.2 about 84% of the hemoglobin is in the form of HHb, whereas only about 23% of the oxyhemoglobin is $HHbO_2$. Of the total oxyhemoglobin that loses O_2 to become reduced hemoglobin, 23% was aready combined with H^+, 16% will not combine with H^+, but 61% will take up H^+ from solution before a pH decrease occurs. Thus, an important consequence of the isohydric shift in the systemic capillaries is that if 0.7 mM of CO_2 enters the blood for every 1.0 mM of oxyhemoglobin reduced (metabolic respiratory quotient = 0.7), all H^+ produced by this quantity of CO_2 are buffered (no blood pH decrease) by the reduced hemoglobin just formed without dependence on the other blood buffer systems. Over the physiologic range of pH, the titration curve of oxyhemoglobin is *almost* a straight line. This line has a slope of about 2.54 mM of H^+ per pH unit.

The most interesting buffer system for the respiratory physiologist is the carbonic acid-bicarbonate system (CO_2 system). Carbon dioxide combines with water to form carbonic acid, which then dissociates into bicarbonate ions and hydrogen ions:

$$CO_2 + H_2O \underset{\substack{\uparrow \\ \text{Carbonic} \\ \text{anhydrase}}}{\rightleftharpoons} H_2CO_3 \rightleftharpoons H^+ + HCO_3^- \qquad (4)$$

This reaction is catalyzed by an enzyme, carbonic anhydrase, which is found in red blood cells, renal tubules, gastric mucosa, and the eye. This enzyme speeds the reversible reaction of CO_2 with H_2O to produce H_2CO_3 by a factor of approximately 7,500. Carbonic acid is a rare and transitory intermediate between CO_2 and HCO_3^-. Because of this fact, CO_2 itself is usually treated as if it were the proton donor. When this is done, the *apparent* pK_1, termed pK_1', is about 6.11 and the Henderson-Hasselbalch equation for plasma at 38° C is written* as follows:

---

*The pK_1 of H_2CO_3 is about 3.4. At pH 7.4 the ratio of $[HCO_3^-]$ to $[H_2CO_3]$ is about 10,000:1. Physiologically, however, CO_2 is a much more useful quantity, since it is about 500 times as abundant as H_2CO_3. If we pretend that it is CO_2 and not H_2CO_3 that dissociates yielding H^+, we can use the ratio of $[HCO_3^-]$ to $[CO_2]$, but we must correct the pK_1 by the equilibrium constant of 500. This *apparent* pK_1, the pK_1', which goes with the apparent ratio of $[HCO_3^-]$ to $[CO_2]$, has a value of about 6.1. *Note that it is incorrect to use this pK_1' of 6.1 with the ratio of $[HCO_3^-]$ to $[H_2CO_3]$.*

$$pH = 6.11 + \log_{10}\frac{[HCO_3^-]}{[CO_2]} \qquad (5)$$

This pK_1' is assumed constant because blood temperature, solute concentrations, and acid strength satisfy the necessary conditions. The $[CO_2]$ is expressed as mM/L so that it matches $[HCO_3^-]$ in mM or mEq/L. However, $[CO_2]$ in the denominator may also be expressed as the constant a times P_{CO_2}. The constant a is a proportionality constant relating CO_2 in mM/L to P_{CO_2} in torr and is equal to 0.0301.

GRAPHIC REPRESENTATION OF ACID-BASE PATTERNS

As we have seen, a buffer system involves three variables so that actual measurement of any two permits determination of the third. This determination can be made by arithmetic calculation, or it can be done graphically. In the following section we discuss three of the several possible ways of graphing the Henderson-Hasselbalch buffer equation.

The Henderson-Hasselbalch equation for the carbonic acid–bicarbonate buffer system lends itself readily to two-dimensional graphic representation and solution. Any pair of the three variables can be plotted on cartesian coordinates against one another, with the third variable then portrayed as a family of isovalue lines or curves. One of these representations plots HCO_3^- concentration as a function of pH, with P_{CO_2} appearing as a family of isobars (Figs. 11-1 to 11-3). As P_{CO_2} is increased or decreased, the values for pH and HCO_3^- concentration describe a nearly straight line, termed the *blood buffer curve*. The shaded vertical bands in Figs. 11-1 to 11-3 indicate the approximate range of normal arterial blood pH and emphasize the basic fact that the various homeostatic mechanisms function to maintain normal pH. The points marked N in all six acid-base diagrams in this chapter indicate normal values for healthy, resting subjects acclimatized at sea level.

It is difficult to overestimate the significance

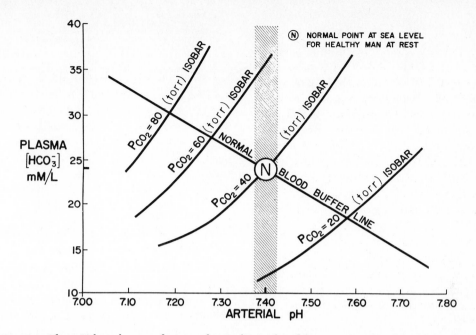

Fig. 11-1. The pH-bicarbonate diagram for analysis of acid-base status. (Modified from Davenport, H. W.: The ABC of acid-base chemistry, ed. 4, Chicago, 1958, The University of Chicago Press.)

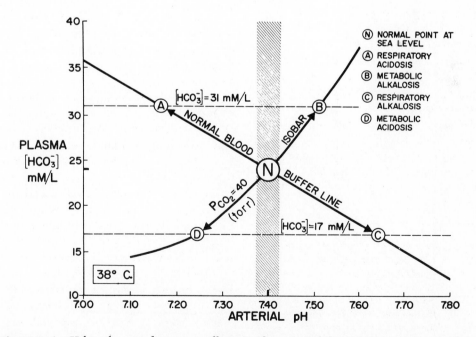

Fig. 11-2. A pH-bicarbonate diagram to illustrate the impossibility of distinguishing acidosis from alkalosis with only one kind of CO_2 content information. (Redrawn from Davenport, H. W.: The ABC of acid-base chemistry, ed. 4, Chicago, 1958, The University of Chicago Press.)

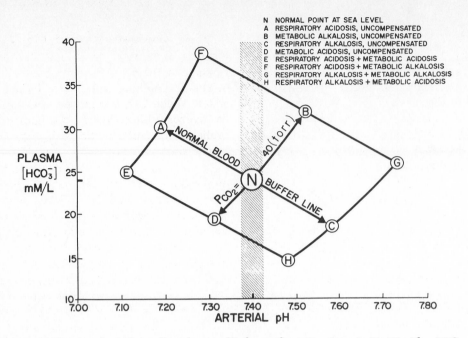

Fig. 11-3. Pathways of acid-base disturbance. (Redrawn from Davenport, H. W.: The ABC of acid-base chemistry, ed. 4, Chicago, 1958, The University of Chicago Press.)

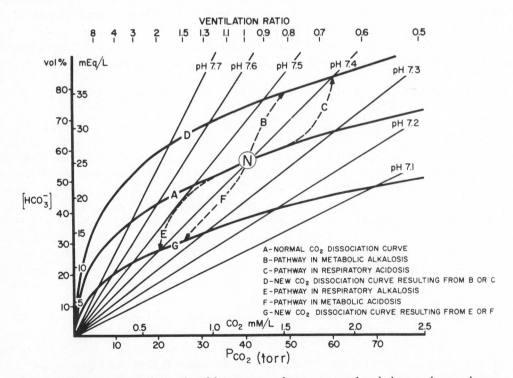

Fig. 11-4. Diagram for analysis of acid-base status, showing normal and abnormal true plasma CO_2 dissociation curves.

of the basic algebraic fact that if any two variables in the Henderson-Hasselbalch equation are measured the third can be calculated, but that *one alone* does not suffice. This point is illustrated in Fig. 11-2.

Technically speaking, the term *CO₂ content information* may include both HCO_3^- and total CO_2 concentrations. If both of these are known, the P_{CO_2} can be calculated from the equation

$$[HCO_3^-] = [\text{Total } CO_2] - a \times P_{CO_2} \qquad (6)$$

and the acid-base status is determined. Furthermore, it should be emphasized that if total CO_2 concentration instead of HCO_3^- concentration is plotted on the vertical axis, a different linear scale must be used and the P_{CO_2} isobars will then need to be recalculated.

Another graphic solution of the Henderson-Hasselbalch equation plots the ratio $[HCO_3^-]/[CO_2]$ (Fig. 11-4). When temperature and consequently pK_1' are constant, this ratio is the pH. The pH is about 7.4 when the ratio is 20:1, 40:2, 60:3, or 80:4. It is about 7.1 when the ratio is 10:1, 20:2, 30:3, or 40:4. These and other pH lines radiate from the origin of the graph. This representation is particularly useful for the respiratory physiologist because P_{CO_2}–$[HCO_3^-]$ dissociation curves can be superimposed on the graphic solution of the Henderson-Hasselbalch equation. Ventilation can also be represented, since ventilation is inversely related to P_{CO_2}.

Hyperventilation does not shift the plasma values *directly* to the left on this graph—but rather downward and to the left—along the *CO₂ dissociation*, or *blood buffer, curve*. Underbreathing shifts the plasma values to the right and somewhat upward along the CO_2 dissociation curve. The HCO_3^- concentration changes with ventilation because alterations in P_{CO_2} shift the equilibrium of equation 4:

$$\underset{\substack{\uparrow \\ \text{Carbonic} \\ \text{anhydrase}}}{}$$

$$CO_2 + H_2O \rightleftharpoons H_2CO_3 \rightleftharpoons H^+ + HCO_3^-$$

During any second, many CO_2 molecules combine with water to form HCO_3^- and H^+. But during the same second, an equal number of HCO_3^- combine with H^+ to form CO_2 and water. When CO_2 is removed from this system by overbreathing, fewer CO_2 molecules are available for combination with water to form HCO_3^- but as many HCO_3^- and H^+ move to form CO_2 as before. Hence, overbreathing not only reduces CO_2 but also reduces the populations of HCO_3^- and H^+. This illustrates the chemical principle of driving an equilibrium reaction to one side by removing one of the reactants (CO_2) from that side. The diagram shows this not only by the slope of the CO_2 dissociation curve but also by departure from the pH 7.40 line in the direction of a higher pH. This is alkalosis. Since it is generated by a change in respiration, it is *respiratory* alkalosis.

Underbreathing out of proportion to CO_2 production produces effects that are opposite to those of overbreathing. Carbon dioxide accumulates, more CO_2 is available to form HCO_3^- and H^+, and the populations of both of these ions increase. In the diagram this corresponds to a rightward movement along the CO_2 dissociation curve, involving an increase in HCO_3^- and a lower pH. This is acidosis—in this case, *respiratory* acidosis.

The quantitative aspects of respiratory acidosis and alkalosis are more fully appreciated if there is some notion of the relative abundance of the molecular species involved. When metabolizing tissue cells produce CO_2, some of this CO_2 moves into red blood cells, where carbonic anhydrase converts most of it to HCO_3^- and H^+. The H^+ thus produced are largely removed from solution by combination with hemoglobin, oxyhemoglobin, intracellular and plasma proteins, polypeptides, and amino acids. Thus, when CO_2 is stored in body fluids as HCO_3^-, most of the H^+ produced with the HCO_3^- are buffered and eventually excreted in the urine. When mixed venous blood encounters the lower P_{CO_2} in the lungs, dissolved CO_2 quickly leaves the blood, forcing combination of HCO_3^- with H^+, and producing more dissolved CO_2. Most of the H^+ that enter into this union did not exist as free H^+, having come from blood buffers.

If arterial plasma has a pH of 7.40 and contains 24 mEq/L of HCO_3^-, the following approximate populations exist:

$$\underset{\text{(each}\ \times\ 10^{-8}\ \text{mole/L)}}{\underset{120{,}000\quad\quad\quad 240\quad\quad 4\quad\quad 2{,}400{,}000}{CO_2\ +\ H_2O \rightleftharpoons H_2CO_3 \rightleftharpoons H^+\ +\ HCO_3^-}} \tag{7}$$

Carbonic anhydrase ↓

Any shift in equilibrium, to either left or right, has a much greater proportionate effect on H^+ than on HCO_3^-. But the availability of buffers, where H^+ may be either stored or retrieved, changes this picture. Even though the H^+ concentration is only 4×10^{-8} mole/L, H^+ are replaced as soon as they combine with HCO_3^-.

The *Siggaard-Andersen curve nomogram* is another graphic representation of the Henderson-Hasselbalch equation. It was widely used in the clinic with the Astrup tonometer micromethod for blood-gas and pH analysis. It involves the following definitions:

Acidosis and *alkalosis* are defined in terms of pH. Blood pH is *plasma* pH. *Respiratory* acidosis is the result of increased arterial P_{CO_2}, whereas *respiratory* alkalosis is the result of decreased P_{CO_2}. *Metabolic* (nonrespiratory) acidosis is an acidosis that is reflected in a decrease of standard bicarbonate, whereas *metabolic* alkalosis is an alkalosis that is reflected in an increase of standard bicarbonate. *Total CO_2 content* is the total content of CO_2 in plasma separated from the cells at the actual P_{CO_2}. *CO_2 combining power* is the total content of CO_2 in plasma separated from cells at the actual P_{CO_2} and then equilibrated to a P_{CO_2} of 40 torr before analysis. *Standard bicarbonate* is the *plasma* bicarbonate ion concentration measured under the standard conditions of 38° C, $P_{CO_2} = 40$ torr, and full oxygenation of the hemoglobin. It thus expresses the *metabolic* aspect of acid-base balance only and is normally 24 mEq/L. Standard bicarbonate is estimated on the Siggaard-Andersen curve nomogram by intersection of the $P_{CO_2} = 40$ torr line with the pH-log P_{CO_2}, or blood buffer, line. The term *buffer base* is used as defined in 1948 by

Singer and Hastings as the sum of the cations corresponding to the buffer anions, including the cations corresponding to the hemoglobin anions. Thus, an anemic patient can have an abnormal buffer base value without *any* actual abnormality of acid-base chemistry. The value of the buffer base concept has accordingly been questioned.

The pH–versus–log P_{CO_2} plot, or blood buffer line, is *linear* in the physiologic region. This line is determined by equilibrating aliquots of a blood sample at two different P_{CO_2}'s and then measuring the two resulting pH values. It is usual clinical practice to determine this line by means of only two points. The exact values of P_{CO_2} to which the two aliquots are equilibrated are not critical, but they must be precisely known and equlibration must be complete. The actual pH of the blood sample is also determined, and its P_{CO_2} is then estimated from the blood buffer line. Blood buffer capacity, or the slope* of the pH–log P_{CO_2} line, is largely a function of hemoglobin concentration. However, it is only *approximately* proportional to hemoglobin concentration because blood contains other buffers. NBB on the curve nomogram means *normal buffer base*. The pK of reduced hemoglobin is 7.93, whereas the pK of oxyhemoglobin is 6.68. Oxygenation of hemoglobin is thus an important variable. If a blood sample is 100% saturated, as assumed in the Siggaard-Andersen curve nomogram, then this method will easily predict hemoglobin concentration within the stated ±3 gm/dL range. Siggaard-Andersen and Engel determined the base excess curve empirically by adding known amounts of acid or base to various blood samples.

As the fundamental relationship of acid-base chemistry, the Henderson-Hasselbalch equation is used in many ways—in tables, nomograms, slide rules, and computers, as well as in each of the three possible two-dimensional cartesian graphs just described. Although these devices generate data, they are neither intel-

---

*Δ log P_{CO_2}/Δ pH.

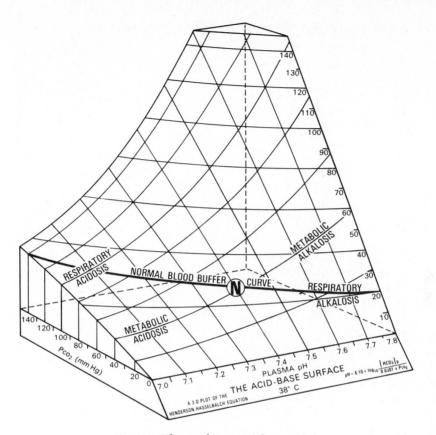

Fig. 11-5. The Acid-Base Surface model.

lectually satisfying nor especially successful in providing the conceptual model necessary for comprehension and analysis of acid-base information. The Acid-Base Surface model (Fig. 11-5) is a three-dimensional plot of the Henderson-Hasselbalch equation. The three continuous variables—pH, P_{CO_2}, and $[HCO_3^-]$—are represented on a triaxial rectangular cartesian coordinate system with scales and ranges so chosen that the three-dimensional surface is inscribed within the physiologically relevant acid-base cube. The Acid-Base Surface is thus a unifying synthesis of the three two-dimensional representations of this equation, all of which are in current use. Although a three-dimen-

sional surface is inherently no more *accurate* than the projection of that surface onto a two-dimensional coordinate system, such a projection results in a complex distortion of the three-variable relationship and is incapable of showing the true *continuous* nature of the third variable. Three-dimensional visual presentation of a three-variable problem thus yields a complete model that is conceptually simpler.

Clinically, acid-base status is usually well characterized by plotting an arterial point on a graph such as Fig. 11-6. However, it is sometimes also necessary to measure blood electrolyte concentrations and the pH of other body fluids. In actual practice the clinical diagnosis

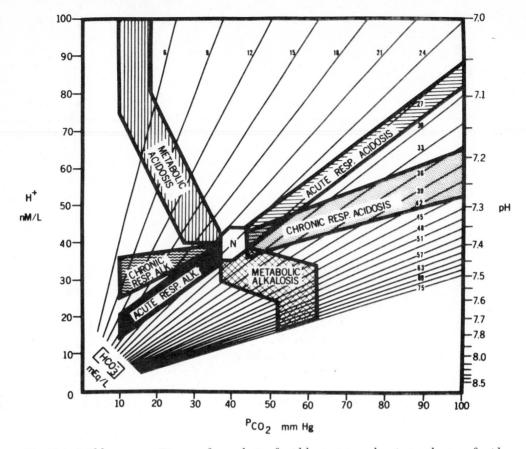

Fig. 11-6. Acid-base map. Diagram for analysis of acid-base status, showing pathways of acid-base disturbance. The map contains information from the Hendersen-Hasselbalch buffer equation, a normal whole-body CO_2 titration curve, and empiric ranges of data found in acid-base disturbances. The area of normal values is labeled N. The numbered lines are isopleths of plasma bicarbonate ion concentration in mEq/L. Plot arterial blood pH and P_{CO_2}. It may be occasionally necessary to extrapolate to a lower pH or to a higher P_{CO_2}. (From Goldberg, M., and others: J.A.M.A. **223**: 269, 1973.)

of acid-base disturbances is usually also based on the history, physical examination, and clinical laboratory data.

CARBON DIOXIDE TENSION AND THE RENAL EXCRETION OF BICARBONATE

The kidney is the key to compensation for initial respiratory changes. It is now known that renal HCO_3^- retention or excretion de-

pends not on HCO_3^- concentration nor on pH, but rather on the P_{CO_2}. Bicarbonate ion concentration is high in both metabolic alkalosis and uncompensated respiratory acidosis. In the latter situation HCO_3^- is retained by the kidney; in the former it is not. Bicarbonate ion concentration is low in both metabolic acidosis and uncompensated respiratory alkalosis. In the latter HCO_3^- is excreted by the kidney, taking the concentration still lower; in the former it is not.

It is the cells of the distal convoluted tubule of the kidney that excrete or retain HCO_3^- in relation to the P_{CO_2}. These cells are rich in the enzyme carbonic anhydrase. When P_{CO_2} is normal, HCO_3^- and H^+ are rapidly formed. The filtrate at this level contains not only Na^+ but also HCO_3^-, in the same concentration as plasma. The cell walls lining this tubule appear to have a cation exchange mechanism, or pump, on the tubular side that exchanges H^+ and K^+ within the cells for Na^+ in the lumen of the tubule. When H^+ reach the tubule by this route, they are free to combine with HCO_3^- in the tubule to form CO_2 and water. The HCO_3^- formed within the cells by the action of carbonic anhydrase moves, along with Na^+, across the opposite wall of the cell and into the capillary.

Why do H^+ and HCO_3^- combine freely to form CO_2 and water in the renal filtrate, whereas the enzymatic action of carbonic anhydrase is necessary in the renal tubular cells and red blood cells? There are two possible answers. Either the reaction proceeds slowly without catalysis, but the filtrate remains in the tubule for some time; or red blood cells are being continually destroyed, their contents entering the circulation and the smaller molecules passing through the glomerulus. Small amounts of carbonic anhydrase may pass through the glomerulus and be present in the filtrate at the level of the distal tubule.

What happens to the CO_2 produced from union of H^+ and HCO_3^- in the filtrate? Carbon dioxide diffuses readily through cell walls. If a CO_2 gradient is established from the lumen of the tubule to the renal cells and blood, CO_2 diffuses toward the region of lower concentration.

Why does the high P_{CO_2} of respiratory acidosis "save" HCO_3^-? There is a P_{CO_2} concentration gradient from plasma to renal tubular cells. As a result of this gradient, CO_2 moves

quickly into these cells and shifts the reaction

$$\overset{\text{Carbonic}}{\underset{\downarrow}{\text{anhydrase}}}$$

$$CO_2 + H_2O \rightleftharpoons H_2CO_3 \rightleftharpoons H^+ + HCO_3^-$$

to the right, producing more H^+, which exchange with more Na^+ and combine with more tubular HCO_3^-, preventing this latter ion from being excreted.

Why does the kidney excrete HCO_3^- when P_{CO_2} is low, as it is in respiratory alkalosis? Carbon dioxide moves from the cells, including renal tubular cells, into the blood. The preceding reaction is shifted to the left, depleting the H^+ population of these cells. Fewer H^+ exchange with Na^+; therefore, fewer H^+ are available to combine with HCO_3^- in the filtrate, and more HCO_3^- is excreted.

What is the effect of renal retention or excretion of HCO_3^- on the acid-base picture? If respiratory acidosis persists, the high P_{CO_2} will cause the kidney to retain HCO_3^-. This HCO_3^- retention results in an upward shift (pathway C in Fig. 11-4) away from the CO_2 dissociation curve and in the direction of normal pH. If the condition persists, there will be complete *compensation* to pH 7.40. If respiratory alkalosis persists, the low P_{CO_2} will force renal excretion of HCO_3^-, moving the plasma values down from the normal CO_2 dissociation curve until pH is again 7.40 (pathway E in Fig. 11-4). In either case a new CO_2 dissociation curve applies. Any further respiratory change will move the plasma values along that new curve.

What makes the kidney stop manipulating HCO_3^- once normal pH has been reestablished? In compensated respiratory acidosis the high P_{CO_2} continues to force H^+ into the filtrate, but the concentration of filtered HCO_3^- is high because of the high plasma level. With this high HCO_3^- level in the filtrate, some escapes combination with H^+ and is excreted in the urine. In compensated respiratory alkalosis the level of filtered HCO_3^- is so low that little of it escapes the tubular H^+, even though their level is also low.

Infusion of acid into the blood quickly drives the reaction

$$CO_2 + H_2O \overset{\text{Carbonic}}{\underset{\text{anhydrase}}{\downarrow}} \rightleftharpoons H_2CO_3 \rightleftharpoons H^+ + HCO_3^-$$

to the left, depleting HCO_3^- and stimulating the peripheral chemoreceptors to increase breathing. The CO_2 thus produced is quickly blown off by the acid-induced hyperventilation. This sudden drop in HCO_3^- concentration is seen in pathway F in Fig. 11-4 as an abrupt downward departure from the normal CO_2 dissociation curve to lower HCO_3^- and pH levels. But in contradistinction to renal compensation, respiratory compensation is rapid. Hyperventilation accompanies downward departure from the normal CO_2 dissociation curve. This reduces P_{CO_2} so that the direction (Fig. 11-4) is downward and to the left at the same time. In contrast to renal compensation, respiratory compensation is *incomplete;* pathway F does not terminate on the pH 7.4 isopleth. Excess H^+ increase breathing. If compensation to pH 7.40 were complete, there would be no excess H^+ and thus no drive for hyperventilation.

Removal of acid (as by vomiting or aspiration of stomach contents) or addition of base (such as HCO_3^-) is seen as abrupt upward departure from the normal CO_2 dissociation curve to higher HCO_3^- levels and higher pH values (pathway B in Fig. 11-4). This is metabolic alkalosis. Except by renal removal of excess HCO_3^-, compensation for metabolic alkalosis is the poorest of those for any of the four primary acid-base disturbances; it succeeds in restoring the afflicted subject's plasma only about one third of the distance back toward normal pH, as pathway B indicates. Compensation is by hypoventilation, which elevates P_{CO_2}. This compensation is poor because only a small fraction of normal ventilatory drive is caused by H^+ in the blood. Reduction or even removal of

this small stimulus does not reduce breathing drive very much. Because breathing is not reduced very much, P_{CO_2} does not rise very much.

Changes in pulmonary ventilation change P_{CO_2} and shift plasma values along the CO_2 dissociation curve (Fig. 11-4). Whenever such changes are transient (measured in minutes), the normal CO_2 dissociation curve continues to apply. However, when ventilatory changes persist for hours or days, the kidney retains or excretes HCO_3^- and a new CO_2 dissociation curve applies. If HCO_3^- has been retained, this new dissociation curve is higher than the old one. If HCO_3^- has been excreted, the new curve is below the old one. When a HCO_3^- shift establishes a new CO_2 dissociation curve, subsequent changes in ventilation will then move the plasma values along that new curve. When renal compensation is complete, the new curve intersects the pH 7.4 line at whatever resting arterial P_{CO_2} level the ventilation has set.

How do we know whether the CO_2 dissociation curve has been shifted up or down? We equilibrate a *blood* sample with a gas mixture that has the composition of resting, sea-level, alveolar gas (P_{CO_2} = 40 torr, P_{O_2} = 100 torr)* and analyze the *plasma* for its bicarbonate content; this is the *standard bicarbonate*. A high value indicates a high CO_2 dissociation curve; a low value indicates a low CO_2 dissociation curve. A primary metabolic disturbance shifts the CO_2 dissociation curve up or down immediately. Ventilatory changes shift plasma values along the CO_2 dissociation curve.

It is sometimes helpful in understanding acid-base disturbances to consider the ratio of $[HCO_3^-]$ to $[a \times P_{CO_2}]$. If the primary disturbance is in the numerator, it is metabolic. If HCO_3^- concentration increases, there is metabolic alkalosis. If HCO_3^- concentration de-

---

*If the P_{O_2} of this equilibration gas mixture is high or low, the Haldane effect will produce a different CO_2 dissociation curve.

creases, there is metabolic acidosis. If the primary change is in the denominator, the disturbance is respiratory. In respiratory acidosis an increased P_{CO_2} decreases the ratio and lowers the pH. If the P_{CO_2} decreases, thus increasing the ratio, the primary disturbance is respiratory alkalosis. The abnormality can be related to the Henderson-Hasselbalch equation as follows:

$$pH = pK + \log \frac{renal}{respiratory} \qquad (8)$$

ACID-BASE PATTERNS IN VARIOUS PHYSIOLOGIC STATES

Metabolic acidosis almost always produces hyperventilation. The H^+ stimulus increases ventilation as the acidosis develops so that partial compensation for the primary disturbance is present almost from the start. However, exercise severe enough to incur a sizable O_2 debt produces a metabolic acidosis (as a result of lactic acid accumulation in muscle and blood) that is uncompensated. Despite large increases in CO_2 production, arterial P_{CO_2} remains essentially normal. Compensation would require that the arterial P_{CO_2} decrease. Without such compensation the accumulation of a given quantity of lactic acid during exercise produces a greater drop in pH than would the same quantity of lactic acid infused at rest.

Gastric mucosa has the capacity to concentrate H^+ 1 million times. The production of HCl (hydrochloric acid) in quantity depletes the blood and the rest of the body of H^+. This depletion, which follows the ingestion of large meals, is reflected in the *alkaline tide,* a blood pH shift to the alkaline side, or temporary metabolic alkalosis. Pancreatic juice is highly alkaline, containing bicarbonate and phosphates. It neutralizes acid stomach contents, which pass into the small intestine. The intestinal reabsorption of gastric contents restores blood pH to normal. Loss of gastric contents through vomiting or gastric aspiration produces metabolic alkalosis.

During sleep metabolic rate decreases.

There is also reduced sensitivity to CO_2. Accordingly, arterial P_{CO_2} increases slightly, producing slight respiratory acidosis. Overnight renal compensation for this respiratory acidosis is presumably incomplete. Patients with chronic diffuse obstructive bronchopulmonary disease may accumulate considerable CO_2.

Acid-base disturbance and compensation

Biochemical correction of acid-base disturbances should never be undertaken without thorough knowledge of the acid-base status, as well as knowledge of the significance of existing compensatory changes.

Metabolic acidosis occurs physiologically during exercise but is also observed during periods of low cardiac output, such as during surgical procedures involving cardiac bypass by means of a pump-oxygenator or resuscitation after cardiac arrest. Uncontrolled diabetes mellitus is a common clinical cause of ketosis and metabolic acidosis. Metabolic acidosis is also an aspect of the clinical syndrome *uremia,* which occurs when failure supervenes in the course of chronic diffuse renal disease. Ammonium chloride tablets are often used to produce metabolic acidosis for clinical purposes.

Chronic diffuse bronchopulmonary disease is an increasingly common clinical cause of respiratory acidosis. The sequence of events as pulmonary failure supervenes is invariably hypoxemia, CO_2 retention, and finally frank respiratory acidosis. What are critical acute changes in pH, P_{O_2}, and P_{CO_2} in respiratory failure? Although no rigid criteria can be defined, an arterial blood pH less than 7.25, a P_{CO_2} greater than 60 torr, and a P_{O_2} less than 50 torr are considered urgent indications for treatment.

Hypokalemic metabolic alkalosis

Potassium depletion and alkalosis generally result from renal, adrenal, or gastrointestinal causes. Significant deficit of total body K^+ and alkalosis can also occur in patients with chronic diffuse bronchopulmonary disease and cor pulmonale. The occurrence of metabolic alkalosis caused by hypokalemia and/or hypochloremia is so frequent in such patients as to require special emphasis. The mechanism probably includes hyperaldosteronism secondary to cardiac insufficiency, reduced dietary intake of K^+, and the kaliuretic (increasing urinary K^+ excretion) effects of diuretic or glucocorticosteroid medications. Depletion of body K^+ and alkalosis may exist despite the fact that serum K^+ levels are within normal limits. Although K^+ depletion is associated with an extracellular alkalosis, an intracellular acidosis is simultaneously present.

Potassium depletion and alkalosis in patients with chronic diffuse bronchopulmonary disease and CO_2 retention may exert a very deleterious effect. Alkalosis itself reduces ventilatory drive, thus aggravating hypoxemia and CO_2 retention. These changes in turn further increase the pulmonary arterial pressure and work of the right ventricle. Alkalosis also shifts the oxyhemoglobin dissociation curve to the left, thereby diminishing the O_2 dumping effect that normally occurs in the tissues. Adequate replacement with potassium chloride is the treatment of choice. Replacement by nonchloride potassium preparations is often inadequate.

Diuretics and metabolic alkalosis

In general, intermittency in the administration of diuretics is a clinical point of considerable value, enhancing therapeutic efficiency while minimizing the possibility of overtreatment.

Various potent diuretics have the capacity to produce serious electrolyte and pH disturbances, especially in patients with impaired pulmonary or renal function. Sometimes the combination of low-sodium diet and potent diuretics results in severe hyponatremia (low blood Na^+ concentration) and the *low-salt syndrome*. Thiazide diuretics, as well as glucocorticosteroids, produce metabolic alkalosis. Un-

compensated alkalosis in patients with chronic diffuse bronchopulmonary disease reduces ventilatory drive, aggravating both hypoxemia and hypercapnia.

Acetazolamide (Diamox) is an inhibitor of the enzyme carbonic anhydrase. One important effect of acetazolamide is to decrease renal reabsorption of HCO_3^-, producing metabolic acidosis; another, through its action in erythrocytes, is to cause CO_2 retention and respiratory acidosis. Large doses of acetazolamide increase brain tissue P_{CO_2}.

The prototype thiazide compound, chlorothiazide (Diuril), was introduced in 1958 as a result of the search for improved diuretic agents similar in structure to the sulfonamide carbonic anhydrase inhibitor, acetazolamide. Chlorothiazides are commonly used in the treatment of cardiac insufficiency, including that associated with cor pulmonale. They act by increasing urinary excretion of water, Na^+, Cl^-, and, to a lesser degree, K^+ and HCO_3^-. Consequently, hyponatremia, hypokalemia, and hypochloremic alkalosis may occur. Patients already liable to hypokalemia or those receiving concomitant glucocorticosteroids or digitalis must be watched closely during thiazide therapy. Daily ingestion of foods high in K^+, such as orange juice, or supplemental KCl should be considered.

Tromethamine (THAM®, or TRIS)

Tromethamine, or tris(hydroxymethyl)aminomethane, is a white, crystalline, water-soluble, organic alcohol amine of empiric formula $NH_2C(CH_2OH)_3$. It was first used to postpone the death of fish in transport, which die as a result of CO_2 accumulation and acidosis. It is an interesting experimental agent and has occasional clinical use in the therapy of respiratory acidosis.

Tromethamine is a weak base, or proton acceptor, which after injection (usually intravenous) into the circulation becomes a component of a buffer system. A 0.3-molar solution contains 36 gm/L, is iso-osmotic with plasma, and has a pH of 10.2 at 38° C. After tromethamine has reacted with H^+, it forms salts with the associated anions, which are then excreted by the kidney. Tromethamine is an osmotic diuretic, increasing both urine flow and urine pH. At pH 7.40 tromethamine is 30% un-ionized. The un-ionized form can diffuse from its extracellular location into the cells, where it combines with the anions of intracellular fluids. The reaction of tromethamine with acids may be represented as:

$$(CH_2OH)_3CNH_2 + HA \rightleftharpoons$$
$$(CH_2OH)_3CNH_3^+ + A^- \quad (9)$$

Alkalinizing agents, such as bicarbonates and tromethamine, are occasionally useful in treatment of the acid-base disturbance of respiratory failure. Their use is limited to cases in which arterial pH remains less than 7.25 after partial or complete restoration of arterial P_{CO_2} to normal or cases in which arterial P_{CO_2} remains high despite vigorous treatment of airway obstruction, hypercapnia, and hypoxemia.

Tromethamine overdosage* depresses respiration by reducing P_{CO_2} and increasing pH, an unusual example of respiratory alkalosis. Hyperventilation is the fundamental cause of respiratory alkalosis, a term that refers to the acid-base picture after excessive CO_2 has been ventilated away or otherwise removed. Emotional stress is the most common cause of hyperventilation. Acetylsalicylic acid and other salicylates increase ventilation out of proportion to metabolic rate, causing respiratory alkalosis; however, in large doses they produce metabolic acidosis as a result of interference with carbohydrate metabolism.

---

*Large doses have been reported to cause hypoglycemia.

CHAPTER 12

NEUROGENESIS OF BREATHING

The breathing cycle involves successive, rhythmic contraction and relaxation of the inspiratory muscles. Active expiration, when it occurs, involves rhythmic contraction and relaxation of the expiratory muscles. The breathing muscles, which include the internal and external intercostal muscles, the abdominal muscles, and the two hemidiaphragms, have two functions: (1) to make the movements of breathing and (2) to contribute to the maintenance of posture, resisting the effects of gravity on the chest. The fluctuations of breathing are therefore superimposed on the postural tonus of the respiratory muscles. The act of breathing is coordinated in the brainstem; however, the mechanism is not fully understood.

As inspiration begins, inspiratory neurons fire faster—from 5 to 10 per second to 30 to 40 per second. Simultaneously, expiratory muscle tone is inhibited. As inspiration proceeds, additional inspiratory neurons are recruited. Toward the end of inspiration the frequency of inspiratory impulses diminishes. During quiet breathing, inspiratory neuron activity continues into the expiratory phase of the breathing cycle, smoothing the transition from inspiration to expiration. A sudden interruption of all inspiratory effort would allow the thorax to fall abruptly, producing a transient, significant rise of intrapleural pressure. Such a spasmodic breathing cycle would impede venous return to the heart, as well as increase resistance to air flow with every expiration. Thus, gradually decreasing inspiratory tone normally allows expiration to proceed without *sudden* alteration of the intrathoracic pressure changes that produce inspiration and expiration.

METHODS FOR STUDY OF THE RESPIRATORY CENTERS

A respiratory center is a region of the central nervous system (CNS) where neuronal activity coincides with the breathing cycle or a region where stimulation of neurons produces responses that are primarily related to breathing. Various technics have been used to localize the respiratory centers of the CNS and to study their function. Early studies involved observing the effects of ablation or transection of precisely located neuron populations or nerve tracts. These technics were superseded by electrolysis or thermal block, which permitted greater control of the intervention. In addition, electric stimulation and chemical injection into selected regions yielded information about the location and characteristics of CNS centers associated with breathing.

Such studies may mislead as well as fail to yield information about *normal* respiratory center activity; it is not known whether fiber tracts or nerve cell bodies are being ablated or stimulated, and electric current may affect adjacent areas of the brain. Thus, the response of a region to an electric current does not guarantee its involvement in the genesis of normal breathing. Furthermore, the introduction of a micropipette for injections can cause damage, and injected material can diffuse to adjacent regions, resulting in unphysiologic conditions.

More recently, electric activity of the brain has been studied using elegant microelectrodes precisely placed in selected brain locations. Newly developed histologic technics have also been used to study the organization of the CNS. The results have forced a reexamination of the mechanisms by which breathing is generated and regulated. Concepts that were widely accepted are now in question and must be replaced by new theories. For example, the long-standing theory that the rhythmicity of breathing results from reciprocal inhibition of inspiratory and expiratory components of the "respiratory center" has been discounted, and another explanation for rhythmicity must be found.

This presentation is synthesized from the reports and reviews of investigators who have spent most of their research careers studying the problem. There is still no consensus that a single theory explains the process; important observations are lacking. Furthermore, there may be disagreement on the interpretation of observations. Our description of the genesis of breathing and the regulation of pulmonary ventilation is presented in that context. It may be superseded by a better one at any time, or other currently proposed mechanisms may become accepted as more valid on the basis of new information.

It may be surprising to the reader that, even with the obvious large gaps, breathing is one of the few brain functions being studied on the basis of brain cell organization and activity and interrelationships among localized groups of neurons. Although progress has been made, much more research is still required.

MEDULLARY RESPIRATORY CENTER

Under proper conditions, with the medulla isolated from the cranial nerves entering at that level and from the rest of the brain above it (transection at the lower pontine level), the medullary center still drives the muscles of breathing. It may require an input to the brainstem of random, non–respiratory-related impulses to produce a "local excitatory state" and allow the generation of a central rhythm for breathing. In the experience of some investigators, the rhythm is "ataxic" rather than smooth; that is, it consists of gasps alternating with small breaths and may exhibit an irregular pattern, but it can nonetheless be recognized as a pattern of breathing.

Until recently it was taught that the medullary respiratory center consisted of an inspiratory and an expiratory component and that the rhythmicity of breathing resulted from reciprocal inhibition between the two components. This concept has been modified (although not necessarily clarified) because of recent observations based on histologic studies and the recording of neural activity with microelectrodes.

Although the concept of two regions of respiratory neurons in the medulla remains valid, description of their interrelationships has changed considerably. A diagram representing the new concept of the CNS respiratory "centers" is show in Fig. 12-1.

A group of cells active during inspiration (inspiratory neurons) is located in the nucleus of the tractus solitarius (NTS); this group is termed the *dorsal respiratory group*. In addition to having an internal network of synapses, neurons in this group receive afferent connections from the ninth and tenth cranial nerves. These nerves transmit sensory impulses from the lungs, pharynx, larynx, and peripheral chemoreceptors. Thus, this region appears to receive and integrate sensory information and to generate and initiate a motor response.

Some of the neurons (called Iα) in the dorsal respiratory group are inhibited by lung inflation, while others (Iβ) are excited. Opinions differ regarding the relationships between these neuron types and their role in the genesis of rhythmicity, but many investigators be-

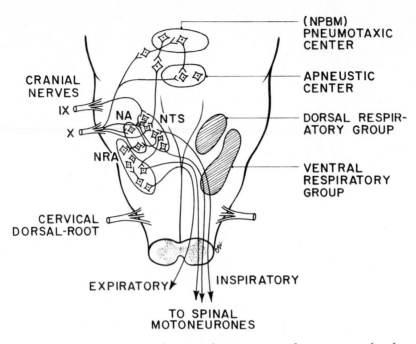

Fig. 12-1. One scheme proposed for the central organization of respiratory-related groups of neurons. (See text for discussion.)

lieve that the dorsal respiratory group is the site of origin of breathing rhythmicity.

Axons from the inspiratory neurons of the dorsal respiratory group project to the contralateral spinal cord and probably innervate the diaphragm through the phrenic nerves. They also project to the ventral respiratory group and drive neurons there.

Neurons in the caudal portion of the nucleus ambiguous (NA) and in the nucleus retroambigualis (NRA) comprise the second region of the medulla with a concentration of respiration-related neurons. This region contains both inspiratory and expiratory neurons and is termed the *ventral respiratory group.*

Rostral neurons in the NA are vagal motoneurons. They serve auxiliary muscles of inspiration through the recurrent laryngeal nerve. The rostral neurons in the NRA tend to be inspiratory, whereas caudal neurons in that nucleus are expiratory. The expiratory neurons

project contralaterally and descend in the cord, terminating at levels from the first thoracic to the third lumbar segments. This suggests that they drive expiratory (internal) intercostal and abdominal respiratory muscles. Inspiratory neurons from the ventral respiratory group appear to drive the inspiratory external intercostal muscles, as well as the diaphragm through its phrenic nerves.

Thus, the major function of neurons of the ventral respiratory group seems to be that of augmenting inspiration and serving expiration when it is active. Neurons in this group are driven by the dorsal respiratory group; rhythmicity and the integration or processing of afferent (sensory) information does not occur in the ventral respiratory group.

Most spinal projections from both the dorsal and the ventral respiratory groups cross the midline in the region of the obex and descend in the ventrolateral columns. There is a spatial separation for both the crossing and the descent of inspiratory and expiratory axons. Furthermore, there is a separation of the descending tracts serving respiration (which originate in the medullary respiratory groups) from the descending tracts originating in the cortex. Patients have been described who had spinal lesions causing paralysis of the trunk and limb muscles and rhythmic breathing but who could not voluntarily change their breathing pattern. The converse also occurs. Bilateral cervical ventrolateral cordotomy for relief of pain may accidentally interrupt descending respiratory tracts as well as ascending spinothalamic pathways, resulting in long periods of apnea even though the patient could breathe voluntarily. This condition is called "Ondine's curse" by Severinghaus and Mitchell, after the German legend in which the water nymph, Ondine, who was jilted by her mortal husband, took away his automatic body functions. He had to remember to breathe, and when he finally fell asleep, he died. Ondine's curse may also result from other conditions that cause primary hypoventilation, chronic hypoxia, and hypercapnea.

PONTINE RESPIRATORY CENTERS

The pons is not necessary for rhythmic breathing; hence, it is not involved in the genesis of rhythmicity. However, neurons in the pons have an important effect on breathing. Transection at midpontine level results in apnea under certain conditions in deep inspiration (apneusis). This was formerly considered to be evidence of a rostral expiratory center called the *pneumotaxic center* and presumed to be reciprocally related to a caudal inspiratory center called the *apneustic center*. However, when the pons is isolated from the rhythm induced by the medulla, no periodic activity is seen in either group of neurons. The so-called pneumotaxic center is made up of two nuclei: the nucleus parabrachealis medialis (previously PNC, now NPBM) and the Kölliker-Fuse nu-

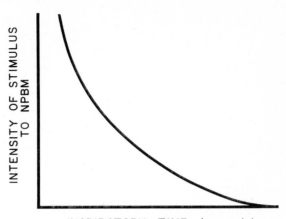

Fig. 12-2. The threshold for termination of inspiration, determined by the duration of inspiration and the intensity of stimulation of the NPBM in the caudal pons.

cleus. Phasic electrical stimulation of this region causes phrenic activity to synchronize with the stimuli by stopping inspiration. The stimulus intensity required to inhibit inspiration is greater early in the inspiratory effort. This is shown in Fig. 12-2; a gradually decreasing stimulus strength is required to terminate inspiration as the duration of inspiration lengthens.

Of course, there is a similar relationship between stimulus strength required to reach threshold and the inspired volume during an inspiration; activity from pulmonary stretch receptors appears to be involved. More evidence for this concept comes from the fact that whereas neurons of the NPBM are tonically active when the vagus nerve is intact, output from the NPBM is phasic with lung inflation after the vagus is cut. This can be interpreted to mean that without vagal input, the NPBM is affected by activity from the medullary inspiratory center and that this effect is attenuated (or abolished) when afferent impulses from lung stretch receptors reach the pons through the vagus nerve. This is not caused by a *direct* effect of the vagus on the NPBM; possibly, vagal afferents inhibit presynaptic impulses going to the area from the medullary inspiratory center.

As indicated, our understanding of the relationship between the NPBM and vagal afferent activity remains incomplete. It has been taught for many years that NPBM activity and/or vagal impulses inhibit the apneustic center and that without at least one of these sources of inhibition, apneusis (sustained inspiratory effort) results (Fig. 12-1). However, lesions involving the NPBM can cause apneustic breathing in patients who had no vagus nerve involvement. Furthermore, it has been demonstrated that cats can survive NPBM lesions and subsequent bilateral vagotomy. However, these animals, like most, developed apneusis after anesthesia. These reports complicated our understanding of the NPBM and its effect on breathing rhythmicity but also indicated that higher centers (depressed by anesthesia) may play a role in the maintenance of rhythmic breathing.

Although we cannot describe the function of the NPBM with certainty, it appears to provide a tonic input to a region that serves to "turn off" inspiration.

Inspiratory "off-switching"

The pattern of impulse discharge for breathing is generated in the medulla (probably in the dorsal respiratory group of neurons) and is typical if not modified by a phasic input associated with inspiration. It consists of a gradual crescendo of impulses, which is terminated by the central generator of the inspiratory pattern. The increasing intensity of discharge is reasonably linear, its cessation is abrupt, and its activity is followed by a silent period. There is no significant discharge of expiratory neurons during quiet breathing; hence, expiration is passive.

Phasic sensory neuron activity reaching the CNS via the vagus nerve, in turn activated by pulmonary stretch receptors, shortens the *duration* of inspiration. It has no effect on the *rate* of phrenic discharge. Thus, vagal activity does not affect the inspiratory effort or inspiratory flow rate but only acts to stop an otherwise unaffected inspiration.

The lung volume needed to terminate an inspiration varies, depending on the phase of inspiration. The pattern of the threshold for terminating inspiration (Fig. 12-2) can be duplicated by artificially increasing lung volume with a ventilator instead of stimulating the NPBM. This is diagrammatically presented in Fig. 12-3.

The effects of the lung volume change and the level of NPBM tonic activity on inspiratory off-switching are additive; if tonic activity of the NPBM increases, a smaller lung volume change is required to stop inspiration, and vice versa.

The threshold curve for the termination of inspiration is constant under a variety of conditions. For example, increasing P_{CO_2} in the inspired air increases inspiratory effort, and the diaphragm contracts more rapidly. The threshold is reached more quickly, and therefore a higher lung volume is required to stop inspiration (Fig. 12-3). At lower alveolar P_{CO_2} levels the inspiratory drive is less, and the inspiratory flow rate is reduced. The result is that inspiration lasts longer and the threshold level is reached at a lower lung volume. Thus, reduced inspiratory flow rates are accompanied by smaller tidal volumes, and more rapid flow rates result in larger tidal volumes.

According to some investigators, the duration of an expiration is ordinarily a constant proportion of the duration of the preceding inspiration. No such relationship appears to exist between an expiration and the duration of the following inspiration. Although the duration of an expiration can be changed, for example, by occlusion of airways or by use of a ventilator, this does not alter the duration of the following inspiration. Other investigators have separated the duration of expiration and inspiration. They have described a control mechanism for expiratory time that is related to vagal discharge during expiration and have proposed that

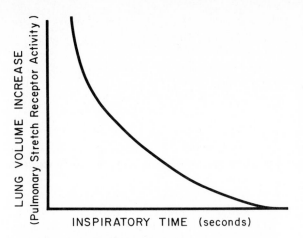

Fig. 12-3. Threshold for termination of inspiration, determined by the duration of inspiration and the increase of lung volume or activity of the pulmonary stretch receptors.

stretch receptor activity during inspiration has little or no effect on expiratory duration. These contradictory reports may be the result of species differences. Considerable differences in these relationships do exist, for example, between dogs and cats. It is not clear which pattern more closely resembles the control system for man.

We can conclude that somewhere in the brain a group of cells generates the impulses that reach the inspiration-terminating threshold. This activity switches off the inspiratory effort when vagal and NPBM input are at a sufficient level. Because the threshold falls, the level is reached at a lower and lower output as inspiration continues.

Persuasive arguments have been made that the vagal afferents are the source of the input and act directly on cells in the dorsal respiratory group, which in turn is the site of inspiratory off-switching. Other investigators propose a separate "off-switch" population of neurons, the site of which is the apneustic center in the rostral pons. It is the site of projection for inputs from both the NPBM and the vagus nerve; thus, apneusis might result when the off-switch is not activated by either vagal or caudal pontine (NPBM) neural activity.

The observation that the pons is not required for rhythmic neuron activity does not invalidate this concept. The central rhythmicity generator might be limited to the medulla, with a cycle duration longer than that ordinarily observed with an intact system. Furthermore, some investigators propose that the dorsal respiratory group has its own automaticity and that the group of inspiratory cells has per se the ability to generate rhythmicity. Such autorhythmicity of neuron groups occurs in invertebrates. It has not been searched for vigorously in vertebrates; indeed, methods in current use for study of the mammalian brain could not identify such a phenomenon if it did exist. This hypothesis may receive more support from future studies.

MODIFICATION OF BREATHING BY HIGHER CNS CENTERS

The breathing pattern can be modified by conscious control originating in the cerebral cortex, for example, voluntary hyperventilation or breath-holding. However, the ability of the cerebral cortex to override the basic rhythmicity of the medullary centers is limited, and most healthy subjects cannot hold their breath to the point of unconsciousness. We alter our breathing pattern voluntarily to speak or to sniff. We are less conscious of some cortically produced modifications such as breath-holding during a brief stint of vigorous physical activity (for example, sprinting). We also modify our breathing pattern and may even hold our breath during the isometric muscular work of supporting heavy objects or straining at stool. Electric stimulation of certain areas of the cerebral cortex modifies the breathing pattern. Most of these areas also subserve other functions, such as emotion (crying, laughing, sobbing), the autonomic nervous system (fright, thermoregulation), special senses (olfaction), or acts that directly control breathing (vocalization, swallowing).

CHAPTER 13

NEURAL REGULATION OF PULMONARY VENTILATION

The previous chapter dealt with the organization of respiratory-related neuron groups in the central nervous system. Theories were presented regarding the neurogenesis of rhythmicity of breathing and certain factors that affect the duration of inspiration and expiration. The ventilatory system also needs some input regarding *effectiveness* (whether lung volume is *actually* changing) and *efficiency* (how much energy is being expended to accomplish the task) of breathing. The most efficient combination of tidal volume (V_T) and breathing frequency (f) is automatically and unconsciously selected for any given level of ventilation and for any given set of mechanical variables, such as lung compliance and respiratory resistance. How is this accomplished?

GAMMA-EFFERENT SYSTEM

A feedback system that is integrated in the spinal cord adjusts the pattern of breathing to the mechanical state of the lungs and chest. It is not unique as a regulator of muscle activity but is a special case of the generalized servo-controlled mechanism involving muscle spindles. The γ-efferent system that responds to changes of the mechanics of breathing does not involve the vagus nerves.

There is some difference between the muscle spindles located in the intercostal muscles and those in the diaphragm. The muscle spindles in the intercostals are in parallel with the α-fibers, which are active in the shortening process. In the diaphragm they are in the tendon, in series with the α-fibers. This means that when the intercostal α-fibers shorten, the spindle fibers are stretched less, and when diaphragmatic α-fibers shorten, muscle spindle fibers are under more tension. The γ-efferent system appears more important for control of the intercostal muscles than the diaphragm; for this reason we will describe the system involved in controlling the strength of intercostal muscle contraction (Fig. 13-1).

Two types of motoneurons exist in the anterior horn of the spinal cord. The α-neuron serving the active muscle fiber has an axon of large diameter, whereas the γ-neuron going to the muscle spindle has an axon of small diameter. The γ-efferent fiber innervates the intrafusal fibers, which are muscle fibers within the spindle, in series with a spiral stretch receptor. Activity of the γ-efferent neuron stimulates the intrafusal fibers to shorten. This stretches the spiral receptor, stimulating neuronal activity, which reaches the cord via the dorsal root. Such impulses stimulate the α-motoneurons, causing the muscle to contract. This in turn relieves the tension on the spiral stretch receptor in the muscle spindle.

It is proposed that the γ-efferent system adjusts the breathing pattern by contracting *in concert* with the α-motor fiber system. If shortening is appropriate for the motor output, the tension on the spiral receptor follows an appropriate pattern, for example, remaining constant if both elements shorten to the same degree. If compliance decreases, for example, so that muscle shortening meets resistance, the γ-efferents shorten the intrafusal fibers disproportionately and stimulate the ventral horn moto-neurons through the γ-efferent neuron, thus increasing α-fiber shortening. If the *effort* required to shorten the intercostal muscles is too great for the actual degree of shortening, the sustained or increased γ-afferent activity affects the upper centers, causing early cessation of inspiration. Although this system is conjectural,

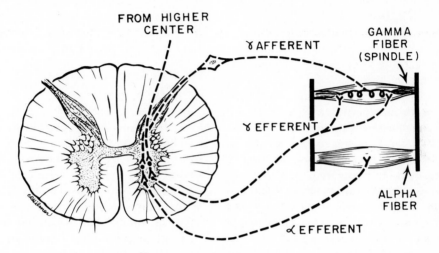

Fig. 13-1. The extravagal γ-efferent system is a feedback system that modifies the breathing pattern.

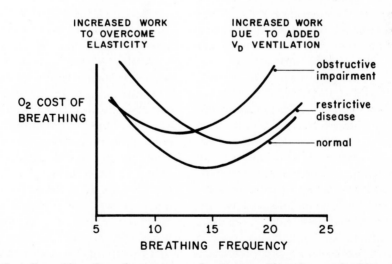

Fig. 13-2. The effect of breathing frequency on the O_2 cost of breathing in healthy subjects, patients with obstructive impairment, and patients with restrictive disease. The curves are not from actual data.

it fits observations about the spinal integration of the breathing pattern, according to theories proposed by Howell and Campbell.

Fig. 13-2 shows the relationship between altered lung mechanics and the efficiency of various breathing patterns. Assuming that alveolar ventilation rate remains unchanged, a lower f is associated with a larger V_T and a higher f is associated with a smaller V_T. Note that as f increases, dead space ventilation rate ($\dot{V}_D$) also increases; thus, *total* ventilation ($\dot{V}_E$) increases at higher breathing frequencies, maintaining alveolar ventilation rate.

Fig. 13-2 is not from actual data but illustrates the findings reported for patients who have altered mechanics of breathing. With normal compliance and resistance, the most efficient f (based on the O_2 cost of breathing) is 12 to 15 breaths/min. At lower frequencies, V_T increases and more of the lung volume relates to a flatter part of the compliance curve. As a consequence, greater effort is required to inflate the lungs and efficiency decreases. If f increases so that $\dot{V}_D$ is greatly increased, $\dot{V}_E$ increases and efficiency again decreases.

These two factors affect the position of curves for patients who have altered mechanics of breathing. Patients who have obstructive lung disease must work more to increase pulmonary ventilation rate because airway resistance (R_{aw}) is high. This condition is even worse at high flow rates associated with increased $\dot{V}_E$. Such patients breathe more efficiently if they breath slowly and deeply. Furthermore, compliance is usually increased, which means that larger tidal volumes do not require high energy expenditures. Patients who have obstructive lung disease do indeed breathe with deeper tidal breaths; the γ-efferent system may provide feedback information for regulation of such a pattern.

In restrictive lung disease, increased effort is required to inflate the lungs. The inappropriate degree of shortening in relation to the applied motor neuron activity probably activates the γ-afferent neurons, which in turn signal the CNS to stop inspiration at a reduced V_T. The reduced V_T is compensated for by increased f. Since R_{aw} is normal, at least in *pure* restrictive disease, the cost of increasing $\dot{V}_D$ is less than the cost of a large V_T; thus, less energy is expended at higher breathing frequencies. Patients who have decreased compliance (or other factors that limit V_T) unconsciously select a breathing pattern of low V_T and high f, probably aided in this selection by the γ-efferent system in the intercostal muscles and diaphragm.

PROPRIOCEPTIVE REFLEXES

The lungs and chest wall contain the receptors of a number of proprioceptive reflexes that affect breathing. At least eight kinds of receptors have been identified on the basis of structure, location, and afferent nerve type. The afferent, or sensory, pathways of most of the pulmonary reflexes are in the vagus nerves. We will describe three of these pulmonary reflexes in some detail but do not wish to imply that other reflexes are unimportant for the breathing pattern.

Hering-Breuer inspiratory reflex

Perhaps the most familiar of the pulmonary reflexes is the Hering-Breuer reflex, which affects the depth of inspiration. Lung inflation stimulates pulmonary stretch receptors, which in turn influence central respiratory center activity. As discussed in the previous chapter, vagal afferents go to the dorsal respiratory group of neurons in the medulla, as well as to the pons (probably to the apneustic center). There is not yet a consensus as to whether the pulmonary stretch receptors influence the medullary center directly or indirectly via "off-switching" neurons located elsewhere (perhaps in the apneustic center).

In 1868 Hering and Breuer demonstrated that breathing can be interrupted by increased intratracheal pressure or by tracheal occlusion at the end of a normal inspiration (blocking expiration). Increased intratracheal pressure distends the airways and increases transpulmonary pressure. Airway distention is the apparent stimulus of the Hering-Breuer reflex, which originates in slowly adapting receptors located in the bronchi and bronchioles. Bilateral vagotomy abolishes this reflex.

After discovery of the inspiroinhibitory Hering-Breuer reflex, it was proposed that V_T is controlled on a breath-by-breath basis. This concept prevailed for more than 70 years, although rhythmic breathing was observed to resume despite continued vagal stimulation. Fig. 12-3 in Chapter 12 shows the effect of vagal activity stimulated by lung inflation on the threshold required to stop inspiration. Its interrelationship with other inputs, such as tonic NPBM (nucleus parabrachealis medialis) activity, that act on the apneustic center has been demonstrated. After transection of the brainstem between the apneustic center and the medullary center, neither vagal section nor vagal stimulation affects medullary rhythmicity. On the other hand, after transecting the pons between the apneustic center and the NPBM, intermittent vagal stimulation can produce rhythmic breathing movements. After the same transection with vagi sectioned but unstimulated, apneustic breathing occurs.

Hering-Breuer receptors adapt slowly; impulses continue for a relatively long time if intratracheal pressure remains increased. Because changes of the mechanics of the lung-chest system affect the sensitivity of this reflex, factors that decrease lung compliance or increase R_{aw} sensitize these receptors. Veratrum alkaloids also increase the sensitivity of the Hering-Breuer reflex, probably by direct action on the receptors.

Species vary in the sensitivity of their Hering-Breuer reflexes; some physiologists have suggested that man has lost this reflex. However, in the study of this reflex the importance of lung geometry has been underestimated. Most studies have considered the relationship between intratracheal pressure and the ratio of breath-holding time to the breathing cycle interval. What would the *relative* species sensi-

tivity be if pressure per unit lung volume or pressure per unit cross-sectional area of the airway were plotted against the number of suppressed breathing cycles?

Paradoxic reflex of Head

If the Hering-Breuer reflex is blocked by cooling the vagus nerve to 8° C, hyperinflation of the lungs causes an additional inspiratory effort that tends to inflate the lungs further. This inspirostimulatory reflex is the opposite of the inspiroinhibitory Hering-Breuer reflex. The receptors for this reflex are in the lung parenchyma. They adapt rapidly, which means that they are mainly stimulated by rapid volume changes; they cease firing promptly after a volume change occurs. The reflex of Head may help to maintain hyperventilation that involves a large V_T, as during exercise, or it may be involved in gasping or sighing. The sensitivity of this reflex in man is not known. Sectioning the vagus nerves abolishes this reflex.

Deflation reflex

A third reflex, the deflation reflex, increases the force and frequency of inspiratory effort as the lungs are deflated by "negative" pressure or during lung collapse. This phenomenon is not the simple absence of the inspiroinhibitory Hering-Breuer reflex. The receptors for the deflation reflex, located in bronchi and bronchioles, function below 8° C, unlike those for the Hering-Breuer reflex. Vagotomy abolishes this reflex. The deflation reflex may be involved in the hyperpnea of chest compression as well as in pneumothorax. The role of the vagi in producing hyperventilation during pneumothorax remains undefined. The deflation reflex is basically nociceptive (responding to injury) and is not involved in the normal process of breathing.

Other vagal reflexes

There is a ventilatory reflex response to pulmonary embolism—a rapid, shallow breathing pattern that is abolished by vagotomy. Pulmo-

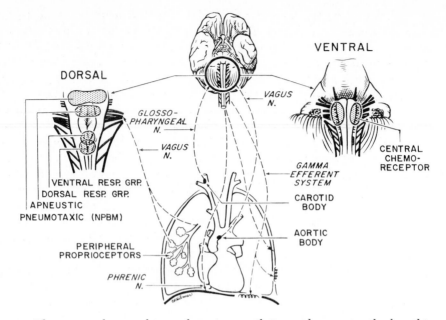

Fig. 13-3. The system that regulates pulmonary ventilation and generates the breathing pattern.

nary capillary distention stimulates juxtapulmonary capillary receptors (J receptors), which in turn produce tachypnea. The receptors have not been identified but are probably responsible for the response to pulmonary vascular congestion and perhaps for some of the pulmonary ventilatory response to exercise. Chemically stimulated receptors respond to a variety of drugs, such as serotonin and antihistamines. Irritants stimulate receptors in the lower airway, whereas mechanical stimulation of the upper airway modifies the breathing pattern. Pulmonary blood pressure changes that modify breathing when the vagus is intact are ineffective after vagotomy. Increasing inspired air P_{CO_2} decreases V_T and increases f by modifying the sensitivity of the pulmonary stretch receptors that serve the Hering-Breuer reflex.

It is not known whether the vagal reflexes are separate from each other or whether several of them involve stimulation of the same receptors. Carbon dioxide sensitization of pulmonary stretch receptors is an example of such an interrelationship. The system that regulates pulmonary ventilation and generates the breathing pattern is shown in Fig. 13-3.

OTHER FACTORS AFFECTING VENTILATION
Blood pressure

An increase of systemic arterial blood pressure causes hypoventilation, and a decrease produces hyperventilation. This reflex originates in the aortic and carotid sinus baroreceptors. At normal arterial blood pressure, tonic baroreceptor activity inhibits ventilation. Baroreceptors in the walls of the atria and great veins, sensing increased blood pressure, may stimulate breathing, an action opposite to that of the systemic (aortic and carotid) baroreceptors. The physiologic importance for respiration of the atrial baroreceptors remains unclear.

Hormones

Certain physiologic states affect breathing; some of these, such as pregnancy, involve hormonal mechanisms. Characteristic respiratory changes occur during pregnancy. Progesterone stimulates ventilation and is probably responsible for the hyperventilation associated with pregnancy. As a result of chronic hyperventilation, pregnant women have a respiratory alkalosis (arterial P_{CO_2} decreases 6 to 8 torr) that is compensated for by HCO_3^- excretion and metabolic acidosis. Indeed, the lowest arterial P_{CO_2} values in healthy, resting individuals are found in pregnant women at high altitude. Respiratory changes also occur during the luteal phase of the menstrual cycle. Arterial P_{CO_2} decreases 3 to 4 torr by the time of ovulation, a change that is also caused by progesterone. This hormone also produces hyperventilation in healthy men, causing P_{CO_2} decreases that are comparable to those observed in women.

EMOTIONS AND RESPIRATION

Asleep or awake, man's breathing reflects his emotional state. If something absorbs his interest, his breathing reflects his excitement. The anticipation of physical or sexual activity greatly increases ventilation *before* such activity begins. When he walks, runs, or climbs, breaths synchronize with steps. That various intense emotions affect breathing is a common observation. Indeed, the respiratory system is a major mode of expression for a variety of feelings. The breath-holding of temper tantrums or anger, the singing, humming, or whistling of happiness, the sighing of passion, and the sobbing and crying of sorrow or grief are only a few examples. On occasion, cough is a symptom of psychogenic origin.

At any given time the emotional state of an individual is a mixture, blend, or "paint-pot" of various feelings. Correlations with breathing are accordingly difficult. Occasionally, however, certain feelings intensify and predominate to such an extent that their relationship to breathing becomes obvious; for example, panic-level anxiety produces hyperventilation.

Depression, which usually involves guilt,

grief, and self-hatred, produces hypoventilation. Anger produces respiratory irregularities, including hyperventilation and breath-holding. Intense grief produces sighing respirations and a sensation of throat tightness or choking. Crying is a complex emotional expression, involving especially the expiratory phase of breathing.

Anxiety produces hyperventilation and increased cardiac output with relatively slight increase of O_2 uptake. Hyperventilation is of practical importance for the performance of demanding tasks; the hypocapnia and respiratory alkalosis it produces are associated with a series of physiologic responses: decreased systemic arterial blood pressure, cerebral vasoconstriction, blurred vision, dizziness, numbness and tingling, increased susceptibility to fainting, impaired psychomotor function, tetany, and carpopedal spasm that produce a performance decrement. The hyperventilation of aircraft pilots to the point of psychomotor impairment is well documented. The spirographic sign of emotional stress pattern (Fig. 17-4) involves hyperventilation and appreciable moment-to-moment variation of rate, depth, and respiratory level. Such hyperventilation is less regular than that of nonemotional origin. Hysterical hyperventilation is a syndrome of extreme hyperventilation of sudden onset and incapacitating degree that is associated with episodes of intense panic-level anxiety. Air hunger occurs in psychogenic hyperventilation despite slight hyperoxia and appreciable hypocapnic alkalosis.

The emotional factors in asthma are a frequently discussed example of psychogenic factors in respiratory disease. There is no doubt that emotionally induced hyperventilation aggravates the symptoms of any obstructive airway problem. In addition to this mechanism, airway constriction, hypersecretion, and edema may be of emotional origin in certain patients; and as if this were not sufficiently complex, intense emotion can trigger allergic phenomena, for example, hives at a funeral.

ABNORMAL BREATHING PATTERNS

A variety of abnormal breathing patterns are related to CNS changes or malfunctions that interfere with the neurogenesis of normal breathing or with the interrelationships among regions that control or affect breathing.

Vagal breathing is the slow, deep pattern observed in anesthetized animals after section of both vagus nerves. It is caused by interruption of proprioceptor afferent impulses from receptors in the lungs and chest wall, modifying the activity of the pontine apneustic center. This breathing pattern is sometimes presented as the result of interference with the Hering-Breuer reflex, but this is probably an oversimplification, since the vagi contain the afferents from many receptors. Furthermore, the concept that the Hering-Breuer reflex exerts a breath-by-breath effect on the breathing pattern is no longer widely accepted.

Apneustic breathing is characterized by sustained, cramplike, inspiratory efforts relieved irregularly by brief expirations. As previously described, this pattern is attributed to a loss of the normal inhibition of the pontine apneustic center, allowing its inspirostimulatory effect to be manifest. Apneusis is thus inspiratory apnea.

Biot's breathing is characterized by irregular periods of apnea alternating with periods in which four or five breaths of identical depth are taken. It is seen in patients who have increased intracranial pressure and is sometimes associated with midbrain lesions. A more specific description of its origin and significance is usually not attempted.

Coupled breathing, or *grouped breathing*, is a pattern in which breaths appear in pairs or triads separated by periods of apnea that last for several seconds. This pattern occurs in situations where the CO_2 level differs from the normal CO_2 threshold. Newcomers to high altitude frequently experience this pattern, accompanied by a dyspnea that is relieved only after the second deep breath. In healthy man at high altitude, breathing pure O_2 abolishes this pattern. Coupled breathing occurs spontaneously in anesthetized dogs, where anesthesia has raised the CO_2 threshold. The stimulus for this pattern of breathing is probably chemical, but the changes in sensitivity or the central changes that result in the prominence of the chemical drive are not understood.

Cheyne-Stokes breathing is a form of periodic breathing characterized by cycles of gradually increasing frequency and increasing V_T, followed by a gradual decrease in both frequency and depth of breathing—a *crescendo-decrescendo* pattern. It is usually seen in patients who have brain damage or who are terminally ill. It is also seen in infants and in some healthy people during sleep, particularly at high altitude. It occurs in patients who have increased circulation time between lungs and carotid chemoreceptors (and brain), for instance, those with cardiac insufficiency. The mechanism is related to the delay between hyperventilation-induced hypocapnia and decreased CNS drive to ventilation, as well as between hypoventilation-induced hypoxia and the ventilatory response mediated by the peripheral chemoreceptors. It is commonly seen after peripheral chemoreceptor denervation when the negative feedback system consists only of CO_2 acting through the central mechanism, which has a longer feedback delay than the peripheral chemoreceptors. When circulation time is normal and there is no apparent chemoreceptor impairment, Cheyne-Stokes breathing may result from midbrain lesions.

Hyperventilation of neural origin

Patients who have decreased lung compliance, such as those with pulmonary fibrosis, exhibit sustained hyperventilation, as evidenced by decreased arterial P_{CO_2}. They may also have moderate arterial hypoxemia but, even if that is relieved by breathing supplemental oxygen, hyperventilation continues, showing that it is not from lack of O_2. The hyperventilation probably results from vagal reflexes initiated by stimulation of the J receptors in the alveolar walls.

Persistent hyperventilation in patients who have cerebrovascular disease suggests that the process involves the pons, where the NPBM and apneustic center are located. By contrast, hemorrhage into the region of the apneustic center occasionally causes apneustic breathing (prolonged inspiratory pauses).

Fever shortens the duration of inspiration and increases f. Vagotomy does not abolish this pattern, suggesting that it involves the CNS.

Hyperventilation may be associated with body position. Tachypnea (rapid breathing) that occurs in the supine position is probably the result of hypoxemia produced by early airway closure and pulmonary congestion that stimulates the J receptors.

Hypoventilation of neural origin

Although it is most often seen in patients who have obstructive lung disease, hypoventilation occasionally occurs in subjects with healthy lungs. In such cases it may result from lesions of the medulla, infection, or cerebrovascular disease.

Narcotic addicts undergoing treatment with methadone sometimes hypoventilate. Narcotics depress sensitivity to both hypoxemia and hypercapnia; the cause is probably direct CNS depression.

The condition called "Ondine's curse" was described in Chapter 12. In this condition the patient can maintain adequate ventilation while awake but hypoventilates severely when asleep. This unusual syndrome probably results from a lesion in the respiratory motor neuron pathways from the medulla or pons. The alternate motor pathway from the forebrain is unaffected, allowing conscious control of breathing.

Seizures may produce apnea in infants. These are sometimes provoked by extreme hypoxemia and are demonstrable by electroencephalography.

CHAPTER 14

CHEMICAL REGULATION OF PULMONARY VENTILATION

CHEMICAL FACTORS AFFECTING VENTILATION

There are situations in which ventilatory drive is purely chemical; however, waking ventilation, at rest or during exercise, is almost certainly driven to some extent by nonchemical factors. Certain patterns of ventilation have no positive chemical component. Indeed, some patterns, such as maximal voluntary ventilation, have a negative chemical component (hypocapnic alkalosis).

Metabolic changes produce changes in CO_2 production, in O_2 consumption, and in the pH of body fluids. Chemical inputs affecting pulmonary ventilation are integrated with other inputs in the CNS. Because breathing is a vital function responsive to a variety of changing internal and external conditions, we are not surprised to find a complex interaction of driving factors and a complex integration of their inputs.

After artificial hyperventilation to reduce P_{CO_2} and elevate P_{O_2}, anesthetized animals undergo a period of apnea during which CO_2 rises and O_2 falls. Following voluntary hyperventilation, conscious physiologists* may wait to feel subjectively a certain level of stimulus before

---

*We have observed a tendency in our respiratory physiologist friends to use themselves as "healthy, objective subjects" in respiratory experiments when they may actually be neither healthy nor objective.

they resume breathing, demonstrating the apnea they have observed in anesthetized animals. However, conscious human subjects who do not know the purpose of this experiment resume breathing immediately without a period of apnea. Following hyperventilation, conscious human subjects exhibit a token breathing pattern of normal rhythm and frequency but ineffectual depth. Whether one does or does not experience apnea following hyperventilation probably depends on the level of excitation. Psychogenic ventilatory drive readily supercedes chemical drive in most individuals who are awake and aware.

It has long been known that both hypercapnia and hypoxia are respiratory stimulants; hypercapnia is more potent than hypoxia. In 1911 Winterstein proposed a unified concept involving the final common path of increased H^+ concentration in the cells; metabolic acids and respiratory acidosis (caused by CO_2 retention) produce H^+, whereas hypoxia favors accumulation of acids resulting from anaerobic metabolism. The discovery by Heymans in 1927 that hypoxia acts through peripheral chemoreceptors required revision of this theory, since it was known that CO_2 acts directly on the CNS. More recent evidence indicates that the increased P_{CO_2} of respiratory acidosis stimulates breathing through effects on cerebrospinal fluid, which is relatively inaccessible to the H^+ changes of metabolic acidosis. This evidence necessitated yet other changes in the theory. We still do not know whether molecular CO_2 acts independently and directly or whether its effect is mediated only via pH.

In his *multiple factor theory* of the chemical regulation of pulmonary ventilation, Gray analyzed and quantified the chemical input to the brainstem. He added the ventilatory drives from CO_2, O_2 lack, and H^+ algebraically to obtain the total chemical drive for pulmonary ventilation. In this scheme hypoxic drive may assume prominence, depressing P_{CO_2} by hyperventilation; however, CO_2 drive is not abolished and continues to exert a partial effect on ventilation.

Carbon dioxide

Increased arterial P_{CO_2} is the most potent naturally occurring stimulus to ventilation. Fig. 14-1 shows a plot of ventilation as a function of inspired CO_2 concentration. Ventilatory response increases gradually up to a CO_2 concentration of 8% to 10%, after which the increase of ventilation is nearly linear. The response flattens slightly near the peak and falls off at about 20% CO_2. The relationship between alveolar ventilation and arterial blood P_{CO_2} is lin-

ear during much of the ascending portion of the curve. The sensitivity of the ventilatory response to hypercapnia is so great that a mere 2-torr change in arterial P_{CO_2} produces a measurable effect.

Central chemoreceptor response to CO_2. In dogs and cats chemoreceptors for hypercapnia are located on the ventrolateral surfaces of the medulla near the exit of the ninth and tenth cranial nerves; these are presumed to be present also in man. Local application of H^+, CO_2, acetylcholine, or nicotine stimulates breathing within a few seconds. As an uncharged molecule, CO_2 diffuses freely from the blood across the blood-brain barrier into the cerebrospinal fluid (CSF), where it reacts with H_2O to form HCO_3^- and H^+. The H^+ thus produced stimulate the central chemoreceptors, which in turn affect the medullary respiratory center, probably the dorsal respiratory group, increasing pulmonary ventilation. This ventilatory response is characterized initially more by tidal volume increase. As CO_2 levels continue to rise, increased breathing frequency contributes to the ventilation increase.

The blood-brain barrier is relatively impermeable to H^+, HCO_3^- and other ions. As a

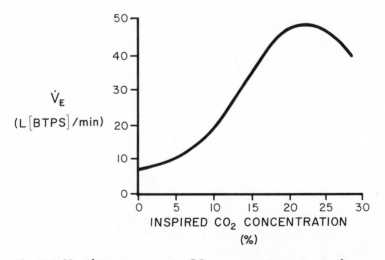

Fig. 14-1. Ventilatory response to CO_2 concentration in inspired gas.

result, a local respiratory acidosis in the central chemoreceptors is not quickly compensated and the CSF remains acidic until blood P_{CO_2} falls. Since blood P_{CO_2} is in equilibrium with CSF P_{CO_2}, increased alveolar ventilation reduces P_{CO_2} in both, returning CSF pH to normal. When *prolonged* hyperventilation lowers blood P_{CO_2}, CO_2 leaves the area of the central chemoreceptors, reducing H^+ concentration and producing a local respiratory alkalosis of the CSF. Chemoreceptor drive decreases until HCO_3^- can trickle through the blood-brain barrier from the CSF into the blood, compensating the local respiratory alkalosis of the central chemoreceptors.

The CSF pH may explain the hyperventilation or hypoventilation of patients when arterial blood analysis does not. Furthermore, the adverse effects of excessively rapid therapeutic correction of acid-base disturbance can sometimes be understood in terms of central chemoreceptor physiology.

CSF has a lower buffer capacity than blood. The buffer capacity of blood results mainly from its protein content, especially hemoglo-bin. Because CSF is low in protein, its pH changes considerably more for a given P_{CO_2} change than does blood pH. CSF contains little, if any, carbonic anhydrase. Therefore, the reactions involving CO_2, carbonic acid, HCO_3^-, and H^+ proceed slowly; there may be a considerable delay before incoming CO_2 produces appreciable quantities of H^+. Is CSF a homogeneous fluid of identical chemical composition everywhere, even at the various sites of formation?

The physiology of the medullary chemoreceptors determines the low threshold and high sensitivity of pulmonary ventilation to P_{CO_2}. Regulated pulmonary ventilation is essential for the maintenance of a proper CO_2 and pH environment for the brain. Thus, for the respiratory system, CSF is the essence of the *milieu intérieur*.

Cerebral blood flow also affects the milieu intérieur and arterial P_{CO_2} strongly affects cerebral blood flow. This effect is so profound that hypocapnea-induced vasoconstriction can cause cerebral hypoxia and deficiency of glucose and other nutrients. At an arterial P_{CO_2} of

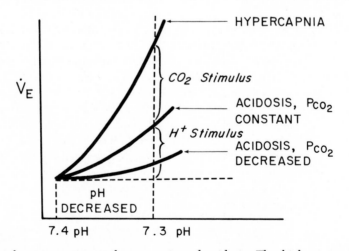

Fig. 14-2. Ventilatory response to hypercapnia and acidosis. The highest curve shows the effect of hypercapnia (increased P_{CO_2} and decreased pH). The lowest curve shows the effect of acidosis (low P_{CO_2} as a result of hyperventilation). The middle curve shows the response to acidosis alone (P_{CO_2} was kept constant by adjusting the CO_2 content of inspired gas).

about 20 torr, induced by hyperventilation, the cerebral vessels constrict maximally, affecting brain pH and P_{O_2}. Maximal vasodilation occurs at an arterial P_{CO_2} of about 120 torr.

Arterial P_{CO_2} oscillates slightly with breathing. These oscillations increase greatly during exercise, when venous-to-arterial CO_2 difference and tidal volumes are large. These oscillations affect the output of the sinus nerve, which serves the peripheral chemoreceptors. Analysis of the pattern of nerve discharge suggests that the output is related to the *rate of change*, as well as the *magnitude*, of P_{CO_2}. Larger oscillations of sinus nerve output increase ventilation for any given level of arterial P_{CO_2} in experimental animals. Such a response has not been unequivocally demonstrated in man.

Peripheral chemoreceptor response to CO_2. Arterial chemoreceptors in the angle of the bifurcation of the common carotid arteries and at the level of the aortic arch respond to hypercapnia. CO_2 stimulates the chemoreceptors when the perfusing blood has a P_{CO_2} greater than 30 torr. As P_{CO_2} rises, the frequency of nerve impulses increases. Because the sensitivity of the central mechanism is greater, peripheral chemoreceptors probably play only a minor role, estimated to be 20% to 30%, in the response to hypercapnia. Perfusion of the brain with hypercapnic blood produces a greater ventilatory response than such perfusion of the peripheral chemoreceptors. The sensitivity of the peripheral chemoreceptors for CO_2 increases during hypoxemia. Peripheral chemoreceptor response to hypoxemia is likewise affected by arterial blood P_{CO_2}. Indeed, this may be the most important physiologic effect of CO_2 on the peripheral chemoreceptors.

Hydrogen ions

Rapid intravenous injection of an acidic solution causes hyperventilation, whereas injection of dilute NaOH solution causes hypoventilation or even apnea. Hyperventilation occurs in metabolic acidosis even with the decreased arterial P_{CO_2} that partly compensates for the acidosis. Thus, increased H^+ concentration directly stimulates pulmonary ventilation.

Ventilation is considerably less sensitive to pH change than it is to P_{CO_2} change. pH must decrease by 0.05 to 0.1 unit before ventilation responds significantly. However, if arterial P_{CO_2} is held constant by adjusting inspired CO_2 concentration to prevent the hypocapnia of acid-induced hyperventilation, a greater ventilatory response is observed for a given pH change.

The relative sensitivity of ventilation to P_{CO_2} and to H^+ is shown in Fig. 14-2. The steep rise in ventilation caused by hypercapnia is a combination of the CO_2 stimulus acting primarily on central chemoreceptors and the H^+ stimulus acting primarily on peripheral chemoreceptors. The middle curve is recorded during an acidosis in which the P_{CO_2} is kept constant by adjusting inspired P_{CO_2}, and it is thus caused only by the stimulus of H^+. The lower curve represents acidosis in which the induced hyperventilation is allowed to decrease P_{CO_2}. Concomitant hypocapnia inhibits much of the response to H^+.

In an animal with denervated peripheral chemoreceptors, the injection of an acidic solution increases ventilation; thus, acidosis stimulates ventilation through some other mechanism. Since blood pH change does not easily affect the CSF surrounding the central chemoreceptors, one must consider some other mechanism, such as a nonspecific excitatory state or a specific effect on medullary respiratory center activity. Thus, acidosis probably stimulates central respiratory centers.

Lack of oxygen

Although hypoxia stimulates pulmonary ventilation, the threshold for this effect is high and unpredictable. Decreasing inspired O_2 does not reliably stimulate ventilation until O_2 concentration falls to 12%, arterial P_{O_2} falls to 50

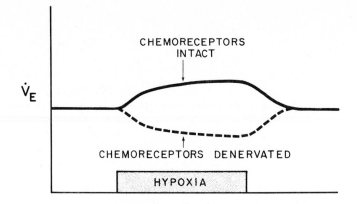

Fig. 14-3. Effect of chemoreceptor denervation on the ventilatory response to hypoxia.

or 60 torr, and oxyhemoglobin saturation falls to about 80%. The normoxic levels of healthy resting subjects acclimatized at sea level are probably not directly involved in the physiologic regulation of pulmonary ventilation.

The hyperventilation induced by hypoxia is a direct effect of decreased arterial blood P_{O_2} and only indirectly a function of decreased arterial blood O_2 content. This fact is supported by two observations: (1) at altitude, where P_{O_2} is low, hyperventilation occurs despite the normal blood O_2 content resulting from increased hemoglobin concentration; and (2) during carbon monoxide intoxication, ventilation does not increase, arterial P_{O_2} is normal, blood O_2 content is low, and O_2 availability is even less.

If P_{CO_2} is held constant by adjusting inspired CO_2 concentration, hypoxia produces a larger ventilatory response than occurs with spontaneous air breathing. This is because hypoxia-induced hyperventilation with air reduces P_{CO_2}, which in turn inhibits the ventilatory response to hypoxia.

In contrast to CO_2, which acts at several sites, hypoxia stimulates breathing only through the peripheral chemoreceptors. However, hypoxia also has a central depressant effect that tends to reduce sensitivity to itself. Thus, hypoxia stimulates ventilation if the pe-

ripheral chemoreceptors are intact, but it depresses ventilation if they are denervated (Fig. 14-3).

There is a tonic level of peripheral chemoreceptor discharge during normal spontaneous air breathing. The large P_{O_2} decrease required to raise the level of chemoreceptor discharge significantly suggests that either there are two kinds of receptors or that other factors, central or peripheral, affect the response to hypoxia. The potent CO_2 effect on ventilation complicates the interpretation of studies of hypoxia. If healthy resting subjects acclimatized at sea level breathe pure O_2, ventilation usually decreases slightly and transiently, but as P_{CO_2} increases, ventilation rises slightly above the pre–oxygen control level.

INTERACTION OF CHEMICAL FACTORS AFFECTING VENTILATION

In the course of chronic diffuse bronchopulmonary disease, arterial hypoxemia always precedes hypercapnia. Thus, hypoxemia occurs without concomitant hypercapnia, but the reverse is true only in patients with CO_2 retention who are receiving O_2 therapy. Alveolar ventilation is the most important determinant and prime regulator of arterial P_{CO_2}, whereas pulmonary blood flow is the major determinant

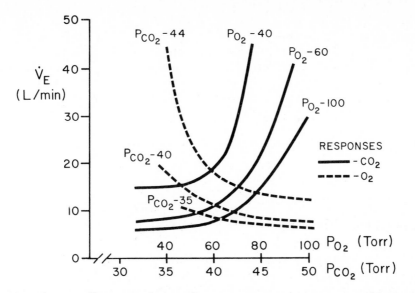

Fig. 14-4. Set of curves illustrating the ventilatory response to hypercapnia and hypoxia. The curves were constructed from published data. The solid lines represent the ventilatory response to P_{CO_2} at constant P_{O_2}. The broken lines represent the response to P_{O_2} at constant P_{CO_2}.

of arterial P_{O_2}. It follows that arterial P_{CO_2} reflects the adequacy of alveolar ventilation with more fidelity than does arterial P_{O_2}.

It may be confusing to discover that P_{CO_2} and alveolar ventilation are *directly* related in some situations but *reciprocally* related in others. However, the paradox is only apparent. Carbon dioxide is only one of several ventilatory drivers. If another drive increases alveolar ventilation, expelling CO_2 more rapidly than it is produced, arterial P_{CO_2} falls. The withdrawal of CO_2 as a ventilatory stimulus diminishes the net response to the other drive. This situation is shown in Fig. 14-2, where the non–CO_2 ventilatory driver is acidosis.

The relationship between hypercapnia and hypoxia as drivers of ventilation is complex. Some interesting observations can be made by studying Fig. 14-4, which is an idealized set of curves constructed from published data. The greater sensitivity of ventilation to CO_2 than to O_2 is evident because equivalent distances

along the horizontal axis represent a 4-torr change of P_{O_2} but only a 1-torr change of P_{CO_2}.

The relationships of pulmonary ventilation to both CO_2 and O_2 pressures are nonlinear. A P_{O_2} isopleth (line of constant P_{O_2}) indicating the CO_2 effect on ventilation reveals that when P_{CO_2} falls below the level of 35 to 38 torr, it no longer affects ventilation. Above that level pulmonary ventilation increases as P_{CO_2} increases. As P_{O_2} falls, CO_2 threshold decreases and CO_2 sensitivity increases. Thus, hypoxia shifts the curve for P_{CO_2} upward and to the left.

The relationship of ventilation to P_{O_2} is also nonlinear. A P_{O_2} decrease from 60 to 40 torr has a greater effect on the response to P_{CO_2} than a P_{O_2} decrease from 100 to 60 torr. Cross-circulation and chemoreceptor denervation studies suggest that the effect of P_{O_2} on the sensitivity of ventilation to P_{CO_2} is probably mediated through the peripheral chemoreceptors.

The ventilatory response to hypoxia when

P_{CO_2} is held constant is also nonlinear (see P_{CO_2} isopleth). Again, a strong interaction between P_{CO_2} and P_{O_2} is evident, since hypercapnia decreases the hypoxia threshold and increases the sensitivity to hypoxia. Since hypoxia depresses ventilation after denervation of the peripheral chemoreceptors, it is likely that the CO_2 effect is mediated primarily through them, although a convergence of two separate effects within the CNS is possible.

In summary, the important *interaction* between hypercapnia and hypoxia in the regulation of pulmonary ventilation should not be underestimated. During air breathing, for which the regulatory system evolved, hypercapnia is always preceded by hypoxemia. Therefore, as P_{CO_2} increases, the actual ventilatory response curve shifts upward and to the left to isopleths of progressively greater hypoxia. This suggests that hypoxia plays an important role in the physiologic regulation of ventilation, and because it affects the response to CO_2, hypoxia may also play an important role in the regulation of ventilation in patients with pulmonary insufficiency.

Breath-holding and rebreathing

Breath-holding is voluntary apnea that persists until ventilatory drive exceeds the cortical inhibition a subject will or can exert. The length of time that the breath can be held depends on P_{CO_2}, P_{O_2}, pH, lung volume, level of physical activity, prior hyperventilation, level of CO_2 acclimatization (tolerance), motivation, and self-discipline.

The study of breath-holding and rebreathing throws some light on the regulation of pulmonary ventilation. Everyone who holds his breath experiences a desire to breathe. This sensation of air hunger, having both intensity and quality, is the cortical appreciation of several factors, including the brainstem excitation that results from chemical factor input. Resumption of breathing provides prompt and total relief from this distress.

If at the breaking point of breath-holding a subject blows the gas then present in his lungs down a long tube, the gas trapped in the proximal end of this tube is alveolar gas (Haldane-Priestley alveolar gas sample). This forced expiratory alveolar gas sample is analyzed for its content of O_2 and CO_2. If a practiced breath-holder repeatedly holds his breath under the same conditions, his alveolar P_{CO_2} and P_{O_2} values are remarkably consistent at the breaking point. The values of alveolar P_{O_2} and P_{CO_2} thus obtained at the breaking point are plotted on an O_2-CO_2 diagram for graphic display and analysis (Fig. 14-5). If the subject was breathing a gas other than air, the values of P_{O_2} and P_{CO_2}, as well as their relationship, may be different at the breath-holding breaking point. If we obtain a subject's breaking-point values for each of an array of different gas mixtures, we can construct a breath-holding, breaking-point curve by joining the breaking points plotted for each mixture. When the O_2 content of the inspired gas mixture is initially high, hypoxia exerts littler influence on the breaking point and the influence of CO_2 is dominant. However, when breath-holding lowers P_{O_2} to severely hypoxic levels, the role of CO_2 in terminating breath-holding is less important. The breath-holding, breaking-point curve demonstrates a smooth transition from the extreme of almost pure hypoxia effect as the major chemical factor, ranging through synergism of hypoxia with CO_2, to the extreme of almost pure CO_2 effect as the overwhelming chemical influence on the breaking point.

During breath-holding, molecules of O_2 move from lungs to blood at a relatively constant rate that is a function of cardiac output. Lung volume decreases, passively increasing the fractional concentrations of the remaining lung gases (N_2 and CO_2). Thus, alveolar P_{CO_2} would increase even if no CO_2 were to enter the lungs from the blood.

The rate of O_2 uptake from the lungs is constant when metabolic rate is constant. If initial lung volume is low, a constant rate of O_2 uptake rapidly changes the proportion of gases re-

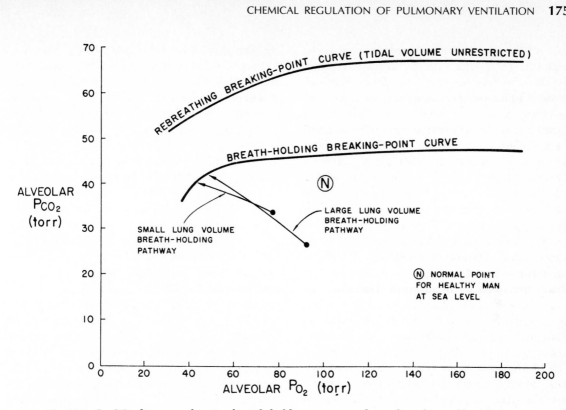

Fig. 14-5. O_2-CO_2 diagram, showing breath-holding as opposed to rebreathing of healthy man acclimatized at an altitude of 1 mile (1.6 km).

maining in the lungs, the breaking-point curve is rapidly approached, and breath-holding time is relatively short. When metabolic rate is high, the rate of O_2 uptake and CO_2 production is also high. A combination of low initial lung volume and high metabolic rate results in an even more rapid rise of alveolar P_{CO_2} and fall of alveolar P_{O_2}; the breaking-point curve is even more rapidly approached, and breath-holding time is even shorter. Prolonged breath-holding requires a combination of large initial lung volume and low metabolic rate.

Is it more comfortable to hold one's breath at a volume somewhat less than full inspiration or at the volume of maximum inspiration? If a breath-holder relaxes against a closed glottis at full inspiration, the high relaxation pressure impedes venous return to the right side of the heart, decreasing cardiac output and cerebral

blood flow. An inspiratory effort against the closed glottis facilitates venous return, increasing cardiac output and cerebral blood flow.

Brief periods of intense hyperventilation lower alveolar and arterial P_{CO_2} but only slightly affect body stores of CO_2. However, moderate hyperventilation for several minutes significantly reduces body CO_2 stores, lowering the level of the CO_2 reservoir in which metabolically produced CO_2 can accumulate during subsequent breath-holding. If a subject hyperventilates breathing O_2 immediately prior to breath-holding, the initial alveolar gas concentrations are remote from the breath-holding, breaking-point curve, and breath-holding time is correspondingly long.

Blood leaving the pulmonary capillaries returns to the left side of the heart and traverses a segment of the systemic arterial circulation before the peripheral chemoreceptors can sense its composition. This delay is usually about 5 seconds but varies slightly. Furthermore, a subject requires about a second to exhale an adequate alveolar gas sample into a Haldane sampling tube when the breath-holding breaking point is reached. Consequently, the composition of the alveolar gas analyzed for a breath-holding, breaking-point curve reflects a longer breath-holding time than the arterial blood chemical factors that are actually involved in producing a breaking point. One reason that breath-holding during exercise penetrates the resting breath-holding, breaking-point curve is that, despite decreased systemic arterial transit time, alveolar gas composition changes more rapidly. During exercise, breath-holding time may be decreased by incompletely adapted pulmonary stretch receptors.

Breath-holding breaking points are protective. Most subjects are unable to lose consciousness during either breath-holding or rebreathing; for them it is physiologically impossible and psychologically intolerable to penetrate the breaking-point curve. However, individuals who are acclimatized to high CO_2 or who have unusually powerful cortical inhibition (self-discipline or volition) can achieve unconsciousness as a result of simple breath-holding.

During tantrums small children sometimes hold their breath to unconsciousness, the cyanosis of lips and nails suggesting that hypoxemia is involved. Hypoxic unconsciousness can also cause drowning accidents among overly enthusiastic underwater swimmers. After extreme hyperventilation to supress CO_2 drive, a breath-holding Valsalva maneuver, together with an increased rate of O_2 consumption, produces unconsciousness from cerebral hypoxia before CO_2 accumulates sufficiently to reach the breaking-point curve. Such loss of consciousness differs from that caused by simple breath-holding in that it involves initial hypocapnia and an increased metabolic rate.

Holding a musical note to endurance while singing involves a breaking point. Sometimes this occurs because the singer has completely exhaled, but low-intensity note-holding when initial lung volume is high may last long enough to produce discomfort of chemical and other origin, particularly if the singer is also dancing or otherwise physically active.

Rebreathing is significantly different from breath-holding. If one rebreathes gas from a closed system, he reaches a breaking point at which further breathing from the system becomes intolerable, and he rips the apparatus from his face. If before he gasps for fresh air, the subject can be persuaded to exhale into an alveolar sampling tube, the gas can be analyzed and the results plotted on an O_2-CO_2 diagram. When rebreathing and breath-holding, breaking-point curves for the same subject are plotted on the same diagram, it is seen that rebreathing penetrates the breath-holding, breaking-point curve at all points (Fig. 14-5). Rebreathing renews vagal inhibition with each breath, whereas in breath-holding the slowly adapting pulmonary stretch receptors have adapted for many seconds and have little or no inhibition left to contribute.

Rebreathing from systems of varying volume dramatically demonstrates the effect of breath size on the inhibition deriving from pulmonary stretch receptors. As we decrease the lung volume a subject is permitted to attain, the rebreathing breaking-point curve shifts down and to the right until, if the subject is forced to breathe only in his expiratory reserve volume, alveolar P_{O_2} and P_{CO_2} at the breaking point are only slightly higher and to the left than at the starting point.

If a person takes half-sized breaths for 1 or 2 minutes from an open system in which CO_2 does not accumulate, he feels a sensation that may be termed air hunger and becomes very uncomfortable. However, if he inspires deeply, activating the slowly adapting stretch receptors, even though the inspired gas is pure nitrogen, he is suddenly and dramatically relieved.

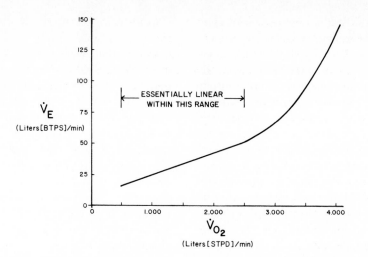

Fig. 14-6. Expiratory minute volume as a function of metabolic rate during physical exercise. Curve is constructed from published data.

HYPERPNEA OF EXERCISE

The hyperpnea of exercise has fascinated generations of physiologists. It was once thought that this hyperpnea is the result of elevated blood P_{CO_2}, since exercise generates large amounts of CO_2. We know that this hyperpnea keeps arterial P_{CO_2} at a precisely constant level over a wide range of metabolic rates. However, this linear relationship between metabolic rate and pulmonary ventilation* fails at both ends of the metabolic spectrum (Fig. 14-6). During rest and very mild exercise, pulmonary ventilation is greater than that predicted by the central linear relationship because of psychogenic ventilation. During exhausting exercise, ventilation outstrips the metabolic rate and may under these conditions actually exceed the maximal voluntary ventilation!† Note that the disporportionate increase

of pulmonary ventilation with respect to O_2 uptake begins at 2.5 L (STPD)/min. This is about 62.5% of peak O_2 uptake or slightly less than the value (70%) above which an exercising subject cannot achieve a steady physiologic state.

The precise matching of pulmonary ventilation with O_2 uptake and CO_2 production has led some to postulate the existence of hypoxia or CO_2 receptors upstream from the alveoli in the pulmonary artery, right side of the heart, or great veins. Such receptors would detect venous or mixed venous P_{CO_2} and "tell" some respiratory center how much pulmonary ventilation is necessary for homeostasis. Although postulated, such P_{CO_2} receptors have not been identified, and perfusion of upstream areas with CO_2-enriched blood does not increase pulmonary ventilation.

The precision of the relationship between metabolic rate and pulmonary ventilation also led to the notion that something senses metabolic rate and regulates ventilation to match it. Crossed perfusion experiments during which a thyromimetic drug was given indicated that ventilation responds to metabolic rate increase even when the only connection between CNS and the region of increased metabolic rate is

---

*A linear relationship also holds for metabolic rate versus heart rate.

†This apparent contradiction results from physiologic airway dilation and possibly also from reflex achievement of a better balance between breathing frequency and tidal volume during exhausting physical work. The administration of bronchodilator drugs to healthy, resting subjects also produces some airway dilation.

neural. Muscle perfusion with CO_2-enriched blood does not stimulate the "metaboreceptors"; apparently CO_2 per se is not the stimulus. There is some evidence to suggest the existence of metaboreceptors in muscle; however, such receptors have not been identified either, and other evidence is contradictory.

Passive movement of the limbs causes hyperventilation. The magnitude of this response correlates well with the number of limbs or joints involved and with the frequency of joint movements. Joint denervation abolishes this effect. As discussed in Chapter 12, certain nonrespiratory inputs increase pulmonary ventilation by altering the "local excitatory state" of the central respiratory centers. However, joint receptor activity produces a larger ventilatory response than would be expected as a nonspecific effect. Evidence suggests that joint receptors specifically stimulate pulmonary ventilation and that this effect contributes to the ventilatory response of the exercising intact animal.

Pending further evidence, it is attractive to attribute the hyperpnea of exercise to the additive effects of several inputs, including metabolic rate, limb movement, and CNS threshold changes; but, in truth, the regulation of pulmonary ventilation during muscular exercise remains a mystery.

CHAPTER 15

RESPIRATORY PHYSIOLOGY OF THE NEWBORN

One of the most fascinating achievements of the biologic world was the evolutionary transition of animal life from an aquatic to a terrestrial environment. The amphibia, able to survive in either environment, gradually became less dependent on the aquatic environment and simultaneously more dependent on the gaseous atmosphere.

In contrast to phylogenetic development, the environmental change is sudden and dramatic when a baby is born. The fetus, comfortably surrounded by and physiologically adapted to the liquid amniotic fluid, must begin to breathe air, exchanging O_2 and CO_2 with the environment. Ordinarily, no amphibious period intervenes during which placental and pulmonary gas exchange overlap. Rather, with the onset of effective air breathing, placental function normally ceases, the transition between the two conditions occurring within seconds, and the adaptation usually reaching completion within hours.

There is great variability in the degree of maturity at birth of different species. The human infant, as well as certain other vertebrates, is born relatively helpless and unprotected; others, such as the lamb and foal, can function independently at birth. The latter have well-developed coats of wool or hair, can walk, and are aware of a special relationship with their mothers. Despite such variability at birth, all mammals and most other vertebrates have fully regulated circulatory and respiratory systems. This implies a significant degree of maturity in this aspect of physiology because they must respond to widely varying metabolic demands. For example, the metabolic responses to environmental temperature changes are large and more demanding for the small, naked, newborn rat or rabbit than for the larger, well-insulated (at least when dry) newborn lamb.

The respiratory and circulatory systems are so closely interrelated that it is difficult to consider the responses of one without the other. This is particularly true for the changes that occur at birth. It is necessary to understand the fetal circulation and circulatory changes that occur at birth, as well as the physiologic factors that suppress breathing in utero but initiate it at birth, when breathing is vital for gas exchange to continue.

RESPIRATORY PIGMENTS

Joseph Barcroft, who studied fetal physiology for nearly 40 years, demonstrated that fetal hemoglobin (Hb F) has an increased affinity for O_2 and that this increase is accompanied by a decreased O_2 affinity of maternal hemoglobin. The leftward shift of the fetal oxyhemoglobin dissociation curve is caused by Hb F, described in Chapter 10. The rightward shift of the maternal oxyhemoglobin curve probably reflects metabolic acidosis and increased intraerythrocytic 2,3-diphosphoglycerate (2,3-DPG) concentration.

It has been demonstrated that adult Hemoglobin (Hb A) and Hb F have essentially the same dissociation curves after hemolysis and dialysis against the same buffer solution. The differences in the dissociation curves of maternal and fetal blood are therefore related to intracellular electrolyte concentration or to differences in the effect of 2,3-DPG on the two types of hemoglobin.

We must examine the *slope* of the oxyhemoglobin dissociation curve in the physiologically relevant range to understand how this affects the supply of O_2 to the fetus. Although umbilical arterial and venous P_{O_2} are both comparatively low, the dissociation curves in Fig.

15-1 show that both arterial and venous fetal blood contain more O_2 than maternal blood at the same P_{O_2}. Although more saturated with O_2 in the placenta, Hb F releases less O_2 to the fetal tissues (change of percent saturation) as a result of the shift of the oxyhemoglobin dissociation curve. Furthermore, increased oxyhemoglobin saturation in both arterial and venous blood reduces the amount of CO_2 transported as carbaminohemoglobin, favoring fetal acidosis. Thus, although an interesting physiologic phenomenon, the oxyhemoglobin dissociation curve shift during fetal life is less important than once thought and may actually work against the fetus. 2,3-DPG is rather ineffective in shifting the oxyhemoglobin dissociation curve of Hb F. Thus, 2,3-DPG plays little role in the transport and release of O_2 in fetal blood.

The following considerations further support this deemphasis of the importance of the shift of the oxyhemoglobin dissociation curve. The amount of material that moves across a membrane, such as O_2 moving across a placenta, depends on the rate of supply of fresh material brought to the membrane (flow dependence) as well as on the ease with which the material moves across the membrane (diffusion coefficient). Both maternal and fetal blood flow rates are high enough to ensure the fetus an adequate O_2 supply, even though oxyhemoglobin saturation is low by adult standards. The O_2 consumption of the fetal lamb does not rise when its oxyhemoglobin saturation is increased by administration of O_2 to the mother. It is of further interest that if temperature remains constant, O_2 consumption does not change after birth, despite increased P_{O_2}.

Since CO_2 diffuses easily in the tissues, transplacental P_{CO_2} and pH differences are likely to be small, and the fetus is usually neither hypercapnic nor acidotic unless the mother is. Normal acid-base values and P_{CO_2} measurements have been found in the fetal arterial blood of animals and in that of human infants during intrauterine exchange transfusions.

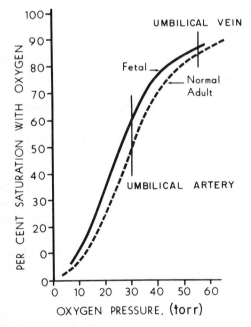

Fig. 15-1. Oxyhemoglobin dissociation curves for fetal hemoglobin (solid line) and adult hemoglobin (broken line). The curves show that fetal hemoglobin holds more O_2 but releases less to the tissues.

THE PLACENTA AND GAS EXCHANGE

Considerable heterogeneity exists between maternal and fetal blood flow in the placenta. The most efficient system for the transfer of large amounts of solute and dissolved gases, with minimal concentration gradient at the final equilibration point, would be the countercurrent system. This is present in the kidney and other organs that effectively transfer materials but is not an important placental mechanism.*

Anatomic and histologic studies suggest that maternal arteries and veins serve and are served by an *intervillous space,* in which *cross-current* flow is prominent. There is not complete agreement on this point because the pattern of maternal blood flow in the intervillous space has not yet been clearly described. The more efficient countercurrent arrangement may be unnecessary in the placenta because total equilibration may be unnecessary. It may be more efficient for the maternal blood flow to remain high so that it does not require continuous subtle regulation in response to metabolic changes of the fetus. If that is so, equilibration of gases and solutes across the placenta is unnecessary.

There is a longer diffusion path for gas transfer in the placenta than in the lung. A greater distance for diffusion reduces gas transfer and the transfer of other materials as well, but the effect is offset by a larger area for diffusion; hence, total transfer is adequate.

A relatively large P_{O_2} difference exists between maternal placental venous blood and umbilical arterial blood. There is some species difference, but it is generally agreed that a pressure difference of about 20 torr exists in

---

*Early work by prominent investigators suggested that the countercurrent mechanism was involved in the anatomic arrangement of placental blood vessels. Since 1950 histologic as well as gas-transfer studies have been interpreted to suggest that a countercurrent system is not a prominent factor in the exchange of materials across the placenta.

man. Since countercurrent flow is not important for placental gas exchange, it is likely that total equilibration is not achieved during a single passage of blood through the placenta. There is also increased likelihood of uneven perfusion/perfusion ratio (analogous to the $\dot{V}/\dot{Q}$ ratio in the lung), which would contribute to a reduced P_{O_2} in umbilical arterial blood even if equilibration were achieved in each capillary.

Placental O_2 consumption also could contribute to a reduced umbilical arterial P_{O_2}. Such an effect has been demonstrated experimentally and accounts for a significant part of the P_{O_2} difference. Placental O_2 consumption, together with the shape of the oxyhemoglobin dissociation curve, can explain the observation that a large increase of maternal P_{O_2} (from breathing pure O_2) results in only a modest increase of umbilical arterial P_{O_2}. It also helps to explain the relatively small decrease of fetal P_{O_2} during maternal hypoxemia.

PERINATAL CIRCULATION

Normal fetal development depends on the placenta as the organ for gas exchange, a function that is transferred to the lungs at birth. The dramatic circulatory changes that occur at birth are matched at no other time in life. Contrary to earlier belief, the transition from fetal to adult circulation is gradual rather than abrupt, requiring hours to days.

In the fetus, the right and left sides of the heart pump blood in parallel from the vena cavae to the aorta. Since resistance to blood flow in the pulmonary circulation is high and the ductus arteriosus is a bypass, most of the output of the right side of the heart shunts directly to the aorta instead of unnecessarily burdening the left side of the heart, which already receives venous blood through the open foramen ovale.

The pattern of circulation through the fetal heart is shown in Fig. 15-2. The most oxygenated stream of blood in the fetal circulation

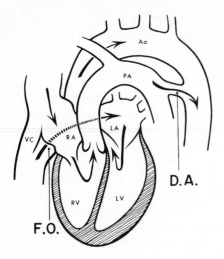

Fig. 15-2. Pattern of circulation in the fetal heart, showing the preferential shunting of blood from the placenta through the foramen ovale *(F.O.)* and the shunting of blood through the ductus arteriosus *(D.A.)*, bypassing the pulmonary circulation.

comes from the placenta and lower part of the body. This comprises about 75% of the venous return. About 85% of the total venous return shunts preferentially through the foramen ovale into the left atrium. The concept of a streaming pattern of blood flow through the right atrium derives from comparison of the O_2 content of blood in the carotid artery with that in the descending aorta; blood in the carotid artery has the composition of left ventricular blood (62% saturated with O_2), whereas that in the descending aorta (58% saturated with O_2) is a mixture of blood from the left ventricle with that shunted through the ductus arteriosus from the right ventricle. This circulatory pattern preferentially perfuses the brain, heart, and liver with blood of the highest systemic O_2 content.

This pattern of blood flow must change quickly at birth to that of the adult system, in which the two sides of the heart work in series,

with the lungs in the circuit between the right and left sides.

This profound transition requires regulation of the pulmonary circulation, with suitable response to neural and/or chemical stimuli. Such a concept is accepted for the adult pulmonary circulation and is also true for the pulmonary circulation of the fetus and newborn.

The response of the pulmonary circulation to hypoxia in both adult and fetus is an increase of pulmonary arterial pressure, resulting from pulmonary artery constriction. The response occurs even in isolated perfused lungs, indicating that it is a local response to reduced P_{O_2}. In fetal lambs pulmonary artery pressure is higher than aortic pressure, with most of the right ventricular output flowing through the ductus arteriosus to the aorta.

At birth, blood ceases to flow through the placenta, a large peripheral vascular bed that had received more than one half of the cardiac output, and arterial pressure increases. High left ventricular pressure increases left atrial pressure. Simultaneous lung inflation reduces pulmonary vascular resistance, decreasing right ventricular pressure and, secondarily, right atrial pressure. The left-right atrial pressure difference closes the foramen ovale in the interatrial septum. Since this pressure difference is small, some right-to-left shunt may persist for 24 hours or longer.

Inflation of the lungs at birth decreases pulmonary vascular resistance, as already indicated. Although some of the decrease results from lung expansion, which pulls vessels open by stretching the lung parenchyma, an important contribution is the relief of hypoxia-induced vasoconstriction.

Pulmonary artery pressure is high at birth, relative to the normal postadjustment value. In fact, pulmonary artery pressure at birth is not much below aortic pressure and decreases only gradually. We should not be surprised at this; a sudden fall in pulmonary vascular resistance would reverse the flow of blood through the ductus arteriosus before its lumen closes, resulting in a great imbalance of outputs from right and left ventricles.

Closure of the ductus arteriosus eliminates the circulatory shunt that bypasses the pulmonary circulation from pulmonary artery to aorta; hence, all venous blood flows through the lungs after birth. For some time after birth hypoxemia can reestablish a fetal pattern of circulation. This difference in reactivity of the ductus arteriosus and pulmonary arteries assists the hypoxic fetus by increasing effective cardiac output, but this difference is a liability to the hypoxic newborn infant because it increases ductal right-to-left shunt and further decreases O_2 uptake.

The umbilical vein joins the portal vein and forms the ductus venosus just below the liver. It runs forward (around and through the liver) to the junction of the hepatic veins with the inferior vena cava and thereby permits more than 10% of the umbilical venous blood to bypass the liver. This vein is probably not of great physiologic importance, at least near term, since it has already disappeared in some animals prior to an equivalent stage of fetal development. The ductus venosus closes off at birth, although there is still no agreement on the mechanism of closure. Consequences of delayed or incomplete closure are not clear, although it eliminates a potential shunt (around the liver) from the portal vein to the inferior vena cava.

PRENATAL RESPIRATORY EFFORTS

Since Vesalius, who first described rhythmic breathing movements of the fetus, further observation has revealed that the normal fetus, at least near term, rarely makes respiratory movements unless subjected to asphyxia. The rapidity of such movements (40 to 80 per minute) when they do occur probably precludes much fluid movement through the small airways. Be-

cause of the relatively solid lung and soft chest wall, diaphragmatic gasps would suck little fluid into the lung but instead would probably collapse the chest. However, suspensions of radiopaque thorium oxide or india ink injected into the amniotic sac gain access to the fetal lung, indicating that aspiration can occur.

Consideration of prenatal lung movements brings to mind the presence of fluid in the air spaces, its source during fetal life, and its fate at birth. How does the presence of this fluid affect the expansion of the lungs at birth and the ease with which the lungs can begin their gas-exchange function? Early work suggested that the lung fluid derived from aspirated amniotic fluid and that its occurrence was a dangerous complication of birth. However, recent work indicates that the presence of this fluid is a normal condition and that the lung itself is the source of the fluid during the last half of gestation. For example, analysis of blood, tracheal fluid, and amniotic fluid after injection of radioisotopes into fetal blood suggests that the lung fluid comes from the fetus, not from the amniotic sac. Tracheal fluid, with its higher Cl^- and H^+ concentrations but lower protein and CO_2 levels than amniotic fluid, probably does not originate from the fluid surrounding the fetus. Rather, the lung fluid is an ultrafiltrate of blood plasma modified by subsequent selective reabsorption of some materials.

Surfactant is a phospholipid produced by pulmonary alveolar cells called *pneumonocytes*. It is not found until after lamellar inclusion bodies appear in the alveolar cells. Normal surface tension is found in extracts of the lungs of fetuses as small as 200 gm. Surfactant is ordinarily present by the 23rd week of human gestation; the rate of phospholipid synthesis increases with gestational age. Full development of biosynthetic pathways is achieved sometime during the third trimester of pregnancy. There is considerable variability in the capacity of surfactant to lower surface tension in the fetus. Its *presence* by 23 weeks does not mean that it can form an effective lining layer. On the other hand, some infants who are premature by many weeks and who weigh as little as 675 to 900 gm have enough surfactant for effective lung function.

In those infants born with an adequate surfactant supply, the rate of secretion increases after birth with the onset of breathing. As air replaces the fluid that filled the airways and alveolar spaces, surfactant is incorporated into the lining layer of the alveoli and small airways.

STIMULUS FOR THE FIRST BREATH

Near term the fetal animal responds poorly to the chemical stimuli of acidosis, hypercapnia, and hypoxemia; however, younger fetuses respond to hypoxia with intrauterine gasps. Functional carotid chemoreceptors are present in the fetus, but for unknown reasons they are not generally active. However, it has been shown repeatedly that infants are responsive to chemical respiratory stimulants immediately after birth. It is not clear as to why there is a sudden and profound change in the breathing control system at birth. The barrage of input signals faced by the newborn infant makes it difficult to sort out the fundamental stimulus or stimuli responsible for the initiation of breathing and which stimuli change the thresholds for the usual regulators of ventilation. However, research has provided some information regarding the onset of breathing.

Although a degree of asphyxia usually precedes the first breath, neither hypoxemia nor hypercapnia is the primary stimulus for the first breath. Arterial P_{O_2} may be as low as 25 to 30 torr and P_{CO_2} may be as high as 45 torr without stimulating fetal breathing. Breathing is stimulated by umbilical cord occlusion in the absence of other stimuli, but a minute or so of occlusion is required, resulting in more severe asphyxia than normally occurs. Furthermore, these conditions do not duplicate the environ-

ment at birth, when (along with an ordinarily mild degree of asphyxia, if it occurs) there is thermal insult, tactile stimuli caused by squeezing and handling, and a barrage of new light, sound, and postural stimuli. Studies of peripheral chemoreceptor sensitivity show that the fetus has a markedly attenuated response to hypoxia and hypercapnia, as judged by afferent activity of the carotid nerves arising in the region of the chemoreceptors. Interestingly, the effect of hypoxia on the response to hypercapnia is opposite in premature infants and those born at term. Hypoxia potentiates the response to hypercapnia in term infants but reduces the sensitivity of the ventilatory system to hypercapnia in preterm infants. This may indicate that peripheral chemoreceptors have a reduced effect in the fetus and that in the fetus the effect of hypoxia is only one of CNS depression, depressing the response to the stimulus of hypercapnia.

The responsiveness of the peripheral chemoreceptors to both hypoxemia and hypercapnia changes after birth and the onset of breathing. This threshold change may relate to an increased level of general autonomic nervous system discharge. This may be a direct effect or the result of local catecholamine release.

Tactile or painful stimuli do not produce fetal breathing efforts. Furthermore, when painful stimuli do produce breathing efforts, such efforts are limited to gasps if other stimuli are excluded. Rhythmic, sustained breathing is not established by tactile stimuli alone; as soon as the stimulation ceases, the fetus stops all breathing and gasping movements. However, these stimuli do stimulate breathing in the newborn after ventilation is established and P_{O_2} rises.

Application of cold to the skin is a recognized stimulus to breathing in both adults and infants. Cooling a fetus after surgical removal from the uterus, with the umbilical cord intact and the placenta functional, stimulates breathing. However, it is necessary to cool the body temperature by 3° to 4° C before breathing starts, and this is preceded by shivering in the normal fetus. At or near term, such cooling initiates rhythmic breathing, but the required temperature change is much greater in the fetus than in the infant. Perhaps the threshold decreases at birth by the mechanism proposed for the change of peripheral chemoreceptor sensitivity (increase of general autonomic activity after the onset of breathing).

THE START OF BREATHING

With proper obstetric management most healthy infants begin to breathe within seconds after birth, even before separation from the placenta. This was not the case when heavy maternal sedation and general anesthesia were widely used, causing serious depression of the infant and often requiring vigorous stimulation to start breathing.

The chest wall recoils elastically as the infant emerges from the birth canal, drawing 10 to 40 ml of air into the lungs to replace the fluid squeezed from the air passages during delivery. The glossopharyngeal musculature of some infants forces 5 to 10 ml of air into the trachea by means of "frog-breathing." Neither action is essential for the first breath, however, since babies delivered by cesarean section or those in whom a pharyngeal airway is inserted at birth expand their airways uneventfully.

We will introduce our discussion of the mechanical factors associated with the initiation of breathing with a description of the relationship between pressure change and volume change in the thorax, as shown in Fig. 15-3. Intrapleural pressure is atmospheric before the first breath inflates the lungs. This fact, of considerable functional significance, indicates that the chest does not recoil outward until after birth. If the fetal chest recoiled outward, as it does in extrauterine life, one of two conditions would result:

1. The opposing recoil of the fluid-filled fetal lung would be small because of the lack of sur-

face tension normally provided by an air-liquid interface. The two sets of opposing forces would balance at a large lung volume, and the lungs would then contain a larger fluid volume at birth (particularly with cesarean section); rapid initiation of effective breathing would require a different mechanism.

2. If the lung did not follow the chest wall, intrapleural pressure would decrease and liquid would fill the pleural space. This would interfere with expansion of the lungs at birth.

The mechanism of the permanent increase of chest volume that results from the first breath is not understood. It is described as a "plastic-like" phenomenon. Whatever its cause, this expansion sets up the opposing forces between lung and chest wall that produce and maintain a "negative" intrapleural pressure after breathing starts.

During the first breath (Fig. 15-3), intrapleural pressure falls to about -40 cm H_2O, with little volume change during the first 0.5 second or so; the subsequent sudden inflow of air is associated with very little further change of pressure. During expiration, pressure first decreases considerably, after which there is a

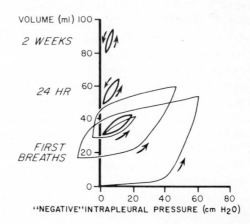

Fig. 15-3. Pressure-volume curves for the initial breaths of a newborn infant. Functional residual capacity and compliance change during the first weeks of life.

rather sudden terminal volume decrease. The lungs do not empty completely during this expiration, thus establishing about one half of the neonatal residual volume with the first breath. Subsequent breaths stabilize a rather constant volume-pressure relationship over the next several hours at a compliance (ease of filling) of 4 to 5 times that at birth and at a flow resistance of one quarter to one half that of the first few breaths. Airway resistance (R_{aw}) decreases because of clearance of fluid from the airways and the progressively more "negative" end-expiratory intrapleural pressure. As functional residual capacity increases, small airways expand.

Since resistance to gas flow through the airways depends on radius, length, and the number of passages, R_{aw} is predictably greater for infants than for adults. If lung dimensions were strictly proportional to body mass, the radius of infant airways would be one twentieth that of adults; the resulting extreme R_{aw} would throttle pulmonary ventilation, since resistance to laminar flow varies inversely as the fourth power of tube radius. It is estimated that the radius of infant alveoli is about one half that of adults and that the terminal bronchioles are about three fourths of adult size. Infant R_{aw} is about 25 to 30 cm $H_2O \times$ liter$^{-1} \times$ second^{-1}, as compared with about 2 cm $H_2O \times$ liter^{-1} $\times$ second^{-1} for healthy adults. Total pulmonary ventilation of infants is about 560 ml/min, as compared with 8 L/min for adults. Thus, total ventilation is 14 times greater in the adult, whereas R_{aw} is about one fourteenth. However, the relationship between R_{aw} and pulmonary ventilation is similar for adults and infants after the first few breaths.

During the first breath, movement of fluid in the airways creates a viscous resistance that contributes considerably to the pressure required to expand the lungs. For example, the viscous resistance to the movement of amniotic fluid in the airways of a guinea pig is 58 cm H_2O at a flow rate of 0.7 ml/sec.

Surface tension forces of the alveolar lining fluid are of great physiologic importance. Pulmonary surfactant affects the ease of breathing, the evenness of ventilation, and the efficiency of gas exchange. These concepts are described in detail in Chapter 6. Because of their importance for neonatal physiology, the reader may wish to review them in connection with this chapter.

REGULATION OF BREATHING IN THE INFANT

It was pointed out in the last section that the threshold for many respiratory stimulants decreases dramatically after breathing is initiated at birth. Regulation of breathing patterns and ventilation are surprisingly similar in the newborn infant and adult.

Measurement of an infant's response to hypoxia is complicated by the influence of other variables, such as pH, P_{CO_2}, and sensory inputs. However, a ventilatory response to hypoxia is seen even during the first day of life. Tonic chemoreceptor activity is transiently decreased by the administration of pure O_2, indicating that the chemoreceptors are still being stimulated by hypoxemia.

There is increasing reason to believe that the sensitivity of the newborn infant to CO_2 is comparable to that of the adult, but it is difficult to compare the ventilatory responses meaningfully. Is it more valid to compare the ventilatory response of infants with that of adults in terms of body weight or on the basis of body surface area? Apparent differences may result from such a choice.

As in the adult, decreased arterial blood pH in the infant is a stimulus to pulmonary ventilation that is independent of CO_2. Thus, metabolic acidosis increases ventilation even in the presence of decreased arterial P_{CO_2}. Temperature also has an important effect on the pulmonary ventilation of infants; ventilation increases in response to modest cooling. More importantly, the sensitivity to hypercapnia decreases greatly during mild hypothermia.

The few studies that have been done with human infants indicate that neurogenic reflexes are active in the newborn. The neural pattern is presumed to be the same as that of adults. Pulmonary stretch receptors are responsive in the fetus; the afferent impulses travel in the vagus nerve. These receptors inhibit the inspiratory activity of the medullary center (Hering-Breuer reflex) presumably by modifying the tonic effect of pontine centers on the medulla.

The paradoxic reflex of Head is an inspiratory gasp in response to a sudden increase of intratracheal pressure that distends the airway or inflates the lung; it is observed in the adult as well as in the newborn human infant. The afferent pathway of this reflex is in the vagus nerve. Except during "frog-breathing" and vigorous crying, the functional significance of this reflex in the infant is unknown.

Subthreshold stimuli establish a "local excitatory state" in the medullary center that is a prerequisite for rhythmic breathing. Both higher and lower nonrespiratory CNS mechanisms are involved. Perhaps the lower threshold of the chemoreceptors and the response to cold, tactile, and pain stimuli in the newborn infant as compared to the fetus, along with the establishment of rhythmicity in the medullary respiratory center, have a common basis in the afferent activity of the autonomic nervous system and the stimulation of sensory receptors in the birth experience. We are just beginning to appreciate the importance of the activity of these systems in establishing and maintaining respiration.

RESPIRATORY DISTRESS SYNDROME

To see the respiratory distress syndrome of the newborn (RDS) is an unforgettable lesson in pulmonary physiology. It occurs in a premature baby, often after a complicated delivery, in which there was a period of asphyxia followed by resuscitation. During the next several hours breathing becomes progressively more labored, and there is retraction of the lower ribs and sternum on inspiration. Breathing frequency increases, sometimes to 120 breaths/min, and tidal volume is small. Cyanosis develops, and the need for O_2 therapy and ventilatory assistance is apparent. The infant appears exhausted, becomes flaccid and unresponsive, and exhibits periods of apnea that increase in frequency and duration. Death often occurs on the first or second day, despite vigorous medical treatment.

RDS is responsible for more pediatric deaths than any other disease. Substantial progress has been made in the treatment of RDS, reducing mortality from more than 80% to a general average of less than 20% and in certain centers less than 10%.

Although much has been learned about this syndrome, our understanding of its pathogenesis remains incomplete. We still cannot clearly distinguish cause from effect. However, the clinical manifestations of RDS are well established and include the following:

1. *Labored breathing.* Surfactant deficiency increases surface tension within the alveoli; hence, a greater transpulmonary pressure is required to inflate the lung. Fig. 15-4 shows an idealized graph of surface tension as a function of area for an extract of normal infant lung compared to that of a lung extract from an infant who died of RDS. Surface tension decreases only slightly as the area of the extract from the abnormal lung decreases. Surfactant system

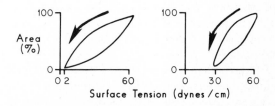

Fig. 15-4. Surface tension as a function of area for surfactant-containing lung extract (left) and surfactant-deficient lung extract (right).

failure decreases compliance, increases work of breathing, causes alveolar hypoventilation, and disrupts ventilation-perfusion relationships.

2. *Impaired gas exchange.* High, unchanging alveolar surface tension produces patchy atelectasis, aggravating alveolar hypoventilation and ventilation-perfusion mismatching. Without surfactant, small alveoli cannot remain open at the relatively low transpulmonary pressures that open and maintain larger alveoli. Hence, small alveoli collapse, shunting blood through lung regions in which gas exchange does not occur. This shuntlike or venous admixture–like effect contributes to arterial hypoxemia, CO_2 retention, and respiratory acidosis.

3. *Increased pulmonary vascular resistance.* Pulmonary vascular resistance increases greatly, presumably as a result of precapillary arteriolar constriction. Increased resistance shunts additional blood through the ductus arteriosus, further aggravating arterial hypoxemia and respiratory acidosis. Systemic hypoperfusion causes tissue hypoxia and metabolic acidosis, complicating the problem even more.

4. *Hyaline membrane formation.* The decreasing size of the collapsing alveoli and increasing surface tension caused by surfactant deficiency unbalance the opposing forces that normally govern the flow of fluid across the alveolocapillary membrane. The high surface tension of the alveolar lining fluid increases the force that drives fluid from capillaries into alveoli, and a plasma ultrafiltrate accumulates. As this ultrafiltrate fills the alveoli, the radius of curvature of the gas-liquid interface shrinks and surface tension becomes even greater (Laplace's law), drawing more fluid into the alveoli.

A specimen of such lung tissue fixed and stained for examination by light microscopy reveals a glassy, pale blue–staining membrane lining the alveoli, hence the term *hyaline mem-*

brane. It was originally believed that the hyaline membrane results from aspiration of amniotic fluid and that the membrane causes the disease.

The primary inciting cause of RDS remains unknown. It usually occurs in premature infants or in infants whose condition is conducive to surfactant destruction (for example, asphyxia during difficult delivery), which has persuaded some scientists that surfactant deficiency is the primary insult. Because surface tension effects increase as the patient's clinical condition deteriorates, other scientists believe that pulmonary ischemia is the initial event. According to this theory, blood coagulation disturbance, autonomic imbalance, persistent patent ductus arteriosus, and/or a vasoactive substance that produces profound pulmonary vascular constriction are the primary causes of the syndrome.

Fortunately, whatever the initiating factor, the treatment of RDS is the same, including all supportive measures required for any premature infant. Normal body temperature is carefully maintained lest metabolic rate and O_2 consumption increase. Oxygen therapy is usually necessary but should be used with caution to avoid O_2 intoxication, which itself destroys surfactant. No level of hyperoxia is both safe and adequate; hence, some compromise is usually necessary. An arterial P_{O_2} of from 50 to 65 or 70 torr, monitored by means of an indwelling umbilical artery catheter, is adequate. Metabolic acidosis is usually treated with infusions of sodium bicarbonate solution, and hypovolemia by transfusions of packed red blood cells. Arterial blood gases and systemic arterial blood pressure are usually monitored through an umbilical artery catheter. Positive end-expiratory pressure (PEEP) may be necessary to prevent lung collapse and improve alveolar ventilation. If respiratory acidosis or apnea develops, mechanically assisted ventilation is required until the patient improves.

CHAPTER 16

RESPIRATORY PHYSIOLOGY IN UNUSUAL ATMOSPHERES AND ENVIRONMENTS

HYPOVENTILATION AND ASPHYXIA

Mammals evolved from life forms that lived at sea level. Survival included the avoidance of asphyxia. These animals survived partly because they developed chemoreceptors that, when excited, increased breathing. Increased CO_2 and decreased O_2 usually occur together and elicit the same qualitative, but not necessarily the same quantitative, responses (Fig. 16-1). Both increase pulmonary ventilation and cerebral blood flow, but CO_2 is more effective. Both increase coronary blood flow, although hypoxia is more potent in this regard. Both cause airway constriction, and both lower body temperature.

Asphyxia can be produced in various degrees by breath-holding, rebreathing from a closed system or in a closed space, breathing through a tube that artificially increases dead space, chest-binding or otherwise limiting tidal volume, interposing an obstruction to breathing, creating a large pneumothorax, opening the chest cavity so that breathing efforts are ineffective, or paralyzing the respiratory neuromuscular apparatus.

Asphyxia, or suffocation, still occurs today in certain situations—infants trapped in bedclothing in their beds or with plastic films over the face that act as one-way respiratory valves, children closed in empty refrigerators, men trapped in ditch cave-ins or avalanches, and strangulation from aspiration of food or from criminal assault.

Hypoxia

The term *anoxia* means no oxygen; *hypoxia* means less than normal oxygen pressure. Anoxia has frequently been used to describe situations that are hypoxic, not anoxic.

Hypoxia may be defined as either insufficient P_{O_2} or insufficient concentration of free O_2 molecules to meet the requirements of aerobic metabolism. *Hypoxemia* means an arterial blood P_{O_2} that is less than the normal value of 100 $\pm$ 10 torr for a healthy resting person at sea level. Arterial P_{O_2} decreases with age and is less at higher altitudes. *Histohypoxia* means a reduced P_{O_2} at the cell level. The function of intracellular enzymes can be impaired in the presence of normal P_{O_2}, or such impairment may even be the result of excessive P_{O_2}, as shown by studies of hyperbaric oxygenation. Thus, a term is needed to indicate all conditions involving impairment of aerobic metabolism. Strughold has suggested the term *hypoxidosis* for this purpose. Hypoxidosis includes (1) hypoxia, (2) lack or dysfunction of intracellular enzymes, (3) lack of energy sources or substrate, and (4) excessive accumulation of metabolites.

Classification of hypoxia. There are four general types of hypoxia, classified in terms of the

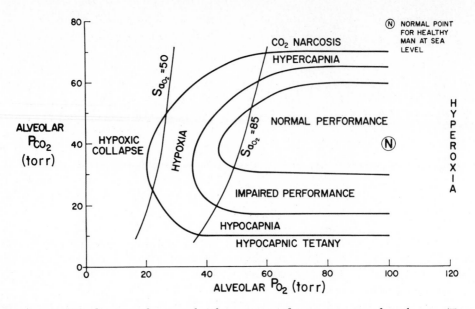

Fig. 16-1. O_2-CO_2 diagram, showing alveolar patterns of respiratory gas disturbance. (From Rahn, H., and Fenn, W. O.: A graphical analysis of the respiratory gas exchange, Washington, D.C., 1955, The American Physiological Society.)

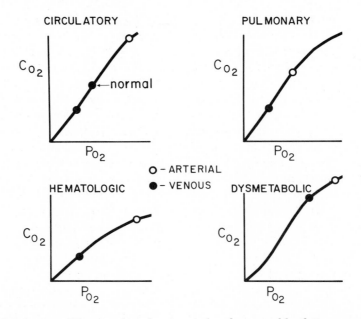

Fig. 16-2. Classification of hypoxia based on arterial and venous blood O_2 content and pressure.

nature of the defect in oxygen supply. These can be identified by blood-gas measurements in arterial and venous samples, as indicated in Fig. 16-2, which shows the relationship between oxygen content and pressure in arterial and venous blood for the four types of hypoxia.

1. *Circulatory hypoxia* (also called *stagnant hypoxia*). This form of hypoxia results from reduced blood flow to the tissues with respect to oxygen need. It may be generalized if cardiac output is low or limited to one region if it results from embolism, atherosclerosis, or blood pooling. It results from *relative* inadequacy of blood flow because of increased tissue-oxygen utilization. An example of this is the hypoxia that occurs during severe muscular exercise. This type of hypoxia causes histohypoxia even when arterial blood is adequately oxygenated.

In circulatory hypoxia arterial blood P_{O_2} and oxygen content are normal, whereas the venous blood has a low P_{O_2} and O_2 content. Thus, arteriovenous blood oxygen difference is increased. The capacity of arterial blood for oxygen is normal in circulatory hypoxia.

2. *Pulmonary hypoxia* (also called *hypoxic hypoxia*). In this type of hypoxia arterial and venous oxygen pressures and contents are low. The arteriovenous oxygen difference is normal or slightly decreased because of increased cardiac output resulting from mild hypoxemia. Blood oxygen capacity is normal; hence, oxyhemoglobin saturation is reduced. This type of hypoxia results from hypoventilation, a decrease of pulmonary diffusing capacity from any cause, right-to-left circulatory shunt, or decreased oxygen pressure in the inspired air. The decreased P_{O_2} may be a result of high altitude, where the barometric pressure is low, or it may be the result of reduced oxygen concentration in the inspired air, as in asphyxia. This is the only form of hypoxia in which insult to the bronchopulmonary system is the primary cause.

3. *Hematologic hypoxia* (also called *anemic hypoxia*). When the P_{O_2} of arterial blood is high but its oxygen content is low, the result is called hematologic hypoxia. The O_2 content of venous blood is proportionately reduced and the arteriovenous blood oxygen (oxygen content) difference is normal. Arteriovenous P_{O_2} difference is increased because arterial blood P_{O_2} is normal and the P_{O_2} of venous blood is low as a result of its low oxygen content. Hematologic hypoxia occurs in (1) anemia, where total hemoglobin concentration is low; (2) carbon monoxide poisoning, where hemoglobin concentration is normal but unavailable for combination with oxygen because of competition by carbon monoxide; and (3) hemoglobin alterations that interfere with the oxygenation of hemoglobin, such as methemoglobinemia. In the latter two cases, it is necessary to recognize the difference between the total hemoglobin present in the blood and the total hemoglobin available for combination with oxygen.

4. *Dysmetabolic hypoxia* (also called *histotoxic hypoxia*). If the cells are unable to utilize oxygen as a result of metabolic derangement, as in cyanide poisoning, arterial blood P_{O_2}, O_2 content, and oxyhemoglobin saturation are increased. There is also high venous P_{O_2} and oxygen content because of the inability of tissues to extract oxygen from the blood. Thus, the arteriovenous blood O_2 difference is low. Dysmetabolic hypoxia is another example of histohypoxia in which arterial blood oxygen is normal.

Aerobic metabolism may be slowed in response to reduced energy requirements, although transport and utilization potentials for O_2 are normal. This type of hypometabolism is termed *hypoxidation* and includes the following: (1) hypothermia, (2) hibernation, (3) the effects of depressant drugs or anesthetics, and (4) hypothyroidism.

Increased tissue O_2 consumption does not produce hypoxia unless capillary blood flow to the metabolizing tissue fails to match the increased requirements. When this happens, the primary site of hypoxia may be considered to be in the capillary; this is an example of circulatory hypoxia. *Inadequate* capillary blood flow is then more descriptive than *decreased* capillary blood flow.

Effects of hypoxia. The response to hypoxia depends on the rapidity of onset and the severity of the hypoxia. The symptoms of acute hypoxia resemble those of alcohol intoxication, whereas chronic hypoxia produces symptoms that resemble fatigue. The symptoms are unrelated to the type of hypoxia; it is the level of histohypoxia that is important.

Fulminating hypoxia results from the sudden removal of oxygen from the inspired air. It occurs during explosive decompression, for example, sudden loss of cabin pressure in an airplane flying at 20,000 feet (6,100 M) altitude. It produces rapid loss of consciousness and collapse. Respiratory and cardiovascular systems are stimulated initially, but as hypoxia becomes more severe and the tissues lose or metabolize their oxygen, the respiratory and cardiovascular systems are depressed. There is a precipitous fall in blood pressure, heart rate, and cardiac output. Breathing ceases shortly before cardiac arrest.

Acute hypoxia results from a relatively rapid decrease in oxygen availability. The change is more abrupt than can be accommodated by physiologic adaptations to hypoxia; an example is an ascent to high altitude. Symptoms of acute hypoxia result from a descending depression of the central nervous system. As hypoxia becomes more severe, there is depression of cortical activity followed by depression of lower centers. Cortical depression gives a false sense of well-being, loss of judgment, unstable emotions, and memory loss. One of the early consequences of hypoxia is a reduction in the acuity of night vision, resulting from inadequate regeneration of visual purple, a pigment in the retinal rods required for sensing low-intensity light. Progressive acute hypoxia leads to muscular incoordination, nausea, vomiting, and convulsions, which occur just before loss of

consciousness. Late in the progression of acute hypoxia, there is usually increased ventilation, heart rate, and blood pressure, but these responses are unpredictable and may not occur.

Chronic hypoxia is long-term exposure to low levels of oxygen. It can result from residing at high altitude or from a chronic lung disease that causes hypoxemia. Compensatory mechanisms usually ameliorate the symptoms of chronic hypoxia; however, there is always a loss of physiologic reserve for physical activity.

Chronic alveolar hypoventilation

Hypoventilation is an important pathophysiologic aspect of certain clinical entities. The term *chronic alveolar hypoventilation* is used to describe this problem, which is an example of pulmonary hypoxia. As already implied, hypoventilation produces both hypoxemia and CO_2 retention. These blood-gas disturbances, if present for months to years, can result in a chain of serious consequences: respiratory acidosis, pulmonary arterial hypertension, and polycythemia. Hypercapnia produces somnolence. Polycythemia increases blood viscosity. Increased blood viscosity combined with increased pulmonary arterial pressure increases the work of the right ventricle, leading to hypertrophy and eventual insufficiency.

Patients with extreme obesity may exhibit this chain of consequences. The symptoms of the fat boy were well described by Dickens and have been termed a "pickwickian syndrome." Another clinical example of chronic alveolar hypoventilation is kyphoscoliosis, in which thoracic deformity prevents adequate pulmonary ventilation.

Snorkel breathing

A snorkel (from German, "little snout") is a tube, or pair of tubes, housing air intake and exhaust pipes that can be extended above the surface of the water for operating submerged craft. The term also refers to a plastic breathing tube with a mouthpiece at one end and a valve at the other that admits air when projected above water but closes when submerged. It is used for swimming near the surface with the head underwater.

What is the maximum length of a snorkel tube through which a person can breathe? Several physiologic considerations are involved.* If the subject inspires through the tube but expires into the water around him, there is no problem of added dead space. However, if he expires through the snorkel tube, respiratory dead space is increased and he always reinspires some of his expired gas. The longer the tube, the more the rebreathing. This phenomenon could be a depth-limiting factor, depending on the volume of the tube.

If the tube is very narrow, the resistance to air flow is so great that adequate ventilation cannot be achieved. Note that the total ventilation requirement is increased by the increased work of breathing and the increased dead space.

Another factor is the maximum inspiratory pressure a subject can exert in sucking in his breath. Beneath the surface the pressure of the water on a subject's chest tends to deflate the lungs. If he dives while holding his breath, intrapulmonary pressure increases to the level of the hydrostatic pressure of the surrounding water as gas in the lungs is compressed. However, in breathing through a snorkel tube, intrapulmonary pressure is essentially the same as ambient pressure at the water surface. Reference to the pressure-volume diagram of chest wall and lungs in healthy man (Fig. 6-3) shows that he can exert, at maximum, an inspiratory pressure of about 100 torr. This is about 54 inches (1,350 mm) of water and corresponds to a depth of about $4^{1}/_{2}$ feet (1.33 M).

The heart is another very important consid-

---

*This problem reminds us of our hero hiding in the water from his enemies. He is completely submerged and quietly breathing through a hollow reed that the film producer has conveniently provided for this purpose.

eration. Since the chest contents are essentially at atmospheric pressure, whereas the body generally is subject to the pressure of the surrounding water, the heart must pump "uphill" into a vascular bed of very high resistance. Increased work of the heart could well be limiting in this circumstance. Lanari and Bromberger studied healthy submerged human subjects who were breathing through tubes; they found showers of ventricular premature systoles.

HYPERVENTILATION AND TETANY

Acapnia means a lack or absence of CO_2. *Hypocapnia* means lower than normal P_{CO_2}. Physiologically, acapnia is unknown. If an infinitely high ventilation rate were possible, it would bring alveolar gas to the concentration levels of tracheal gas and reduce the P_{CO_2} of arterial blood to 0. Hyperventilation moves alveolar and blood-gas tensions in the direction of inspired air (Fig. 16-3). Alveolar and arterial P_{O_2} values increase, but as already implied, no amount of hyperventilation could increase these P_{O_2} values beyond the P_{O_2} of inspired air.

The dizziness experienced on blowing up an air mattress is the result of reduced P_{CO_2}, not increased P_{O_2}. Hyperventilation lowers P_{CO_2}; if the alveolar ventilation rate is doubled, alveolar P_{CO_2} is halved. If alveolar P_{CO_2} decreases to the level of 20 or 25 torr in a sea-level resident, the person experiences dizziness and numbness and tingling of the extremities. Systemic arterial blood pressure falls, and there is cerebral vasoconstriction. A decrease of alveolar P_{CO_2} to a level of 15 or 20 torr may produce tetany. This condition is characterized by increased neuromuscular excitability, muscular tension, spontaneous twitching, and sustained involuntary muscular contractions. It is the result of acute respiratory alkalosis and the related decrease of Ca^{++} concentration. Hyperventilating subjects are prone to develop a particular spasm of the hands and feet, termed *carpopedal spasm*. At P_{CO_2} levels associated

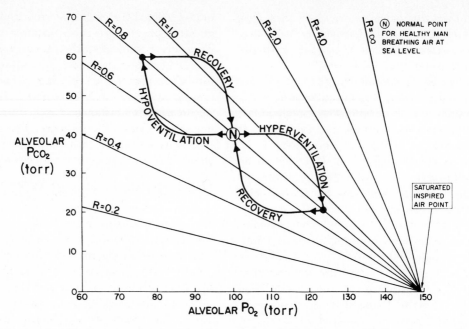

Fig. 16-3. O_2-CO_2 diagram, showing alveolar pathways during hyperventilation, hypoventilation, and recovery. (From Rahn, H., and Fenn, W. O.: A graphical analysis of the respiratory gas exchange, Washington, D.C., 1955, The American Physiological Society.)

with dizziness, numbness, and tingling, there is usually loss of neuromuscular coordination and psychomotor performance. This performance decrement may be a serious matter if the hyperventilating subject is a jet aircraft pilot.

Hyperventilation can evoke abnormal electroencephalographic patterns. It is standard practice for EEG technicians to have their patients perform a hyperventilation test. The 3-per-second dome-and-spike pattern of petit mal epilepsy is sometimes discovered in this way.

Hyperventilation tends to be hypnotic. Some individuals cannot stop, even in tetany, unless commanded to do so. Amateur mountain climbers sometimes continue high ventilation rates into their rest periods. Such ventilation then constitutes hyperventilation because metabolic rate is lower at rest; P_{CO_2} falls, and the

climber feels dizzy. Experienced group leaders carry paper or plastic bags into which hyperventilators can rebreathe; this conserves CO_2, and the dizziness disappears.

Both the hypoxia of high altitude and the increased H^+ concentration of metabolic acidosis increase pulmonary ventilation. This hyperventilation reduces P_{CO_2}. If either hypoxia or acidosis persists, "acclimatization" to low P_{CO_2} occurs. Individuals so acclimatized develop increased resistance to the effects of low P_{CO_2}. After such acclimatization, tingling and dizziness may not occur until alveolar P_{CO_2} falls to a level of 15 or 20 torr; tetany may not occur until alveolar P_{CO_2} drops to 10 torr.

Hyperventilation is an important clinical problem. Aside from its occurrence in acidosis, massive hemorrhage, and salicylism, it commonly indicates emotional stress. Such stress may be of psychoneurotic origin or may occur in relation to the realistic problems of living. Hyperventilation is often observed in visitors to high altitude, where its symptoms complicate the usual responses. Hyperventilation of emotional origin may be sustained or episodic. The episodic type is sometimes of dramatically sudden onset, may involve extreme hyperventilation, and is rapidly productive of distressing symptoms. (See also the discussion of emotional stress pattern in Chapter 17 and the section on emotions and respiration in Chapter 13.)

The symptoms of hyperventilation are often misdiagnosed as serious organic disease. Paradoxically, the patient often complains that he "can't get enough air." Dizziness, hypotension, and cerebral vasoconstriction can produce serious impairment of psychomotor performance, the implications of which should not be underestimated.

If hyperventilation is suspected, the diagnosis is usually simple: (1) measurable, if not perceptible, increase of minute volume of breathing; (2) reproducibility of symptoms by hyperventilation; (3) abolition of symptoms by rebreathing; and (4) arterial blood findings of increased P_{O_2} and pH in association with decreased P_{CO_2} (respiratory alkalosis).

ALTITUDE AND HYPOBARISM

Table A-4 in the Appendix shows the relationship between altitude and barometric pressure. Note that 5,500 M (18,000 feet) corresponds to a barometric pressure of 380 torr, or one half of the sea level value of 760 torr at which altitude atmospheric air is one half as dense as it is at sea level. Another value of particular interest is that at 19,200 M (63,000 feet); the barometric pressure is 47 torr and equals the water vapor tension in the lungs at 37° C.

Responses and acclimatization

Unfortunately, man is not endowed with any sensory mechanism to transduce falling P_{O_2} into

a red alert. This lack is in striking contrast to the alarming dyspnea of rising CO_2 levels. Characteristic features of hypoxic accidents are the insidious onset of impairment and the victim's lack of awareness of danger.* Decompression chamber experiments have shown an interesting pattern of cerebral dysfunction as hypoxia becomes more severe. This pattern involves progressively more frequent and longer periods of cerebral uselessness interspersed between relatively lucid intervals.

If a newcomer to high altitude ascends above a critical level and remains there beyond a critical length of time, he may experience fatigue, headache, irritability, dizziness, palpitation, nausea, loss of appetite, coupled breathing, exertional dyspnea, abdominal cramps, impaired cerebration, insomnia, and, rarely, pulmonary edema (Fig. 16-4). Men are more likely to develop palpitation and dyspnea. A constellation of these symptoms is termed *acute mountain sickness*. The first day and night are usually the worst; after that the newcomer gradually feels better, but it may be many days before he is reasonably comfortable. Many newcomers feel dehydrated initially but have little desire to drink.

Hypoxia causes hyperventilation,† which reduces alveolar and arterial P_{CO_2}, producing respiratory alkalosis. Under the influence of reduced P_{CO_2} the kidney excretes HCO_3^-. However, this compensation is nullified by a further increase in ventilation on the second day. More HCO_3^- excretion is followed by still greater hyperventilation. After 7 to 10 days,

---

*Women are more resistant (as usual) to the effects of hypoxia than men.

†E. B. Brown observed that about 3% of a male military population tended to faint during decompression simulating altitude and used the term "fainter" to describe these subjects. It appears that occasional individuals do not respond to hypoxia with the usual increase in pulmonary ventilation. The mechanism and implications of this observation for altitude acclimatization, anesthesia, and various cardiopulmonary diseases remain unexplored.

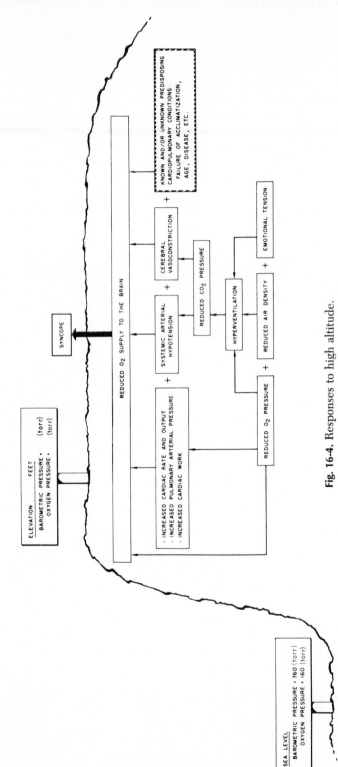

Fig. 16-4. Responses to high altitude.

ventilation no longer increases. The kidney continues to excrete HCO_3^-, and arterial blood pH falls toward normal.

The ventilatory events during altitude acclimatization result from an interplay between the central and peripheral chemoreceptors. Hypoxia initiates hyperventilation, and hyperventilation reduces P_{CO_2}, producing respiratory alkalosis both in blood and in the environment of the central chemoreceptors. The ventilatory drive that normally arises from the central chemoreceptors is depressed so that the chemical drive for breathing is then hypoxia. However, as the respiratory alkalosis of the central chemoreceptors is compensated for by gradual loss of HCO_3^-, ventilatory drive returns over a period of many days, gradually adding to the hypoxic drive to increase total ventilation.

Postulating a CO_2 dissociation curve for the cerebrospinal fluid environment of the central chemoreceptors, we may speculate as follows. Carbon dioxide sensitivity increases as expressed by the new low CO_2 dissociation curve. A given small shift to the right (increasing P_{CO_2}) along this new low curve changes pH more than the same shift along the normal, higher CO_2 dissociation curve. Recovery of the ability to respond to CO_2 despite continuous hyperventilation is an important aspect of altitude acclimatization. After acclimatization the pH of cerebrospinal fluid is normal (7.32) at all altitudes.

When the acclimatized subject descends from altitude, arterial P_{O_2} increases and the hypoxic drive is reduced or abolished. This decreases ventilation somewhat, resulting in a P_{CO_2} increase. However, the P_{CO_2} rise produces respiratory acidosis in the central chemoreceptors, increasing their ventilatory drive. Ventilation does not return to normal until this respiratory acidosis of the central chemoreceptors is compensated for by accumulation of HCO_3^- and associated cations such as Na^+. After descent from acclimatized residence at high alti-

tude, hyperventilation persists for several weeks.

A definite tolerance to low P_{O_2} develops as the newcomer remains at high altitude, and the minimum P_{O_2} that will sustain consciousness decreases. Altitude acclimatization involves acclimatization *both* to low O_2 and to low CO_2, the latter reflecting *sustained* hyperventilation in the successfully acclimatizing individual. Appetite and a sense of well-being gradually return.

Occasionally, a high-altitude dweller stops hyperventilating and may even hypoventilate. P_{CO_2} rises, and P_{O_2} falls to levels inconsistent with useful performance. This has been suggested as an important mechanism in the development of *chronic mountain sickness*.

It is a mistake to assume that metabolic rate decreases on ascent to altitude merely because ambient P_{O_2} is low. Metabolic rate actually increases somewhat because of increased work of breathing, acclimatization to low temperature, and increased sympathetic nervous system activity. In a study of the acute effects of exposure to high altitude, Chidsey and Beckwitt found a 10% to 15% increase of basal metabolic rate (BMR). This increase returned to the normal control level at about the tenth day of exposure. Increased O_2 uptake and BMR, norepinephrine, and free as well as total thyroxine were observed. Epinephrine remained essentially unchanged. These data suggest increased sympathetic nervous system activity rather than increased adrenal medullary activity.

Exposure to altitude increases thyroid gland activity. This is presumably caused by increased secretion of pituitary thyrotropic hormone (TSH). Under conditions of actual exposure at high altitude, therefore, the combined effects of hypoxia and cold probably both play a role in elevating the level of thyroid function. Experimental evidence suggests that hypothyroidism protects against the effects of altitude, presumably because it reduces the O_2 requirement of experimental animals. Hyperthyroid rats are more susceptible to the effects of high altitude than normal rats. Glucocorticosteroids (GCS) also protect against the effects of altitude; smaller doses are necessary for protection of hypothyroid experimental animals.

Ascent to high altitude is associated with a prompt, slight rise of hematocrit, hemoglobin concentration, and erythrocyte count.* In man this increase is probably not a result of splenic contraction, as it may be in the dog. A shift of fluid out of the vascular compartment, producing hemoconcentration, has been postulated.

Increased red blood cell production (erythropoiesis) in the bone marrow is stimulated by the hormone *erythropoietin*, which increases during hypoxia. The resulting polycythemia develops over weeks to months. This polycythemia is marked in young people, is less pronounced among the middle-aged, and may be completely absent in the aged. The erythropoiesis-stimulating hormone, erythropoietin, is governed by P_{O_2}. The polycythemia of altitude acclimatization and the anemia of chronic hyperoxia illustrate this fact.

At one time some physiologists believed that hemoglobin produced at high altitude differs from normal adult hemoglobin (Hb A) because the blood of altitude-acclimatized subjects has a different oxyhemoglobin dissociation curve. However, it is now clear that hemoglobin produced at altitude is the same as hemoglobin produced at sea level. The 2,3-diphosphoglycerate (2,3-DPG) concentration within the erythrocyte increases at altitude, adaptively shifting the oxyhemoglobin dissociation curve to the right.

The myoglobin content and vascularity of muscle increase as a result of exposure to high altitude. Studies of chronically hypoxic rats indicate that this increased vascularity is caused by an increased number of capillaries, rather than simply increased patency of existing vessels. Although examples of anatomic and biochemical responses to altitude are known, much remains to be learned of the biochemistry of hypoxia- and pH-sensing organs, as well as the biochemistry of tissue responses.

During exercise at high altitude, healthy individuals show increased alveolar P_{O_2} but decreased arterial P_{O_2} and saturation. With this in mind, certain athletic teams competing at high altitude have breathed O_2 before performance. This has greater psychologic than physiologic value because the body is poorly equipped to store O_2. The solubility of O_2 at body temperature is low (Table 8). The lungs are the major site of O_2 storage, but they lose their extra supply rapidly as soon as the athlete breathes air. At intermediate altitudes that boast competitive sports, arterial oxyhemoglobin saturation is relatively good—above 90%. Oxygen breathing can increase this saturation, but the volume of O_2 gained is small. Because of the shape of its dissociation curve, myoglobin remains saturated until P_{O_2} falls to extremely low values.

Oxygen breathing during exercise at high altitude has real value. It permits considerably higher metabolic rates than does breathing air at the same altitude. Oxygen breathing after exercise speeds recovery and improves the way an athlete feels.

The significance and extent of acclimatization can be seen from the fact that altitude-acclimatized mountain climbers can climb at ambient P_{O_2} levels that are too low to sustain the consciousness of sea-level residents. Altitude acclimatization, which includes the process of acclimatization to low CO_2 as well as to low O_2, decreases tolerance for high CO_2. After altitude acclimatization the capacity for breath-holding and underwater swimming is therefore greatly reduced.

The hazard of carbon monoxide intoxication

---

*This increase of hemoglobin concentration is similar to the prompt increase observed with exercise, during which increases of 10% may occur within 5 minutes. Thus, determination of hemoglobin concentration and O_2 capacity is relatively meaningless unless the conditions of physical activity and P_{O_2} are precisely stated.

is greater at altitude. It is estimated that for every 1% carboxyhemoglobin present in the blood, altitude tolerance is reduced by about 335 feet (100 M). High-altitude hypoxia also means that internal combustion engines produce larger amounts of CO because of less complete combustion. Smokers are more likely to feel the effects of CO poisoning than are nonsmokers because of both pulmonary dysfunction and their higher initial carboxyhemoglobin levels.

The following observations seem to indicate a relationship between hypoxemia or deficient systemic arterial blood flow and growth failure or weight loss, although the mechanisms are presently unknown:

1. Obesity is quite uncommon at high altitude. Mountaineers sojourning at very high altitude lose weight continuously. The mechanism of this weight loss is uncertain, although hypoxia, anorexia, dehydration, cold, and increased thyroid function probably all play a role. Weight loss may amount to as much as 30 to 40 pounds (13.5 to 18 kgm) during 6 weeks at extremely high altitude.

2. The birth weight of infants born at altitude is less, and the higher the altitude, the less the weight. If we define prematurity as a birth weight of less than $5^{1}/_{2}$ pounds (2,500 gm), then the higher the altitude, the higher also is the prevalence of prematurity.

3. Patients with severe pulmonary emphysema characteristically lose weight.

4. Congenital cardiovascular diseases with decreased cardiac output or with arterial hypoxemia are often associated with growth failure.

Summary of findings at 1-mile (1.6-km) elevation

Many cities are situated at elevations considerably above sea level. In cities at 1 mile (1.6 km) above sea level, such as Denver, Colorado, Albuquerque, New Mexico, and Guadalajara, Mexico, the following physiologic effects may be observed in healthy acclimatized individuals:

1. Inspired P_{O_2} is about 130 torr (dry) instead of 160 torr (dry) as at sea level, resulting in a slightly hypoxemic arterial P_{O_2} of 75 torr. Arterial blood O_2 saturation at rest is therefore 94% instead of 97% as at sea level.

2. There is slight hyperventilation at rest, as well as for any higher metabolic level.

3. Slight respiratory alkalosis results from the chronic hyperventilation. Alveolar and arterial P_{CO_2} values are 36 torr instead of 40 torr as at sea level.

4. There is slight compensatory metabolic acidosis with whole blood total CO_2 content of 19 mM/L instead of 22 mM/L as at sea level.

5. Minute volume of breathing and alveolar ventilation decrease promptly when O_2-enriched gas mixtures are breathed, indicating abolition of tonic peripheral chemoreceptor activity.

6. Total circulating hemoglobin mass and concentration are slightly increased as a result of the hypoxemia.

7. Ventilatory capacity (expressed BTPS) is slightly increased (about 10%) as a result of decreased air density.

8. Visual dark adaptation is slightly impaired as a result of hypoxemia. Aircraft pilots should use supplemental O_2 during night flights above 1-mile (1.6-km) altitude.

9. The mean electric axis of the QRS complex of the ECG shows slight right deviation for subjects of comparable age as compared to data from sea level.

10. The birth weight of infants is slightly lower than at sea level.

Pulmonary arterial hypertension

High-altitude dwellers are said to exhibit low systemic arterial blood pressure; however, significant pulmonary arterial hypertension is found in otherwise healthy individuals living at or above an elevation of 10,000 feet (3,050 M). The mechanism of this hypertension is *hypoxic pulmonary vasoconstriction*. The pulmonary arterial pressure of certain individuals is strikingly high, and during exercise systolic pulmonary arterial pressure may rise to more than 100 torr.

Significant species differences in response to the hypoxia of high altitude exist. Sheep have been found relatively unreactive in contrast to cattle, which resemble human subjects in their reaction.

As already indicated, the mean electric axis of the QRS complex in the frontal plane shows increasing right deviation in populations at progressively higher altitude. Age, somatotype, and functional residual capacity are also factors affecting the electric axis of QRS. This right axis shift quite probably reflects the right ventricular hypertrophy resulting from pulmonary arterial hypertension. The following data show the relationship between altitude and mean QRS axis.

	Altitude (feet)	Mean QRS axis (degrees)
Lima, Peru	500 (152 M)	+55°
Denver, Colorado	5,300 (1,600 M)	+68°
Leadville, Colorado	10,200 (3,100 M)	+84°
Morococha, Peru	14,900 (4,540 M)	+125°

High-altitude pulmonary edema. An acute pulmonary edema may occur in individuals at elevations above 9,000 feet (2,745 M). This condition has been noted to occur especially in those originally residing at high altitude who are returning after an interval at lower elevations. It has been observed in both sexes and in children as young as 5 years of age. It often, but not necessarily, follows exertion at altitude. Patients with high-altitude pulmonary edema should be given supplemental O_2 and removed to a lower altitude as rapidly as possible; the condition is reversible by prompt, vigorous therapy but is occasionally fatal. The clinical findings include pulmonary edema with bilateral patchy infiltrations in the chest roentgenogram, arterial hypoxemia, increased pulmonary arterial pressure, reduced cardiac output, but normal heart size. In fatal cases postmor-

tem examination has shown thrombi in pulmonary capillary and precapillary vessels.

Interval studies have shown normal pulmonary artery wedge, as well as left atrial, pressure. However, Grover found tachycardia in patients subject to high-altitude pulmonary edema. Exercise studies at altitude of such patients showed abnormally large changes in arterial P_{O_2}, alveoloarterial P_{O_2} gradient, and pulmonary arterial pressure when compared with exercise studies of healthy subjects at altitude.

High-altitude disease of cattle. Cattle living at elevations of 10,000 feet (3,050 M) or more often develop a condition termed *brisket disease*, named for the edematous brisket of the affected animal. Pathophysiologically, it is a chronic pulmonary arterial hypertension, resulting in right ventricular failure. Brisket disease is an economically important problem and resembles chronic mountain sickness of human beings in almost all important respects. However, cattle residing at high altitude do not develop appreciable polycythemia and have been reported to show increased clotting time. It is also of interest that cattle fail to sustain hyperventilation at high altitude. Animals vary greatly in their individual response to the same hypoxemic stress, and different species vary even more so. For example, a comparable condition does not occur in sheep living at the same altitude.

Acclimatization as opposed to adaptation

There is no general agreement on terminology to describe the physiologic processes involved when a single individual becomes accustomed to altitude over a period of days to years, as opposed to the tolerance observed in groups of people living at altitude for generations. We will refer to the first process as *acclimatization* and to the second process as *adaptation*. Adaptation includes, among other things, a restoration of fertility (adequately functioning germinal epithelium) that people merely acclimatized to altitude do not recover.

There is evidence that the processes of altitude adaptation, occurring over many generations, result in pulmonary arterial hypertension of somewhat lesser degree.

By far the largest populations at high altitude live in the Andes mountains of South America. Some of these people live at what may be the upper limit for permanent human habitation—a village at 17,600 feet (5,370 M) above sea level. Amerind natives of the high Andes are of short stature but are large chested and able to engage in vigorous ball games. When they act as porters, they run with their loads until tired or winded, then sit down and rest before another cycle of activity.

The Sherpas of Nepal are known for their assistance as pack-bearers in numerous Himalayan climbing expeditions. Indeed, it is no exaggeration to say that without their assistance such expeditions would be impossible. It was Tenzing Norkey, a Sherpa, who together with Edmund Hillary first climbed Mount Everest (1953).

There is a popular belief that residents at high altitude are better equipped than sea-level residents to engage in high-altitude athletics. Although this may be true for altitude-*adapted* individuals, it does not appear to be true for those who are merely *acclimatized* to high altitude. Grover and Reeves arranged for a track team from Leadville, Colorado (altitude 10,200 feet [3,100 M]), to compete first at Leadville and then in Kentucky against a championship Kentucky track team. The Leadville team was defeated as badly in Leadville as it was in Kentucky.

To understand this, a clear-cut distinction must be drawn between those athletic events that are extremely demanding but relatively brief (essentially anaerobic) and those events of longer duration (essentially aerobic). Grover and Reeves showed that exhausting events of less than 1 minute's duration were done as well in Leadville as in Kentucky. However, as the time required for exhausting events increased, performance in Leadville fell progressively below performance in Kentucky.

Subatmospheric decompression and altitude chambers

It is convenient to distinguish two types of decompression—subatmospheric decompression, to which aerospace travellers are exposed, as opposed to the decompression from high pressure down to atmospheric level, to which divers are exposed. Morbid consequences of the former are termed *altitude decompression sickness,** a term for all early sequelae of decompression from atmospheric level down to ambient pressures of 0.5 to 0.6 atm. These sequelae include the prompt effects of expanding gases trapped in body cavities as well as the delayed effects of gases, primarily nitrogen, that evolve from body fluids and tissue, but they do not include the effects of hypoxia. Morbid consequences of the latter are termed *diver's decompression sickness*, or "caisson disease," from the submerged chambers used in underwater construction work.

In 1908 Boycott and Haldane suggested that exposure to ambient pressures of less than 300 torr could cause decompression sickness. During World War I it was speculated that decompression sickness caused by evolved gas could disable a flier. "Bends" precipitated by altitude chamber flights were first described in 1930. Neurocirculatory collapse complicating decompression sickness was first described in 1938, and during World War II aviator's decompression collapse became a well-known entity.

---

*Decompression of this type presents the same problems of aerobullosis, bends, chokes, and possible lung overinflation as does decompression during ascent from a dive. The term *Hypobarogenous aerobullosis* has been suggested by Slonim as more descriptive of what occurs during decompression than the term *aeroembolism*. Actually, embolism is only a part of the pathology of decompression sickness.

Altitude decompression sickness is usually self-limited, responding readily to a return to ground level or to recompression to 1 atm or more of pressure. Physical exertion promotes the appearance and growth of gas bubbles. A given subject tends to show the same pattern of recurrence of bubbles and symptoms if exposure is repeated. Although tissue deformation caused by the changing volume of trapped gases during ascent may cause intense pain and may even be followed by local inflammatory reaction, life itself is not threatened. The same is true for the effects commonly ascribed to evolved gases. Cerebral and coronary vessels usually show a great many bubbles in decompression sickness, so symptoms of myocardial or cerebral ischemia can be expected. If circulatory or neurologic symptoms develop, the term *neurocirculatory collapse* is used to describe the symptom complex. Neurocirculatory collapse occurred 150 times during approximately 1 million altitude chamber exposures, an incidence of 0.015%.

The complications of subatmospheric decompression can be minimized or avoided by preflight denitrogenation, by limiting the duration of exposure at altitudes over 20,000 feet (6,100 M), and by discontinuation of flights as soon as symptoms are identified. The recommended treatment for neurocirculatory collapse complicating altitude decompression sickness is prompt compression to 6 atm of pressure, absolute.

Decompression sickness is readily produced experimentally in dogs and other animals. Extensive decompression results in the appearance of gross bubbles in the venous circulation, pulmonary arterial hypertension, and tachypnea. These objective signs of decompression sickness are reversed in anesthetized dogs by increasing the ambient pressure. Small increases in ambient pressure may be quite effective in reducing severe pulmonary arterial hypertension. The pulmonary arterial hypertension and tachypnea may be the result of simple mechanical blockage of the pulmonary vascular tree by bubbles,* since bubbles appear in the venous circulation before pulmonary arterial hypertension and tachypnea develop; however, pulmonary reflexes may be important.

Behnke cites rapid, shallow breathing, or tachypnea, as a sign pathognomonic of bubbles in pulmonary vessels after decompression. Exposed subjects with tachypnea should be suspected of aeroembolism before a diagnosis of hyperventilation is accepted, especially if other symptoms of decompression sickness are present.

Bubbles do not appear in the arterial system until circulatory collapse is imminent because intraarterial pressure is relatively high and because bubbles tend to form in muscles, which they leave by way of the venous circulation. The high-pressure arterial system and the tissues it supplies are thus naturally protected against bubble emboli.

After decompression an experimental animal may appear perfectly stable for 5 to 30 minutes before showing signs of decompression sickness and then, within a minute, develop bubbles in the venous circulation, severe pulmonary arterial hypertension, and tachypnea.

During recompression, gas bubbles in the venous circulation diminish greatly in size but do not completely disappear, nor do they disappear completely during recompression in vitro.

Altitude or decompression chambers, from which the air can be evacuated, have been constructed in various sizes and shapes. These are used for simulating and testing the effects of altitude. In addition to the convenience that such chambers afford, a much more rapid "ascent" can be made than is possible on a mountain. Some chambers are constructed so that pressure can be reduced with extreme rapidity

---

*Injection of small bubbles into the venous circulation also causes pulmonary arterial hypertension and tachypnea.

to simulate the sudden decompression an aerospace traveller would encounter if his sealed, pressurized cabin suddenly disintegrated. The term *rapid decompression* is more descriptive than its synonym, explosive decompression.

DIVING AND HYPERBARISM

Diving expeditions are constantly extending our experience with the problems of hyperbarism. In one expedition off Cap Ferrat, France, under Jacques-Yves Cousteau, six men remained at a depth of 330 feet (100 M) for 3 weeks, breathing a 2% O_2–98% helium mixture. Decompressive ascent was accomplished during a period of 4 days. Dives without equipment (free dives) to depths greater than 197 feet (60 M) have been recorded.

During a dive, gas volumes are compressed as predicted by the general gas law: PV = nRT—where P is pressure, V is volume, n is the number of moles of gas, R is the gas constant, and T is absolute temperature. At constant temperature if pressure is doubled, volume is halved. If total lung capacity (TLC) is 6 L, a diver who inspires fully at the surface and dives quickly to a depth of 66 feet (20 M) (3-atm total pressure) has only about 2 L of gas in his lungs. If residual volume (RV) occupies 1.5 L of his 6-L total lung capacity, this diver could exhale only 500 ml at the 66-foot (20-M) depth. Actually, he could blow out somewhat less, since gas leaves the lungs for the blood under these conditions of pressure.

A diver who fills his lungs with compressed air under a total pressure of 3 atm has 3 times as many molecules of gas in the lungs as he would have if he filled them at the surface. If he did not allow gas to leave the lungs during ascent, he would be in serious trouble. With open mouth and glottis and with no effort on his part, gas will escape continuously until he reaches the surface. If a diver cannot be certain his glottis is open during ascent, he should assure this by active, slow exhalation.

If a diver whose lungs contain 5% CO_2 holds his breath and plunges rapidly to a depth of 33 feet (10 M) (2-atm total pressure), the lungs still contain 5% CO_2, but since total lung volume is halved, the CO_2 molecules are packed closer together. Although the diver still has 5% CO_2 in the lungs, alveolar P_{CO_2} is doubled. Because the P_{CO_2} of arterial blood is not doubled, CO_2 moves rapidly into the blood, as it would in CO_2 inhalation, and the CO_2 concentration in the lungs decreases.

If the metabolic rate of a diver does not change during a dive, the number of CO_2 molecules entering the venous circulation from the tissues remains constant. During a steady state, which is possible if a diver breathes from a self-contained underwater breathing apparatus (scuba), alveolar P_{CO_2} may be essentially the same as at the surface, but alveolar CO_2 *concentration* may be quite low. A diver at 5-atm pressure may have only 1% CO_2 in the lungs, but the alveolar P_{CO_2} is 0.01 [(5 × 760) − 47] = 37.5 torr.

Divers often show acclimatization to high CO_2 as a result of the increased density and P_{O_2} of breathing mixtures at depth. If they dive without a compressed gas supply, they may also show acclimatization to low O_2 as a result of breath-holding.

As ambient pressure increases, the partial pressure of the constituent gases in a mixture also increases. These increased partial pressures drive more gas into solution in body fluids and tissue than are normally dissolved. During brief exposures, equilibration is far from complete, but as exposure time increases, equilibrium is gradually achieved. The solubility of N_2 in fat is about 5 times as great as its solubility in body fluids, which explains the predilection of gas bubbles for fatty tissue.

The rapidity of safe ascent from depth depends not only on depth but also on the time spent at that depth. The greater the depth, the greater the pressures forcing gases into solution. The longer the time spent at depth, the more nearly the dissolved gases will have achieved equilibrium. If ascent is too rapid, gases expand from wherever they may be, come out of solution,* cause pain and mechanical obstruction, and form emboli in the blood. If bubbles form in the joints, a diver experiences "bends." If they block the pulmonary circulation, he experiences "chokes." If gas bubble emboli coalesce in the left side of the heart or in the great arteries, they may interfere with cerebral or coronary circulation, a sometimes fatal condition.

When compressed air is breathed during a dive, decompression according to the Standard U.S. Navy Diving Tables is recommended. These tables give safe rates of ascent and should be consulted any time that decompression involves a pressure decrease to one half or less of the pressure experienced at depth or for decompression following dives deeper than about 33 feet (10 M). When the pressure decrease exceeds this 2:1 ratio, a diver must decompress gradually by spending time at intermediate depths to allow dissolved gas to come out of solution gradually.

Nitrogen is both relatively insoluble and the major atmospheric constituent. Because of its low solubility it leaves gas bubbles slowly. However, it is a mistake to assume that bubbles emerging during decompression consist of pure N_2. CO_2 and O_2 diffuse into a bubble present anywhere in the body until the partial pressures of the gases in the bubble are in equilibrium with the surrounding fluid or tissue and water vapor saturates the bubble gas. Eliminating N_2 from the breathing mixture minimizes bubble formation. Experimental an-

---

Hypobarogenous aerobullosis is a neologism proposed by Slonim to mean the generalized emergence and growth of gas bubbles from solution in fluids and tissues throughout the body as a result of decompression. This term should be distinguished from aeroembolism, which has been used in this sense, but as the term suggests, aeroembolism should mean the *intravascular* emergence, growth, and *transport* of gas bubbles as a result of decompression.

imals breathing pure O_2 are well protected against bubble formation during decompression from any pressure level, as compared to animals breathing gas mixtures containing N_2; however, if O_2 is substituted for N_2, another serious problem is created.

Recompression is the treatment of choice for victims of decompression sickness. This may be accomplished either in a recompression chamber or by allowing the diver to descend again so that decompression can be accomplished more slowly.

Nitrogen narcosis

Most physiologists believe that "rapture of the deep," an intoxicated condition that a diver may experience, is *nitrogen narcosis*. Although chemically and physiologically inert at ordinary partial pressure, N_2 is narcotic at high pressure. Substitution of helium for N_2 in the diver's breathing mixture precludes this condition.

However, a few physiologists believe that the symptoms attributed to N_2 are actually caused by CO_2 accumulation. The greatly increased density of a breathing mixture at depth increases the work of breathing; for a given effort a smaller volume is ventilated than would be the case if air were being breathed at the surface. According to the CO_2 accumulation theory, it is the increased P_{CO_2} resulting from this hypoventilation that produces the symptoms in question; substitution of helium for N_2 protects against these symptoms because the less dense helium mixture is easier to breathe. Proponents of the nitrogen narcosis theory suggest that if CO_2 accumulation produces lightheaded intoxication at depth, then CO_2 inhalation should produce the same effect in the laboratory—and it does not!

HYPEROXIA

Oxygen therapy is often a lifesaving modality in clinical medicine. In general, O_2 should be used in sufficient concentration to restore arterial blood and tissue tensions to normal or, at most, somewhat higher values.

A gram of hemoglobin can combine chemically with a maximum of 1.36 ml (STPD) of O_2. At a normal P_{O_2} of 100 torr, arterial hemoglobin is 97% saturated, so little additional O_2 can be added to hemoglobin by increasing P_{O_2}. On the other hand, each 100 ml of plasma contains only 0.3 ml of dissolved O_2 at normal alveolar pressures. If exposed to 100% O_2 at 1 atm of pressure, each 100 ml of plasma would dissolve approximately 2.4 ml of O_2, whereas at 3 atm the dissolved O_2 content is more than 6 vol%, exceeding the normal arteriovenous blood O_2 difference of man at rest. Reducing the temperature of plasma would increase dissolved O_2 further for any given P_{O_2}.

Within minutes after a subject starts to breathe an O_2-enriched mixture, such as 60% O_2, there is a decrease of as much as 1 gm/dL in hemoglobin concentration of the circulating blood. Breathing O_2-enriched mixtures decreases cardiac rate, cardiac output, and cardiac work. By direct action increased P_{O_2} produces systemic arterial vasoconstriction, thus increasing diastolic blood pressure. Cerebral vasoconstriction also occurs. As expected, high P_{O_2} also constricts the placental artery, which does not have an autonomic nerve supply. Increased P_{O_2} dilates the pulmonary vasculature, thus exerting an action *opposite* to that which it has on the systemic vasculature. This action is a part of the mechanism that regulates the distribution of $\dot{V}_A/\dot{Q}_c$ ratios in the lung, since it tends to increase perfusion where ventilation is good.

Normobaric and hypobaric hyperoxia

The effect of hyperoxia on the living cell is biochemical and must be understood in biochemical terms. Hyperoxia inhibits a number of intracellular enzymes, including succinic dehydrogenase, catalases, hydrogenases, urease, arginase, and succinic oxidases. It also inhibits a pyridine nucleotide system, decreasing aden-

osine triphosphate (ATP); sodium succinate appears to protect the ATP supply.

When a sea-level resident breathes pure O_2, ventilation decreases initially but then rises gradually to level off at about 15% above resting, control ventilation. This may occur because the increased amount of *dissolved* O_2 available to and used in metabolism means that less oxyhemoglobin is reduced to hemoglobin to meet the metabolic needs of the peripheral chemoreceptors, more unbuffered H^+ stimulate the chemoreceptors, and breathing increases.

Carbon dioxide narcosis. In patients whose ventilatory drive depends on hypoxia as a result of CO_2 retention and decreased responsiveness to CO_2, pulmonary ventilation may decrease seriously, or such patients may even become apneic when an O_2-enriched breathing mixture is administered. This clinical situation is termed *carbon dioxide narcosis*. The cerebral complications of stupor, coma, and increased cerebrospinal fluid pressure *(pseudotumor cerebri)* are manifestations of increased P_{CO_2}, rather than O_2, and can be relieved by increasing alveolar ventilation to remove CO_2. The term "oxygen poisoning" has been used but is not descriptive and should be abandoned. Carbon dioxide narcosis is never a contraindication for O_2; rather, it is an indication for providing *both* O_2 and the required ventilatory assistance.

Oxygen intoxication. Although pure O_2 at normobaric or hypobaric pressures can be breathed for minutes to hours without *apparent* adverse effects, O_2 is clearly toxic to living cells when they are exposed to more than twice the normal P_{O_2} (more than 40% O_2 at sea level) for considerable periods of time. Indeed, one is tempted to call a discussion of O_2 intoxication "too much of a good thing." Excessive concentrations or, more relevantly, excessive partial pressures of O_2 are already known to have a variety of toxic effects. Toxic manifestations range from mucous membrane irritation, pulmonary congestion, loss of pulmonary surfactant, atelectasis, hyaline membrane formation, ocular damage, and impaired fertility to convulsions and death. Susceptibility to these toxic effects varies with the species, the tissue exposed, and the age. However, the lung, the central nervous sytem, and a CNS ontogenetic derivative, the eye, are particularly susceptible to hyperoxic damage.

Rahn and Farhi kept mice in a 100% O_2 atmosphere at about 200 torr for 60 days, during which time they conceived and delivered apparently normal young. However, there is evidence that the fertility of both male and female mice is impaired by P_{O_2} in excess of 500 torr for 2 weeks. Ulvedal kept roosters at a P_{O_2} of 380 torr for 22 days. Sperm motility, total sperm count, and ejaculate volume decreased during the first week. Spermatogenesis was impaired and testicular atrophy was noted. The mechanism of these changes may be either a direct cytotoxic effect of O_2 or an indirect endocrine effect.

Dogs and other mammals die after normobaric exposure to pure O_2 for $1^{1}/_2$ to 3 days. At autopsy the lungs show vascular congestion and consolidation, and the alveoli are filled with fluid and lined with a hyaline membrane. Animals sacrificed prior to spontaneous death show atelectatic areas in the lungs. These pulmonary findings can be produced unilaterally if one lung breathes pure O_2 while the other lung breathes air. They are prevented or delayed by hypophysectomy or adrenalectomy. These *pulmonary* effects are not observed in animals living in pure O_2 at 0.5-atm pressure.

Guinea pigs and rats show progressive loss of pulmonary surfactant after 5 to 7 days of 100% O_2 breathing at 1-atm pressure. As a result of this loss, surface tension in the alveoli increases, promoting alveolar collapse and progressive atelectasis together with vascular engorgement, pulmonary edema, hyaline membrane formation, and alveolocapillary diffusion block.

The eye is another organ that shows great sensitivity to the toxic effects of hyperoxia. Exposure to 100% O_2 at 1-atm pressure for more than 24 hours depresses the electroretinogram (ERG). Normobaric hyperoxia exerts a selective action on the endothelium of developing retinal vessels but does not affect immature cerebral or meningeal vessels or directly injure other retinal structures. The mature eye is also sensitive, but the visual cells, rather than the vascular bed, are the target tissue.

Retrolental fibroplasia is a clinical example of the toxic action of O_2 on the immature eye. High P_{O_2} causes an arteriolar spasm in the retina of premature infants, which is followed by a retinal fibrosis, termed *retrolental fibroplasia*. This complication of O_2 therapy can be avoided by keeping the inspired O_2 concentration less than 40% (assuming a normal alveoloarterial gradient) and limiting the use of O_2 in premature infants to a maximum of 7 days. However, in the presence of cardiopulmonary disease, such as pulmonary hypoperfusion syndrome, the concentration of inspired O_2 must be high enough to achieve normal arterial blood P_{O_2}.

Some think that high O_2 is less dangerous to man than it is to the more commonly used experimental animals. This idea may be the result of clinical experience with O_2 therapy in which high concentrations are seldom actually achieved and where continuous exposure does not occur. However, human subjects exposed to high O_2 atmospheres show signs and symptoms of toxicity. Pratt observed pulmonary vascular congestion and hyaline membranes at autopsy in patients given 100% O_2 at atmospheric pressure preterminally. Such fluid accumulation impairs gas diffusion and, paradoxically, produces or aggravates hypoxemia. Further study of the effects of long-term exposure to high O_2 atmospheres in man is needed, but such studies inevitably endanger the health of experimental subjects.

Hyperbaric hyperoxia

Hemoglobin becomes almost fully saturated when exposed to a normal P_{O_2} of 100 torr during passage through the pulmonary capillaries. If additional O_2 is forced into the blood at higher tensions, it enters solution in the aqueous or plasma compartment. Because of its relative insolubility at body temperature, O_2 in physical solution increases only 3 vol% in the aqueous compartment of blood for each 1,000-torr rise in P_{O_2}. Nevertheless, more O_2 can be forced into physical solution during practical hyperbaric exposure than the normal volume of O_2 extracted from arterial blood by the tissues. The arterial blood P_{O_2} of normal animals and man breathing pure O_2 at 3 atm of pressure is about 2,000 torr. It should be noted, however, that pulmonary gas exchange is inefficient in the presence of a right-to-left shunt; as a result, the arterial blood P_{O_2} increase is comparatively modest, even at 3 atm.

During hyperbaric hyperoxia, cardiac rate, cardiac output, and regional blood flow to certain organs decrease in normal man; vasoconstriction causes increased peripheral vascular resistance. The content and tension of O_2 rise in venous blood, suggesting that more O_2 is available for utilization despite concomitant vasoconstriction. After total interruption of blood flow to an organ, normal function persists longer if an animal has been hyperoxygenated prior to the induction of ischemia. However, neuropathologic studies suggest that when total circulatory standstill is induced in an animal, hyperoxygenation confers less than 5 minutes of additional protection to the CNS. Furthermore, pathologic evidence shows that despite hyperbaric hyperoxia, an intact circulation peripheral to a nonperfused zone does not prevent necrosis of the adjacent ischemic tissue.

Hyperbaroxic toxicity. When rising O_2 pressure reaches a critical level, convulsions occur. In man this level usually results from breathing pure O_2 at a pressure of about 3 atm. However, symptoms may appear in less than 15 minutes at 4-atm pressure. The clinical sequence includes restlessness, pallor, convulsions, coma, and finally death if exposure continues. Fortunately, prompt and complete recovery follows removal of a victim from the high O_2 pressure environment. The seizures occur at irregular intervals and are of abrupt onset and spontaneous cessation. The frequency of these convulsions increases as the duration of exposure increases. Adding low concentrations of CO_2 to the breathing mixture accelerates the onset of convulsions and potentiates other neurotoxic effects because CO_2 increases cerebral circulation and exposes the brain to higher P_{O_2} levels. However, high concentrations of CO_2 inhibit O_2 convulsions.

Experimental animals breathing 100% O_2 at 3-atm pressure show a loss of pulmonary surfactant after 4 to 5 hours of exposure. Depression of the ERG is maximal after 3 to 5 hours of exposure to 100% O_2 at 3 atm, and irreversible retinal injury occurs regularly after 5 to 6 hours. After exposure to 100% O_2 at 3 atm for more than 4 hours, human subjects show progressive contraction of visual fields and impairment of central vision. In the rabbit, an animal with an avascular retina, death of visual cells occurs.

Dogs exposed to 100% O_2 at 3-atm pressure for more than 4 hours develop a selective retinal lesion termed a *cytoid body*. This lesion consists of segmental degeneration of axons in the nerve fiber layer of the retina around the optic nerve head. They appear similar to the cytoid bodies of the "cotton wool" spot, which are characteristic of human retinal vascular disease. This lesion is not observed in dogs subjected to shorter periods of hyperbaric hyperoxia ranging from $3/4$ to 2 hours. These ocular lesions can be prevented by the use of a 98% O_2–2% CO_2 breathing mixture. However, when this is used, the resulting cerebral vasodilation exposes the CNS to the toxic effects of O_2, as shown by neurologic deficits and neuronal necrosis.

Such high O_2 pressures produce retinal vasoconstriction and decrease retinal blood flow. It is not known whether a hyperoxia-induced ischemia is the paradoxic cause of the damage or whether direct cytotoxic action of high P_{O_2}

together with high tissue susceptibility is the explanation. Although the strong vasoconstrictive reaction of the retina to hyperbaric O_2 suggests the possibility of ischemic damage, it is difficult to accept ischemia as a likely causative mechanism.

Hyperbaric oxygenation. Many medical and research centers in Europe and America now have chambers in which the pressure can be increased to several atmospheres. Small chambers are used for hyperbaric studies of experimental animals, and large chambers accommodate patients who can be given pure O_2 to breathe. Surgery can thus be performed under hyperbaric conditions while a patient breathes O_2 at a pressure somewhat below that which would produce convulsions and while the surgical team breathes the compressed air that fills the chamber. Locks are installed between chamber and outside in which all personnel may decompress.

Hyperbaric oxygenation involves appreciable hazards, not only to the patient but also to the personnel; all are subject to the dangers of toxicity, explosion, decompression, aeroembolism, and nitrogen narcosis. For reasons of safety, hyperbaric pressures in large chambers are usually generated by compressed air. Special respiratory assemblies are then used to deliver pure O_2 to the patient. As already discussed, exposure to O_2 at 3-atm pressure for only 30 minutes can produce convulsions, although this effect appears completely reversible with prompt decompression. However, with prolonged exposure the direct toxic chemical effect of O_2 on the cerebral tissues can lead to permanent CNS damage, paralysis, and death.

There are also difficulties associated with compression and decompression. Rapid pressurization is well tolerated if pressures in the paranasal sinuses and middle ear equalize well. The absorption of gases from any cavity is more rapid when it is filled with O_2 than when it is filled with air. This fact favors pulmonary atelectasis, retraction of the tympanic membrane,

or pain from the gas space beneath a dental filling. If the negative pressure in a closed body space exceeds plasma osmotic pressure, fluid and plasma protein will transude into the space.

To avoid obvious toxicity, hyperbaricists limit uninterrupted therapeutic exposures to 5 hours or less at a P_{O_2} not exceeding 3 atm. Because of the possibility of nitrogen narcosis, physicians should probably not attempt to perform complicated tasks, such as cardiovascular surgery, while breathing air at more than 4 atm. However, this limit can be greatly extended by replacing nitrogen in the inspired gas mixture with helium. The most serious hazard of hyperbaric oxygenation is decompression sickness as a result of rapid decompression. This may occur in a mild form, including arthralgia and transient skin rash, or in a severe form, with neurologic deficit, paralysis, coma, and death. It also carries the risk of arterial aeroembolism resulting from rapid expansion of lung gas if a subject does not exhale during decompression. The risk of serious decompression sickness can be virtually eliminated by application of tested decompression schedules and by prompt recompression should symptoms appear.

Since O_2 is the most flow-limited substance required in cell metabolism, improving O_2 transport to an ischemic organ confers real benefit. The rationale of hyperbaric oxygenation rests on the assumption that exposure to high pressures of O_2 can prevent or reverse tissue hypoxia without inflicting serious damage on a patient. However, the clinical effectiveness of hyperbaric oxygenation is limited by failure to deliver O_2 through defective blood vessels and by the brevity of tolerated exposures.

Clinically, hyperbaric oxygenation appears promising for treatment of circulatory shock, carbon monoxide poisoning, cyanide intoxication, and serious anaerobic infections (as with *Clostridium welchii*) and as a potentiator of ionizing radiation in the therapy of certain malignancies. It may also prove useful in cardiovascular surgery, cerebral ischemic episodes, and circulatory arrest.

Organs that have been harvested for later transplantation lose viability rather quickly because of ischemia. Hyperbaric oxygenation, together with hypothermia, can be used to maintain tissue integrity for longer time periods. Hyperbaric oxygenation is also being evaluated for prevention of ischemic damage to vulnerable tissues during surgical transplantation.

RESPONSES TO ATMOSPHERES CONTAINING CO_2

The excitatory and depressant effects of CO_2 on ventilation were considered in Chapter 14. In concentrations up to about 12% (sea level), CO_2 behaves as a powerful stimulant. Arterial CO_2 pressures above 120 torr inhibit hyperbaric O_2 convulsions. Human subjects breathing 25% CO_2 are conscious but unable to perform simple tasks, such as removing the respiratory valve and mouthpiece from their own mouth. They may think great thoughts but cannot recall these at the end of the experiment. Tunnel vision is common. Recovery from such exposure is accompanied by a variety of psychologic reactions that depend on the personality of the subject. However, most subjects report that the experience is not unpleasant and state that they would be willing to repeat it. It has been reported that brief exposure to high CO_2 may improve reading speed and retention, as well as mathematical computation speed and accuracy, for hours following exposure. However, Porteus' maze test shows decreased ability to plan ahead following CO_2 exposure.

In concentrations of 30% and above, CO_2 is anesthetic. High CO_2 has been used as a somatic therapy in psychiatry for a variety of disorders; however, the extreme subjectivity and the problem of establishing satisfactory controls make the results of such treatment difficult to evaluate.

Because high CO_2 depresses the CNS, its concentration should not be allowed to rise unmonitored in closed spaces where people may be exposed. CO_2 accumulation in coal mines is a well-known hazard. Crashes have been attributed to the use of CO_2 fire extinguishers in pressurized aircraft.

Carbon dioxide produces local vasodilation in denervated areas, but its central action is opposite and dominant. High CO_2 breathing mixtures produce blanched skin through a wide concentration range; conservation of circulation by this mechanism may explain, in part, how CO_2 increases cerebral and coronary blood flow.

Administration of high CO_2 produces a rapid fall of body temperature. Not only is metabolic rate reduced, but shivering also is inhibited and heat loss by evaporation from the upper respiratory tract is increased because of increased pulmonary ventilation. High CO_2 reduces the rectal temperature of rats even when ambient temperature is high. Peripheral vasoconstriction retards heat gain from the hot environment while evaporation of water removes heat from blood perfusing the respiratory tract and the slowly metabolizing body core.

High CO_2 is lethal if breathed for long periods of time; the higher the concentration of CO_2, the shorter the survival time. Carbon dioxide also synergizes with both hypoxia and hyperoxia in shortening survival time. Barley, grown in O_2 in a closed, dark container, dies when the CO_2 concentration reaches 30% (sea level). High CO_2 atmospheres prevent the decay of meat at room temperature.

Acclimatization

Chronic exposure to an atmosphere containing a low concentration of CO_2 results in certain responses that increase tolerance to the effects of this gas. The ventilatory response to CO_2 decreases with such exposure; breathholding time and alveolar P_{CO_2} at the breathholding breaking point are both increased. The initial respiratory acidosis is more rapidly compensated if inspired CO_2 concentration is high than if it is low! Initial euphoria is followed by lassitude and impaired performance, which tend to persist despite acclimatization.

As in altitude acclimatization, an interplay between central and peripheral chemoreceptors during CO_2 acclimatization gradually decreases ventilation and CO_2 sensitivity. Initially, increased P_{CO_2} produces respiratory acidosis in blood and in the central chemoreceptors. Hydrogen ions, and perhaps CO_2, produce a sustained increase in ventilation by stimulation of peripheral chemoreceptors. This is augmented by the respiratory acidosis in the central chemoreceptors. However, as HCO_3^- accumulates in the cerebrospinal fluid, the ventilatory drive of the central chemoreceptors decreases. CO_2 sensitivity is reduced, and the breath-holding, breaking-point curve is elevated because P_{CO_2} increments along the new high CO_2 dissociation curve now produce less pH change than similar increments produced along the normal CO_2 dissociation curve.

Emerging from a CO_2 atmosphere, subjects report a smell of ammonia. Return to air breathing produces respiratory alkalosis in the central chemoreceptors and reduces peripheral chemoreceptor drive. Total ventilation is thus depressed until HCO_3^- loss restores normal central chemoreceptor pH.

SPECIAL ATMOSPHERES
Aerospace cabin and submarine chamber atmospheres

Prolonged exposure to high P_{O_2} atmospheres suppresses erythropoiesis, producing anemia. This fact is of obvious practical importance in selecting atmospheres for aerospace cabins and submarine chambers and in planning routine periodic examinations of exposed personnel. The atmospheres within manned aerospace capsules launched by the United States thus far have consisted of 100% O_2 at 0.34-atm pressure. This means an inspired P_{O_2} of about 250 torr. However, atmospheres consisting of gas mixtures would have certain advantages for prolonged space missions. Along with other inert gases, helium has been considered as a replacement for nitrogen. The advantages of helium include its low density and reduced hazards of aerobullosis and nitrogen narcosis.

Despite their relative chemical unreactivity, the noble gases can exert certain effects on biologic systems. The viability of chick embryos incubated in 21% O_2–79% helium is reduced by 50%. Further tests of appropriate mammalian systems are needed to assess the advisability of using helium as a component of cabin or chamber atmospheres.

A distinct disadvantage of helium is its high *thermal conductivity*. Accelerated heat loss complicates the problem of environmental thermoregulation. Furthermore, because it conducts sound rapidly, helium distorts the voice, making verbal communication difficult in atmospheres containing high helium concentrations.

Artificial gills

The coming exploration and habitation of undersea regions will require devices that permit man to breathe underwater. Perhaps the most attractive answer to this problem involves the efficient and rapid extraction of dissolved O_2 from sea water, although electrolysis also deserves consideration. To accomplish extraction, energy will be required to circulate both water and air. The average O_2 content of ocean water from surface to a depth of 3,300 feet (1,000 M) is about 4 ml/L, whereas below that depth 7 to 8 ml/L are usually present. The partial pressures of O_2 and other dissolved gases increase slightly with depth.

Bodell showed that silicone-rubber membranes (Silastic), which allow diffusion of O_2 and CO_2, can be used to make artificial gills capable of extracting dissolved O_2 from water; 2,000 feet (610 M) of thin-wall, fine-caliber tubing were capable of extracting 136 ml/hr of O_2. An adult rat was sealed in a flask and the atmosphere circulated at a rate of 400 ml/min through the gill tubing, while tap water was circulated over the gill coils at a rate of 4,000 ml/min. Although a control rat that was simply sealed in a flask died in 1 hour, the experimental rat was still living after 25 hours. The flask atmosphere reached equilibrium at a P_{O_2} of 75 torr and P_{CO_2} of 15 torr.

Liquid respiration and submerged survival

Kylstra studied mice and dogs respiring hyperbarically oxygenated electrolyte solutions and demonstrated submerged survival. Chambers containing pools of saline or Ringer's solution were filled with O_2 at several atmospheres of pressure. When the experimental animals sank into the saline, their breathing movements continued and they respired the hyperbarically oxygenated solution. The P_{O_2} of the saline solutions was sufficient to drive adequate volumes of O_2 across the alveolocapillary membrane and into the pulmonary capillaries. Such animals survived the ordeal of breathing hyperbarically oxygenated saline and sometimes the ordeal of emerging to return to air breathing. However, pulmonary complications usually occur within a few days because the aqueous electrolyte solution washes out pulmonary surfactant or because the inhaled saline is contaminated with excreta or bacteria from the body surface. Kylstra suggested that pulmonary gas exchange in liquid-ventilated lungs is diffusion limited. Viscosity and temperature are important variables, as well as the diffusion rates of O_2 and CO_2 through the respired liquid.

O_2 and CO_2 are very soluble in certain organic liquids that have a viscosity near that of water and relative biologic inertness. Clark and Gollan showed that both silicone oils (polymethylsiloxanes) and fluorocarbon liquids (perfluorobutyltetrahydrofurans), equilibrated with O_2 at atmospheric pressure, can support respiration in mice and cats. Arterial P_{O_2} was well maintained, but CO_2 elimination was impaired, with consequent respiratory acidosis. Animals that had breathed silicone oil died shortly after return to air breathing, whereas those that had breathed fluorocarbon liquid survived for weeks. The addition of an anesthetic, Fluothane, arrested the swimming motions of submerged mice, but the animals survived. Pulmonary damage was observed in all animals. They also showed that goldfish can survive under silicone oil for several weeks. The fluorocarbon liquid FC-80 is superior to the silicone oils and has the advantage over aqueous liquids of higher solubility for O_2 and CO_2, higher diffusion coefficients for these gases, and somewhat lower viscosity.

Atmospheric pollution

Of all living things, we alone are in the process of polluting our natural environment; we even have the power to destroy it. Atmospheric pollution is actually only an aspect of the larger problem of environmental pollution, truly one of the pressing health problems of our times. What this exposure lacks in intensity is more than made up for by its chronicity. Where pollution is present, every breath is affected. Atmospheric pollution is largely the result of modern industrial technology and transportation. Motor vehicle fumes and exhausts are a large contributor in many instances.

The chemistry of air pollution is often complex and varies from region to region. Pollutants may be gaseous, liquid, or particulate. The chief noxious ingredients are commonly SO_2, NO_2, O_3, CO, and assorted hydrocarbons, several of which are known to be carcinogenic.

Nitrogen oxides are not only themselves toxic but, with other pollutants, breed ozone. In the presence of ultraviolet radiation, certain hydrocarbons catalyze the oxidation of nitric oxide (NO) to nitrogen dioxide (NO_2), which in turn with ultraviolet radiation dissociates to yield oxygen atoms, or free radicals.* These free atoms combine with molecular oxygen to form ozone as follows:

$$\ddot{O} + O_2 \rightleftharpoons O_3$$

These free atoms also react with hydrocarbons and nitrogen oxides to form peroxyacetylnitrate (PAN), according to the following crude composite equation:

$$\ddot{O} + \text{Hydrocarbons} + NO_x \rightarrow PAN$$

Two simple ways of decreasing the nitrogen oxide effluent from the internal combustion engine are available: (1) recirculation of exhaust through the intake manifold, thus decreasing O_2 concentration, P_{O_2}, and peak combustion temperature or (2) the use of water to decrease combustion temperature.

The catalytic converter recently installed in automobile exhaust systems decreases the emission of pollutants. Operating at high temperature (650° to 980° C), a platinum-based catalyst oxidizes CO to CO_2 and unburned hydrocarbons to CO_2 and H_2O. Unfortunately, the trace of unburned sulfur that is oxidized to SO_2 and SO_3 can combine with water to form sulfurous and sulfuric acids. Nitrogen dioxide, already in a state of oxidation, is unaffected by the catalytic converter. The catalyst is readily poisoned by lead.

Although obnoxious and irritating, urban air pollution is not known to cause a specific disease entity. It does, however, aggravate the symptoms of patients with respiratory tract disease. Under certain conditions, breathing polluted air can impair pulmonary function temporarily or even permanently. Air pollution is probably a significant causative factor in lung cancer and in certain chronic bronchopulmon-

ary diseases. Is prolonged exposure to oxidant air pollutants a cause of the increasingly prevalent bronchitis-emphysema syndrome? Is it a cause of accelerated aging of the exposed respiratory tract?

An important meteorologic phenomenon that can produce sudden increases in the concentration of atmospheric pollutants is the *atmospheric temperature inversion*. When the normal relationship of *warmer, lower* air to *colder, higher* air is reversed, there is little or no tendency for dilution and dissipation of atmospheric pollutants by convection currents. This inverted relationship is known as an atmospheric temperature inversion. Death has occasionally resulted in individuals with chronic cardiopulmonary diseases when atmospheric temperature inversion produced sudden increases in the concentration of air pollutants.

Studies of the effects of air pollution on human populations are necessarily epidemiologic in nature and suffer from the problems and limitations of this approach. The subject is as important as it is complex, and doubtless various synergistic mechanisms will be discovered as research proceeds.

Tobacco smoking

The prevalence of tobacco smoking and its grave impact on human health require a definitive statement. Tobacco smoking is a complex subject that has economic, psychosocial, and medical aspects. It is often oversimplified. However, the *medical* aspects of cigarette smoking are now abundantly clear.

Cigarette smoke is a complex chemical mixture that produces inflammation of the respiratory tract and, in susceptible individuals, allergic disease as well. Regular inhalation of cigarette smoke usually results in gradual loss of all aspects of pulmonary function. The resulting clinical entity is a type of bronchitis-emphysema syndrome. Predictably, owing to bio-

---

*A free radical is an uncharged reactive fragment consisting of one or more atoms.

logic variation, the precise nature and extent of pulmonary function loss vary considerably from individual to individual.

Because cigarette smoke contains a number of carcinogenic chemical substances, as well as radioactive polonium-210, long-term inhalation greatly increases the probability of bronchopulmonary malignancy in any given individual. Because these carcinogenic chemical substances find their way from the respiratory tract into the stomach and urinary bladder, cigarette smokers are also at increased risk of malignancy of these organs.

Acutely, the nicotine in cigarette smoke produces tachycardia and increased systemic vascular resistance, both of which increase cardiac work. Smokers are also at increased risk of certain vascular diseases, including coronary artery disease, peripheral vascular disease, and stroke. As much as 10% of the smoker's hemoglobin combines with CO absorbed from the smoke to form the relatively stable, but physiologically useless, carboxyhemoglobin, a compound that impedes oxygen transport.

Cigarette smoking is a tranquilizer and a neurosis-gratifying, disease-inducing behavior. The smoker trades health for peace of mind. Unfortunately, those who breathe second-hand smoke (passive smokers) trade health merely for the dubious privilege of proximity to the smoker. The habit of smoking cigarettes often becomes deeply entrenched, so that individuals either are unable to stop smoking or find the effort to stop a difficult, continuing struggle.

Marijuana smoking

Cannabis smoke contains many chemical substances, including Δ-9 tetrahydrocannabinol (THC) and products of oxidation and pyrolysis such as carbon monoxide, tars, and polycyclic aromatic hydrocarbons. Acutely, oral or inhaled THC is a dose-related bronchodilator, increases metabolic rate (increases ventilation without changing P_{CO_2} and pH), does not affect the ventilatory response to hypoxia, but increases the beta-sympathetic–mediated ventilatory response to hypercapnia. Regular marijuana smokers develop clinical bronchitis and spirometric evidence of airway obstruction, both of which tend to improve if smoking is discontinued. Experimental animals subjected to chronic smoke inhalation develop bronchitis, bronchiolitis, squamous metaplasia, focal alveolitis, and cholesterol granulomas. The long-term bronchopulmonary effects of marijuana smoking are similar to those of tobacco smoking.

Noxious gases

Ozone. Ozone, or O_3, is a highly reactive oxidant gas of characteristic odor. It is produced in O_2-containing atmospheres by electric discharge or by ionizing radiation and is thus a natural constituent of the atmosphere. The interaction of solar ultraviolet radiation with O_2 in the upper atmosphere produces an appreciable quantity of ozone, which shields the surface of the earth by absorption of certain ultraviolet frequencies. Exposure to ozone is increasing as a result of modern technology. New sources include electric appliances and equipment and artificial ultraviolet light and other ionizing radiation. Commercially available "air purifiers" and "deodorizers" generate sufficient ozone to be hazardous under certain conditions of use, for example, inadequate room ventilation.

Ozone, known to be poisonous since its discovery in 1840, is toxic at levels of less than 1 ppm. In man low concentrations—from 0.6 to 0.8 ppm for 2 hours—reduce both pulmonary ventilatory and diffusing capacity. Industrial exposure to concentrations of 9 ppm has produced severe pneumonia. Thickening of alveolar walls by edema fluid is the most likely cause of this decreased diffusing capacity. In laboratory animals, concentrations of approximately 4 to 30 ppm for 3 to 4 hours produce fatal pulmonary edema. Experimental animals exposed to ozone concentrations of 1 to 50 ppm over many months show atrophy of alveolar walls, especially in alveoli evaginating from respiratory bronchioles and alveolar ducts.

Measurable tolerance to otherwise lethal doses of ozone develops after sublethal exposures. Cross-tolerance between ozone, nitrogen dioxide, and other oxidant irritants also occurs. Tobacco plants show an ozone type of injury when exposed to mixtures of O_3 and SO_2 at subthreshold concentrations, suggesting a synergism between the toxic effects of these two noxious gases.

Cyanide. The main toxic effect of cyanide involves inhibition of the intracellular enzyme cytochrome oxidase. Oxygen transport and O_2 pressures are usually adequate during cyanide poisoning, but the cell utilization of O_2 is diminished (hypoxidosis). The usual treatment consists of amyl nitrite ($C_5H_{11}NO_2$), sodium nitrite ($NaNO_2$), or sodium thiosulfate ($Na_2S_2O_3$).

Sodium nitrite converts hemoglobin to methemoglobin, which then effectively binds cyanide to form the relatively stable cyanmethemoglobin. Sodium thiosulfate is used as a substrate by the enzyme rhodanese, which detoxifies cyanide by converting it to thiocyanate. In mice, sodium thiosulfate, when administered alone, appears more effective than sodium nitrite. In combination the protective effect is additive in mice but synergistic in dogs. Normobaric O_2 and hyperbaric O_2 have been reported to be of some value in cyanide poisoning; ECG changes are reversed by O_2. Although hyperoxia alone has slight effect, striking enhancement of prophylactic protection has been reported when mice given potassium cyanide were treated with hyperoxia plus sodium nitrite and sodium thiosulfate. The optimum O_2 pressure and the biochemical mechanism of action are presently unknown.

CHAPTER 17

CLINICAL EVALUATION OF PULMONARY FUNCTION

What is pulmonary function? In a clinical sense the term *pulmonary function* refers only to the role of the bronchopulmonary system in respiratory gas exchange; it does not refer to the other functions of the lung—metabolic, endocrine, hematologic, immunologic, self-cleansing, and heat-and-water eliminative. Clinical studies of the lungs are of three general types, and pulmonary function refers to the first two: (1) physiologic measurements, which are quantitative, with results averaged (for example, expiratory minute volume under stated conditions); (2) performance, capacity, load, or stress tests, which are quantitative, with best values reported (for example, vital capacity); and (3) diagnostic tests and procedures, essentially nonquantitative, with results interpreted (for example, chest roentgenogram).

Chronic bronchopulmonary diseases are increasing rapidly in prevalence and will continue to do so for the foreseeable future because of age trends in the population and because of the inescapability of noxious respiratory exposures. The importance of pulmonary function evaluation for both clinical diagnostic and research purposes will increase accordingly. Various methods are used to evaluate the pulmonary function of patients with respiratory symptoms. These include the clinical history, physical examination, and, in certain cases, function fluoroscopy. In function fluoroscopy the patient is instructed to perform various res-piratory maneuvers that permit evaluation of thoracic and diaphragmatic structure, mobility, and excursion. Thus, an estimate can be made of ventilatory capacity, and such abnormalities as weakness or paradoxic motion of a hemidiaphragm or trapping of air during forced expiration can be detected. Chest roentgenographic examination with posteroanterior and lateral veiws in both inspiration and expiration often yields important diagnostic information but lacks any appreciable correlation with pulmonary function. Perhaps the most informative examination is the direct observation of a patient during and immediately following exercise. For this purpose nothing more complicated than a well-trained physician, a stethoscope, and a flight of stairs is required.* However, pulmonary function tests are indicated when the symptoms or degree of incapacity are greater than expected on the basis of clinical findings, where the diagnosis seems unsatisfactory or uncertain, and for preoperative evaluation of surgical and anesthetic risk in patients suspected of bronchopulmonary disease.

SIGNIFICANCE OF PULMONARY FUNCTION TESTS

A large number of pulmonary function tests are now available with which to determine the

---

*Of these, the well-trained physician is easily the most complicated.

nature and extent of pulmonary dysfunction. These tests are important both to physiology and to clinical medicine, just as cardiovascular, renal, and hepatic function tests are necessary for understanding and treatment in their respective areas. Pulmonary function tests have made, and continue to make, a valuable contribution in the following five areas: (1) basic physiologic knowledge of pulmonary function in healthy man as affected by sex, size, age, race, and physical training status; (2) information regarding pathophysiology, the natural history of cardiopulmonary diseases, and clinico-pathologic correlations; (3) diverse research, which has important implications for the rational therapy of disease, including the evaluation of various therapies and analysis of the results of surgery; (4) early detection, diagnosis, and differential diagnosis of disease; and (5) guidance for management and therapy of various cardiopulmonary diseases.

All pulmonary function tests are *diagnostic*. They are quantitative measures of the various aspects of bronchopulmonary function by means of which we define normal function and determine the nature and extent of broncho-pulmonary dysfunction. However, pulmonary function tests cannot indicate that a lesion exists, unless it impairs bronchopulmonary function sufficiently to produce clear-cut deviation from normal values; tests cannot tell *where* a lesion is, much less *what* a lesion is; they make neither *clinical* nor *pathoanatomic* diagnoses.

For example, pulmonary function tests can reveal the existence of a right-to-left circulatory shunt but cannot indicate whether such a shunt is intracardiac or intrapulmonary. They can reveal impaired diffusion across the alveolocapillary membrane but cannot distinguish either interstitial edema from intraalveolar fluid, or reduced surface area from lengthened diffusion pathway. Pulmonary function tests cannot detect slight loss of functioning pulmonary tissue or the presence of small regions in the lungs that have neither ventilation nor perfusion.

The tests may, therefore, be within normal limits in patients with minimal or even cavitary pulmonary tuberculosis or pulmonary neoplasm, unless these lesions happen to be strategically located so that they disturb bronchopulmonary function to a measurable extent. To cause detectably diminished *total lung capacity,* disease processes must be either diffuse or advanced. It is thus clear that pulmonary function tests do not reveal dysfunction in all types of bronchopulmonary disease.

Pulmonary function is measured for a variety of clinical purposes (Fig. 17-1). These include medical diagnosis, preoperative surgical and anesthetic risk evaluation, symptom or disability evaluation for legal or insurance compensation purposes, public health survey, and clinical research. Pulmonary function tests are often necessary for clinical evaluation of *symptoms* such as dyspnea, cough, and wheezing; *signs*, such as digital clubbing and cyanosis; or abnormal laboratory and chest roentgenographic findings. The definitive diagnosis of polycythemia always requires information about blood O_2 pressure and saturation and, if arterial hypoxemia is present, evaluation of pulmonary function. It is therefore clear that pulmonary function tests supplement but do not replace other clinical diagnostic procedures.

Quantitative assessment of all aspects of pulmonary function requires a variety of tests. As with physiologic tests of other organ systems, no single pulmonary function test yields all the information desired in every patient, nor are all tests necessary for the management of every patient.

The results of pulmonary function tests may or may not reflect the status of the respiratory apparatus. They do so only if the subject is cooperative and the performance-limiting factors are respiratory. Subjects may fail to cooperate fully because of nonrespiratory factors, such as communication barriers (language, sensory deficit, altered state of consciousness resulting from hypoxia, drugs, psychosis, metabolic dis-

Indications for pulmonary function tests

I. **Medical diagnostic**
   A. To measure effect of any disease on pulmonary function
   B. To follow the course of any disease affecting pulmonary function
   C. Evaluation of symptoms, signs, or laboratory findings
      1. Dyspnea, orthopnea, wheeze, cough, palpitation, chest pain, cyanosis, digital clubbing, polycythemia, chest x-ray, ECG
   D. Physical fitness selection or evaluation
   E. To reassure physician and/or patient

II. **Surgical diagnostic**
   A. Preoperative risk evaluation re anesthesia and surgery
   B. Postoperative evaluation of thoracic surgical results

III. **Disability evaluation**
   A. Rehabilitation
      1. Industrial medical
      2. Vocational rehabilitation
   B. Insurance
      1. Private
      2. Government compensation laws
   C. Legal
      1. Social security
      2. Personal injury lawsuit
      3. Other legal purposes

IV. **Public health**
   A. Epidemiologic survey

V. **Research unlimited**

Fig. 17-1. Classification of indications for referral of patients to a pulmonary function laboratory.

turbances) pain, anxiety, or actual malingering. The desire for financial compensation is an increasingly prevalent factor affecting cooperation. Nonbronchopulmonary, performance-limiting factors include neurologic, muscular, and skeletal disorders and obesity.

Failure of a patient to cooperate results in data that may suggest respiratory dysfunction. The following points are useful in assessing the *validity* of pulmonary function test data that appear to indicate a deficit:

1. The cardiopulmonary technologist's impression and report of the subject's cooperation.
2. The reproducibility, regularity, and maintenance of effort as determined from simple visual inspection of the spirographic record.
3. Internal consistency of the various test results.
4. Spirographic signs, when present.

   a. Elevation of the respiratory level of the spirographically recorded maximal voluntary ventilation.
   b. Airway collapse pattern.
   c. Air-trapping sign.

Pulmonary function tests at altitude require special consideration. Altitude differs from sea level mainly with respect to ambient barometric pressure, oxygen partial pressure, and air density. However, differences with respect to temperature, humidity, concentration, and chemical nature of gaseous and particulate air pollutants, intensity and pattern of solar radiation, and background intensity of ionizing radiation may also be of physiologic importance.

With regard to all tests of ventilatory capacity the following considerations apply. The volumetric flow rate of a gas increases with driving pressure and decreases with resistance. During laminar, or streamlined, flow the rate varies inversely as the gas viscosity. Tracheobronchial gas flow during normal, quiet breathing is laminar in the small airways and turbulent in the large ones. During tests of ventilatory capacity, turbulence increases so that the flow rate is almost directly proportional to the square root of the driving pressure and inversely proportional to the square root of the gas density. Air density decreases with altitude, resulting in both decreased turbulence and increased flow rates for any given driving pressure or effort. Proper use and, even more especially, development of prediction tables for tests of ventilatory capacity at altitude require a good grasp of these considerations.

Pulmonary function tests performed by a well-trained cardiopulmonary technologist on a cooperative subject compare favorably, with respect to both *reproducibility* and *accuracy*, to other routine clinical tests available in a general hospital.

Pulmonary function tests of various racial groups reveal significant differences. Prediction equations must thus take account of race as well as sex, age, body size, and environmental factors such as altitude. When pulmonary function studies are repeated in the same patient within a relatively short period of time, such as 1 month, it is usually proper to use the predicted values that were calculated in relation to the first study for the second study as well. What is usually sought in such instances is a change in *found* values. The use of the same *predicted* values causes the values for *percent predicted* to reflect this information directly.

SPIROMETRY

Spirometry provides information about ventilatory capacity and vital capacity. Although O_2 uptake can also be measured spirometrically, this method is less accurate than the open-circuit expired gas method. Spirographic records of quiet breathing, forced expired and inspired vital capacity, maximal voluntary ventilation, and vital capacity provide a permanent basis for comparison with later studies.

In the sedentary individual, spirometry can detect obstruction to expiration before dyspnea and wheezing are clinically apparent. In this connection the tendency of cigarette smokers to deny symptoms of cough, expectoration, dyspnea, and wheezing is of interest.

Measures of ventilatory capacity

The effect of gas density on all measures of ventilatory capacity requires consideration. Gas density decreases with altitude and may also vary under experimental conditions or in artificial cabin atmospheres. Subjects performing maximal voluntary ventilation efforts where argon or helium has been substituted for atmospheric nitrogen can readily detect the changed respiratory resistance. Increased ventilatory capacity is measurable at elevations of 1 mile (1.6 km) or less above sea level.

Maximal voluntary ventilation (MVV). The MVV is the maximal volume of gas that can be ventilated by voluntary effort during a given number of seconds, expressed as L(BTPS)/min. The subject is instructed to breathe as deeply and rapidly as he can through a low-resistance system for an arbitrarily chosen period of time, ranging from as little as 12 seconds to as much as 30 seconds. This test, also termed *maximal breathing capacity* (MBC), differs from other measures of ventilatory capacity in that (1) it involves both inspiratory and expiratory phases of ventilation; (2) it requires voluntary, sustained, maximal effort; and (3) it requires neuromuscular coordination. The graphic record provided by spirometry permits analysis of breathing frequency, tidal volume, and midposition, or end-expiratory level. The Collins 13.5-L spirometer (Respirometer) is not inferior to low-resistance, low-inertia, open-circuit methods with Douglas-type gas bag or the 120-L Collins Gasometer when used for patients with appreciable ventilatory deficit.

MVV is a valuable test when conscientiously performed and properly interpreted. It is both more complex and less sensitive than the maximal midexpiratory flow rate. It is more liable to both practice effects and fatigue effects.

Thus, the MVV is generally less suitable for evaluating the effects of drugs or other medical therapy as well as for public health screening or survey work. With some asthmatic patients the exertion of the MVV itself produces bronchospasm.

However, the spirographically recorded MVV may reveal breathing patterns of diagnostic value, such as elevation of midposition, or end-expiratory level, and airway collapse pattern. Although the expiratory phase of the MVV is always *some* portion of the forced expired vital capacity, and often an early portion, calculation of the MVV from data such as the forced expired volume at 1 second ($FEV_{1.0}$) obscures more than it illuminates.

Usually, maximal ventilation is only achieved by voluntary effort. However, during exhausting exercise the ventilation rates of healthy, trained subjects may exceed the MVV, probably because of airway dilation associated with the response to stress.

Forced expired vital capacity (FEVC). The FEVC is a simple, rapidly performed, reproducible, quantitative maneuver involving only the expiratory phase of ventilation (Fig. 17-2). From it are derived a number of useful measurements characterizing the process of forced expiration, a process that is commonly affected by diffuse bronchopulmonary disease. The subject is instructed to inspire maximally and then to blow out as hard and fast as he can until maximum expiration is achieved.

Even when diffuse bronchopulmonary obstruction affects the expiratory phase of ventilation greatly, it affects the inspiratory phase only slightly. Sustained elevation of end-expiratory level during the spirographically recorded MVV is a sensitive semiquantitative indicator that a loss of ventilatory capacity is caused by obstruction rather than restriction. Calculation of the MVV from data obtained from the FEVC curve demonstrates a degree of relationship that does indeed exist, but it should be noted that the spirographically recorded MVV provides considerable information of practical value that the FEVC cannot.

Of the entire FEVC curve, the terminal portion is predictably the most sensitive indicator of diffuse obstructive bronchopulmonary dis-

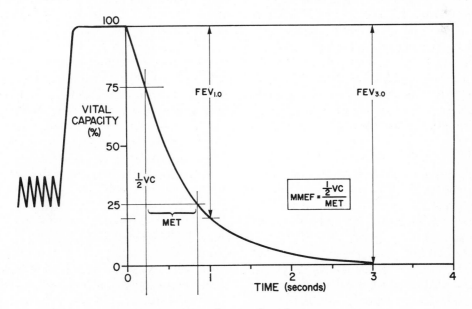

Fig. 17-2. Forced expired vital capacity.

ease. Unfortunately, the terminal portion is also relatively variable because of nonbronchopulmonary factors present during this phase of the expiratory effort. The terminal phase involves neuromuscular factors, such as maintenance and coordination of effort. Similarly, nonbronchopulmonary factors are present during the initial phase of the FEVC curve. The initial phase involves not only neuromuscular factors but also mechanical equipment factors as well, such as inertial distortion. Measurements that avoid both initial and terminal phases of the expiratory effort, such as the maximal midexpiratory flow rate, are therefore the most reliable indicators of diffuse obstructive bronchopulmonary disease.

When patients with chronic diffuse obstructive bronchopulmonary disease have appreciable obstruction to expiration, the FEVC curves are essentially exponential; at any given point in the process of forced expiration the flow rate is directly proportional to the volume. This mathematical characteristic is readily seen when the spirographically recorded FEVC is replotted on a log-linear graph (Fig. 17-3).

Maximal midexpiratory flow rate (MMEFR). The most sensitive quantitative spirometric tests for expiratory obstruction are the MMEFR and midexpiratory time. Although MMEFR is slightly less reproducible than other commonly used measurements of ventilatory capacity, its sensitivity more than makes up for this disadvantage. Indeed, one sees occasional patients in whom MMEFR and MET are clearly abnormal, whereas MVV, $FEV_{1.0}$, and $FEV_{3.0}$ are all within normal limits. This test is also called the forced expiratory flow rate, 25% to 75% ($FEFR_{25\%-75\%}$).

Midexpiratory time (MET). The MET is defined as the time required to expel the middle half of

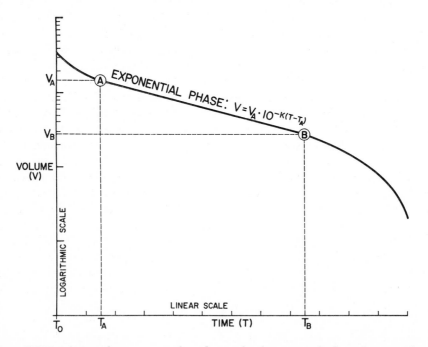

Fig. 17-3. FEVC spirographic curve replotted on a log-linear graph: bronchitis-emphysema syndrome. (An illustrative drawing, not an actual replot of data from a patient's spirographic record.)

the vital capacity during a maximally deep and rapid expiration. MET is both simple and valuable as a test of slowed expiration and is largely independent of body size. However, the MET cannot be fully interpreted without reference to the magnitude of the vital capacity.

A healthy subject can expel the entire vital capacity from the lungs in about 3 seconds and the middle half of the vital capacity in about 0.5 second (MET). In patients with severe obstructive disease the MET may be as long as 8 to 10 seconds.

Vital capacity (VC)

Vital capacity and its subdivisions can also be measured with volume recorders such as the spirometer. Expiratory vital capacity is measured by asking the subject to inspire maximally and then to expire completely into the spirometer. In this test no time limit is imposed on the subject. Unless otherwise stated, the term vital capacity is generally understood to mean *expiratory* vital capacity. In cardiac insufficiency an accentuation of the physiologic reduction of vital capacity on changing from erect to supine position is sometimes observed. Oxygen breathing reduces vital capacity at median and high altitude, probably by dilation of constricted pulmonary blood vessels. In patients with obstructive bronchopulmonary disease who trap air during forceful expiration, inspiratory vital capacity may greatly exceed expiratory vital capacity.

Spirometric signs

Analysis of the spirographic record. Analysis of the spirographic record should begin with simple visual inspection, from which certain inferences may be drawn regarding subject cooperation and data interpretability, and from which an estimate can be made regarding normality or abnormality of ventilatory capacity and vital capacity. In addition to the usual constructions and measurements that are applied to the spi-

rographic record, five spirographic signs containing valuable information can be readily appreciated by simple visual inspection: (1) emotional stress pattern, (2) elevation of end-expiratory level during the spirographically recorded MVV, (3) airway collapse pattern, (4) air-trapping sign, and (5) penmanship sign.

Emotional stress pattern (ESP). Emotional stress, whether realistic or psychoneurotic, produces a hyperventilation characterized by increased rate and depth of breathing, irregularity, and frequent, deep, sighing inspirations, often of inspiratory capacity magnitude. The resulting spirographic representation is termed *emotional stress pattern* (Fig. 17-4). This pattern is accentuated by anything that heightens emotional stress, such as provocative interrogation during a polygraph ("lie detector") test, and is diminished by anything that reduces emotional stress, such as human warmth, or tranquilizers such as meprobamate or promazine. The ESP is an objective spirographic sign containing valuable information, which is readily appreciated by simple visual inspection of the spirographic record.

Elevation of respiratory level (ERL) during the spirographically recorded MVV. The ERL during the spirographically recorded MVV is a valuable spirographic sign of increased respiratory resistance, often obstruction to expiration caused by increased airway resistance (R_{aw}). This can be readily appreciated by simple visual inspection. This elevation occurs during the first few breaths of the patient's MVV effort, and if this effort is vigorous and well sustained, the elevation may be remarkably constant throughout the entire MVV effort (Fig. 17-5). In patients with severe obstruction to expiration, elevation is quite definite and of considerable extent.

Where vital capacity and inspiratory capacity are reduced, there is less room for such elevation to occur and smaller elevations are noted. In such cases each unit of elevation, whether measured in millimeters of spirometer chart

Spirogram—supine

SH:CPL—1600M

Psychoneurosis, symptomatic
Bronchitis-emphysema syndrome, slight
Possible angina pectoris

61 WMM carpenter, height-62, weight 123.
Paroxysmal Dyspnea, 4½ years, episodes
    lasting seconds to minutes
Past history: nasal surgery

MVV_{20}	=	90
MMEF	=	1.627
MET	=	1.08
VC_{I-SU}	=	3.464
RV	=	2.108
TLC	=	5.572
RV/TLC	=	37.8

A   Supine, rest, no medication

B   Supine, awake, 15 min after promazine 25 mgm IV

C   Supine, asleep, 45 min after promazine 25 mgm IV

Collins 13.5 liter spirometer, without
CO_2-absorbing canister or flutter valves

Fig. 17-4. Emotional stress pattern.

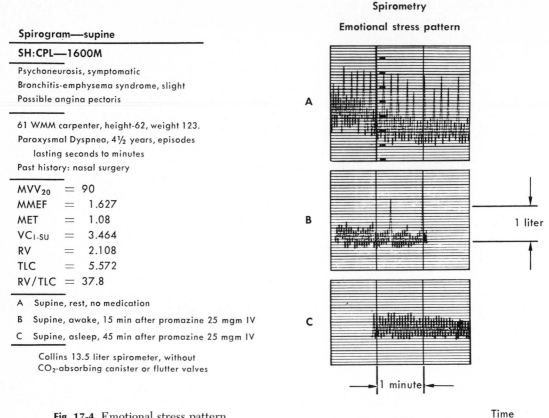

Spirometry

Emotional stress pattern

A

B

1 liter

C

1 minute

Time

paper or in milliliters of lung volume, is more significant of increased R_{aw} than the same unit in patients with normal vital capacity. Indeed, it seems likely that if appropriate correction is made for reduced vital capacity or inspiratory capacity, an appreciable, positive correlation would be found between R_{aw} and the extent of ERL.

During the MVV, ERL results in use of a higher and more favorable portion of the FEVC curve. This gives a better MVV than if ERL did not occur and, at the same time, provides the basis in these patients for comparison of MVV with $FEV_{0.75}$ or $FEV_{1.0}$. The invariably more favorable shape of the early portion of the FEVC curve, together with ERL during MVV, explains why the MMEFR is a more sensitive

measure of ventilatory capacity than the MVV. As a further consequence of ERL, the MVV in terms of percent predicted is always greater than the MMEFR expressed in similar terms, if MVV effort is vigorous and well sustained and if inspiration is not selectively impaired. Conversely, when significant obstruction to expiration is present and MVV in terms of percent predicted is less than MMEFR expressed in similar terms, this indicates failure to produce or sustain the MVV effort for any of various reasons, except in those unusual cases where something selectively interferes with the inspiratory phase of ventilation and diminishes MVV without affecting FEVC and MMEFR. Sustained ERL is a sensitive semiquantitative indicator of expiratory obstruction and in-

Spirogram—erect

RJE: CPL-2186M

Bronchitis-emphysema syndrome

40 WMM Pharmacist, Height-70, Weight-142

Exertional dyspnea
Productive cough
Occasional wheezing

Past history: multiple allergies
Chronic bronchitis

MVV_{20} = 82
MMEF = 1.491
MET = 1.25

VC_{I-SU} = 3.727
RV = 2.736
TLC = 6.463
RV/TLC = 42.3

Spirometry

Elevation of respiratory level

1 liter

2 seconds | 1 minute

Time

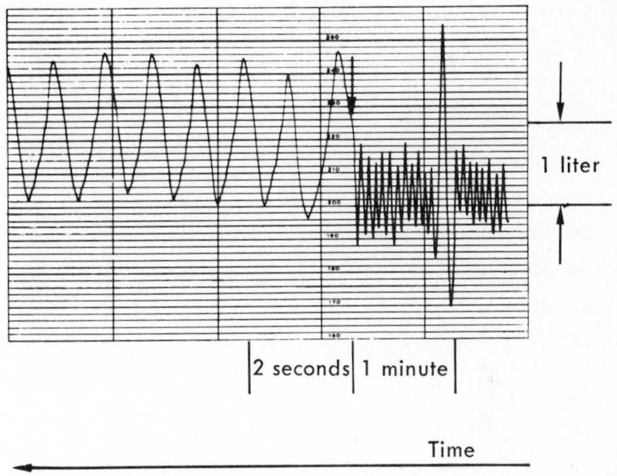

Collins 13.5 liter spirometer, without
CO_2-absorbing canister or flutter valves

Fig. 17-5. Elevation of respiratory level during spirographically recorded MVV.

creased R_{aw} that can be seen when MVV expressed in numerical terms, $FEV_{1.0}$, and $FEV_{3.0}$ are still within normal limits. Patients with restrictive, as opposed to obstructive, ventilatory impairment have abnormal tests of ventilatory capacity but do not show ERL during the spirographically recorded MVV.

Elevation of respiratory level during the spirographically recorded MVV is a simple, objective, reproducible, and valuable spirographic sign of obstruction to expiration and increased R_{aw} that is not easily simulated and that, when present, validates the measures of ventilatory capacity that may appear abnormal solely because of deficient cooperation or actual malingering.

Airway collapse pattern (ACP). The ACP consists of both notching and inflection of the initial expiratory portion of the spirographically recorded MVV and FEVC curve (Fig. 17-6). Occasionally, two or even three notches occur. The notches represent a momentary near cessation of air flow, and the inflection indicates resumption of air flow following collapse at a definitely slower rate. This spirographic pattern results during forceful expiration when the intrathoracic pressure, and therefore transairway pressure difference, becomes supraoptimal and collapses the airway.

Any lack or loss of normal airway support and/or diminution of normal airway stiffness predisposes to airway collapse (Fig. 17-7). Bronchitis-emphysema syndrome of moderate to severe degree is the clinical entity most commonly associated with ACP. ACP is almost always seen with ERL during the spirographically recorded MVV because obstruction to expiration is a factor common to both and is reflected earlier by ERL. Although notching may occur during forceful expiration as a result of supraoptimal force and intrathoracic pressure in healthy subjects, inflection does not.

ACP is a reproducible, valuable sign of chronic diffuse obstructive bronchopulmonary

Spirogram—erect

GRD: CPL-1802M

Bronchitis-emphysema syndrome

Cor pulmonale

Kyphoscoliosis

Fusion of ribs (5), right

33 WMM Guard, Height-65, Weight-123

Dyspnea, wheezing, cough,

expectoration

MVV_{20}	=	53
MMEF	=	0.271
MET	=	5.31

VC_{I-SU}	=	2.651
RV	=	2.067
TLC	=	4.717
RV/TLC	=	43.8

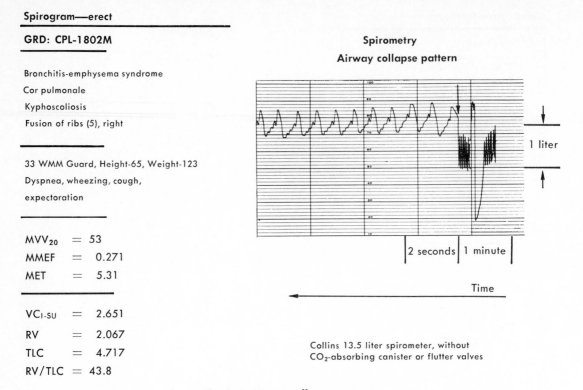

Spirometry
Airway collapse pattern

1 liter

2 seconds | 1 minute

Time

Collins 13.5 liter spirometer, without
CO_2-absorbing canister or flutter valves

Fig. 17-6. Airway collapse pattern.

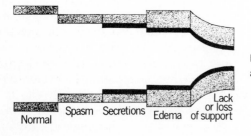

Normal Spasm Secretions Edema Lack or loss of support

Fig. 17-7. Diagrammatic representation of conditions affecting airway.

disease with abnormal airway collapsibility that is readily appreciated by simple visual inspection of the spirographic record. Because it is not easily simulated, ACP yields objective evidence of obstruction to expiration and reduced ventilatory capacity, validating other findings that may be abnormal solely as a result of deficient cooperation or actual malingering.

Air-trapping sign (ATS). The normal mechanics of inspiration and expiration are such that localized or diffuse obstructive bronchopulmonary processes tend to manifest themselves during expiration before inspiration and, first of all, during forceful expiration. When the magnitude of several forced expired vital capacities is clearly less than the magnitude of several ex-

Spirogram—supine, rest

AWS: CPL-1367F

Radiation fibrosis, lungs
sarcoma, epicardium

65 WMF Housewife, Height-58, Weight-87

Dyspnea, cough

Dependent edema

Past history: thoracotomy, Oct. 1964

Medication: prednisone

MVV_{20} = 56

MMEF = 1.845

MET = 0.33

VC_{I-SU} = 1.120

RV = 1.408

TLC = 2.528

RV/TLC = 55.7

Rest: S_{aO_2} = 78

CO_2 = 22.8 mM/L

pH = 7.50

Oxygen: S_{aO_2} = 85

Spirometry

Penmanship sign

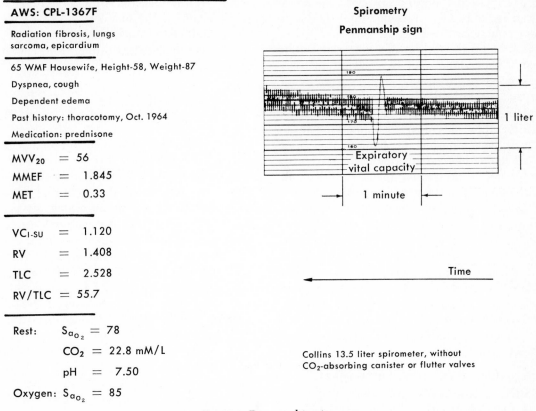

1 liter

Expiratory
vital capacity

1 minute

Time

Collins 13.5 liter spirometer, without
CO_2-absorbing canister or flutter valves

Fig. 17-8. Penmanship sign.

piratory vital capacities performed without regard to time, this disparity is termed *air-trapping sign*. Because ATS is the result of obstructive airway disease, it is almost always seen with elevation of the respiratory level during the spirographically recorded MVV and is often associated with airway collapse pattern.

ATS is reproducible, valuable evidence of air-trapping in the lungs during forceful expiration that is readily appreciated by simple visual inspection of the spirographic record. Because it is not easily simulated, ATS yields objective evidence of obstruction to expiration and reduced ventilatory capacity, validating other findings that may be abnormal solely as a result of deficient cooperation or actual malingering.

Penmanship sign. A spirographic pattern of rapid, extremely regular respirations of low tidal volume is termed *penmanship sign* for its resemblance to a penmanship exercise. It is seen in patients who have greatly diminished vital capacity and diffuse bronchopulmonary fibrosis (Fig. 17-8).

Tests of airway reactivity

It is sometimes desirable to test the sensitivity or reactivity of the airway, often in relation to the clinical diagnosis of asthmatic bronchitis. For this purpose, spirometry is repeated after the administration of bronchodilators such as isoproterenol (Isuprel) or after the administration of bronchoconstrictors such as histamine or acetylcholine. Since these are potent drugs with powerful cardiopulmonary effects, they are always used under the supervision of a physician and only after a specific order by the patient's physician.

Isoproterenol may be administered sublingually, by nebulizer, or by intermittent positive pressure breathing (IPPB) using compressed air instead of oxygen. When isoproterenol is given by IPPB, it should be noted that two things are actually being done to the patient: intrabronchial instillation of a bronchodilator and forced inflation of the lungs. Isoproterenol, as prescribed, together with a suitable volume of sterile water, is administered by IPPB at the required mask pressure, using compressed air, until the entire dose has been given. As in giving medication by any other route of administration, a certain dose is prescribed, and administration should be complete before the postbronchodilator tests are done. Isoproterenol should be administered as quickly as is compatible with the patient's comfort, and spirometry repeated soon thereafter because its effects are transient.

DETERMINATION OF FUNCTIONAL RESIDUAL CAPACITY (FRC) BY THE OPEN-CIRCUIT NITROGEN WASH-OUT METHOD

The *concentration-dilution* principle of elementary chemistry is applied: $C_1V_1 = C_2V_2$ or $V_1 = C_2V_2/C_1$. Lung nitrogen* is washed out (diluted) with almost pure oxygen in such a manner that nitrogen is neither added to nor lost from the system. Initial lung nitrogen *concentration* is assumed, and final lung nitrogen *concentration* (alveolar gas sample) is actually measured. Initial *volume* is FRC, and final *volume* is FRC plus bag volume. Correction is made both for the small nitrogen content of the almost pure oxygen and for the body nitrogen that is brought to the lungs from the tissues by the circulation during the period of oxygen

---

*Actually, *nonabsorbable* gas, mostly nitrogen.

breathing. The result of this process is represented by a simple concentration-dilution equation containing one unknown—FRC, which is accordingly determined.

FRC is calculated according to the following equation:

$$\text{FRC} = \frac{(V_B)(N_B - N_C) - C}{81 - (N_A - N_C)} \times \frac{P_B}{P_B - 47}$$

where FRC is the functional residual capacity in milliliters (BTPS); V_B is the measured volume of gas in the Douglas-type gas bag in milliliters (BTPD); N_B is the measured nitrogen concentration of gas in the Douglas-type gas bag in percent; N_C is the analyzed correction for nitrogen content of the almost pure oxygen in percent; C is the estimated correction for body nitrogen in milliliters (BTPD) brought to the lungs from the tissues by the circulation during 7 minutes of pure oxygen breathing, varying with body size and calculated for the fasting, resting subject from the linear equation $C = (BSA) \times (96.5) + 35$; 81 is the assumed initial alveolar nitrogen concentration of the fasting, resting subject in percent; N_A is the measured nitrogen concentration of alveolar gas after 7 minutes of oxygen breathing in percent; and P_B is barometric pressure in torr.

Methods involving wash-out or wash-in of inert gas measure *communicating* lung volume, as distinguished from the body plethysmograph, which measures total thoracic gas volume. The difference between the two—*noncommunicating* thoracic gas volume—is made up of the volume of any regions in the lung that are not ventilated during the test, plus the volume of any gas that is extrapulmonary but intrathoracic or intraabdominal.

After intensive therapy of diffuse obstructive bronchopulmonary conditions that involve a reversible inflammatory component, inert gas wash-out or wash-in often reveals slightly increased residual volume (RV), total lung capacity (TLC), and RV/TLC ratio. This seeming paradox is explained by the fact that previously obstructed regions of lung are less obstructed following treatment and thus contribute to the volume that is measured by the inert gas methods. Simultaneous measurement of thoracic gas volume with the body plethysmograph shows a larger difference between communicating and noncommunicating lung volume prior to treatment in such cases.

Patients with chronic diffuse obstructive bronchopulmonary disease may trap air to a variable extent during forceful expiration. Spirographic evidence of such air trapping is a useful laboratory sign. However, for calculation of TLC it is best to avoid air trapping by using *inspiratory* vital capacity, rather than the usual *expiratory* vital capacity. FRC is actually greater in the erect than in the supine position because of a shift of the midposition, or end-expiratory level (Fig. 4-2). However, subtraction of the appropriate expiratory reserve volume gives an accurate RV that is almost the same for the two different body positions. The comparative reproducibility of TLC is greater than that for RV because vital capacity with its high reproducibility comprises a large fraction of the TLC.

TESTS USED TO DETECT SMALL AIRWAYS DISEASE

Resistance to airflow in small peripheral airways normally accounts for only one third of the total R_{aw}. Thus, early or regional small airways disease may affect the distribution of inspired gas yet escape detection by conventional spirometry and measurements of total R_{aw}. Small airways involvement occurs early in the course of certain common bronchopulmonary diseases; it is important to detect it early so that diagnosis can be made and appropriate treatment begun.

One of the earliest manifestations of small airways disease detectable by routine pulmonary function testing is increased RV. Unfortu-nately, this increase occurs relatively late in the course of small airways disease. A simple, sensitive, reproducible test to detect increased small airways resistance would be very useful. Five such tests are used for this purpose.

Frequency-dependence of compliance

Use of the frequency-dependence of dynamic compliance to detect small airways disease is discussed in Chapter 6. When small airways (less than 2 to 3 mm diameter) are obstructed as a result of disease or constriction, dynamic compliance decreases as breathing frequency increases. Specifically, if compliance measured at a breathing frequency of 60 breaths/min is less than 75% of that measured at 20 breaths/min, small airways disease is probable, even if total R_{aw} and conventional spirometry are within normal limits.

Flow-volume curves

A graph of the relationship between maximal expiratory flow rate and forced expiratory volume (the flow-volume curve) is considered by some to display information regarding small airways disease more accessibly and usefully than the same information presented in the form of a conventional expiratory spirogram. A flow-volume curve is recorded on rectangular cartesian coordinates (X-Y plot) with maximal expiratory flow rate on the vertical axis and expired volume (after maximal inspiration) on the horizontal axis. If small airways are obstructed, the last part of the vital capacity is expelled at a reduced volumetric flow rate. During forced expiration of the last part of the vital capacity, maximal flow rate reflects the dimensions of airways at points where lateral airway pressure equals intrapleural pressure. As decreasing lung volume approaches RV, the points of equal pressure move into smaller airways. Reduction of maximal expiratory flow rate near the end of the forced expired vital capacity effort reflects increased resistance in small peripheral airways.

Forced expired time (FET)

FET, the time required to expel the entire vital capacity after a maximal inspiration, is a reproducible test that correlates well with the extent of small airways disease. This test is simple and does not need to be corrected for body size (standardized) before comparison with a predicted value. The final portion of the FEVC reflects small airways disease. On the average a healthy subject at sea level can expel 83% of his vital capacity in 1 second, 94% in 2 seconds, and 97% in 3 seconds. Small airways obstruction strongly affects flow rate during the final phase of the FEVC maneuver, thus increasing the duration of the expiratory effort. Measurement of the total time required to perform the FEVC maneuver may be as useful as more complicated tests for detection of early small airways obstruction, even if the early phase of the maneuver is within normal limits.

The fraction of the total FEVC that a healthy subject can exhale in 1, 2, and 3 seconds is well established, as is the average value of 0.5 second for the MET, a sensitive test of small airways disease that excludes the first and last 25% of the vital capacity. Even greater sensitivity could be achieved by examining later phases of the FEVC curve, such as the flow rates between 50% and 90% of the exhaled vital capacity.

Closing volume (CV)

The CV test measures the point during forced expiration at which small airways in the lung bases begin to close. CV is the volume of gas remaining in the lungs at the time of closure expressed as a percentage of the vital capacity. Closing volume is normally greater than RV and less than FRC, but in severe disease it can exceed FRC so that closure occurs at the level of tidal volume during spontaneous breathing.

To understand the significance of this test, one must comprehend both the distribution of inspired gas after a complete expiration and the forces that hold small airways open. During the active expiration of the expiratory reserve volume (below resting midposition level) the lower lobes of the lungs empty more completely than the upper lobes because of chest shape and rib action. Hence, the RV of the upper lobes is *proportionately* greater than that of the lower lobes. During maximal inspiration, proportionately more air goes to the lower lobes than to the upper lobes, a fact that also depends on chest size and rib action. Inhaling a single breath of pure O_2 from a position of complete expiration produces different air/O_2 ratios in the upper and lower lobes. For example, there may be 3 times as much nitrogen in the upper lobes as a result of their proportionately higher RV and lower inspired volume than in the lower lobes. A continuous recording of nitrogen concentration during a steady, slow expiration (not exceeding 0.3 L/sec) after the breath of O_2 shows a sudden increase near the end of the expiratory maneuver that reflects the point at which the lower lobe airways close and at which there is a sudden increase in the proportion of gas exhaled from the upper lobes. The test can also be done by inhaling a bolus of a tracer gas at the beginning of the inspiratory maneuver and monitoring its concentration during the subsequent slowly exhaled breath.

What causes the basilar airways to collapse during a complete expiration? The expiratory flow rate is not high. The answer is that transpulmonary pressure, which maintains the patency of small airways, is lower in the dependent basilar regions of the lungs. This is because alveolar pressure is the same throughout the lungs, but intrapleural pressure is less "negative" at the lung bases, as a result of the weight of the lungs. When lung elasticity decreases and/or when lung volume decreases (as at the end of expiration), the weight of the lung may even produce a supra-ambient (positive) intrapleural pressure at the lung bases, reversing the usual transpulmonary pressure difference. When peripheral airways are smaller as a result of constriction or disease, they close (in conformity with Laplace's Law) at higher transpulmonary pressures, even if intrapleural pressure remains "negative." Thus, CV is affected by peripheral airways disease.

CV of the lungs increases in the following conditions:

1. Age, as a result of progressive loss of lung elasticity.
2. Obesity, as a result of decreased FRC. The latter may be less than the CV, a condition that causes abnormal distribution of inspired gas.
3. Cigarette smoking, which produces small airways disease in many smokers.
4. Disease of the left side of the heart with bronchoconstriction. The latter is often reversible with β-adrenergic bronchodilators.

CV is not measurable if the distribution of inspired gas in severe bronchopulmonary disease is so abnormal that the composition of gas in the upper and lower lobes does not differ significantly. Thus, although CV is usually a sensitive test for small airways disease, it has the disadvantage of being inapplicable to patients who have severe bronchopulmonary disease.

Volume of isoflow (Viso$\dot{\text{V}}$)

During an FEVC maneuver the early flow regime is relatively turbulent and the flow rates are thus strongly dependent on gas density, whereas the final flow regime is relatively laminar and the flow rates are thus almost independent of gas density. The subject performs two FEVC maneuvers—the first after filling the lungs with air and the second after filling the lungs with an 80% helium–20% oxygen gas mixture that is much less dense, but somewhat more viscous, than air. The two FEVC maneuvers are recorded as flow-volume curves and compared. Beyond the point in the two maneuvers where flow has become relatively laminar,

the two curves are almost congruent. The obstruction in small airways disease results in earlier slowing of expiratory flow and thus earlier development of a relatively laminar flow regime. Hence, the lung volume at which the two curves intersect and become congruent (Viso$\dot{\text{V}}$) is larger than that of healthy subjects. This interesting test is being evaluated for use in early detection of small airways disease.

ARTERIAL BLOOD STUDY

Analysis of arterial blood for CO_2, O_2, and pH provides basic information about cardiopulmonary function. Although somewhat more difficult to obtain than capillary or venous samples, arterial blood is essential for this purpose and there is no satisfactory substitute. Arterial blood, with rare exceptions, is a stream of uniform composition. It has the further advantage of reflecting cardiopulmonary function more directly than capillary or venous blood possibly can, since these latter sources are subject to the complicating effects of changing regional and tissue conditions.

Arterial puncture and placement of an indwelling cannula is a procedure that requires aseptic technic and involves the potential hazards of hematoma, nerve trauma, and infection. Obviously, this is a procedure for the physician. With proper technic, complications are extremely rare and almost never constitute a contraindication to this vital source of information.

Principles of blood-gas and pH analysis

It must be stressed that collection, storage, and analysis of blood for CO_2, O_2, and pH present unique problems that are not encountered when blood is used for other clinical chemical determinations. Competency in clinical blood chemistry does not necessarily imply competency in blood analysis for CO_2, O_2, and pH. Indeed, familiarity with clinical blood chemistry often breeds contempt for the necessary precautions that are termed *anaerobic technic.* Anaerobic technic is based on knowledge of the physical chemistry and physiology of blood as a tissue. This technic comprises all those methods and devices that ensure that blood composition, with respect to the interdependent parameters of CO_2, O_2, and pH, does not suffer violence from the time of withdrawal from the circulation to the time of analysis. Time and again, individuals without adequate instruction or understanding of the relevant principles collect, prepare, or store blood samples in such a manner that they are totally worthless.

Blood samples should be drawn with the least possible traction, suction, or pulling force. Evacuated containers that draw blood samples into a vacuum are worthless for this purpose. In drawing systemic arterial samples, it is often possible to avoid traction completely. Blood samples with air bubbles should be discarded. Blood samples should be analyzed immediately. If this is impossible, maximum immersion of the syringe up to but not above the flange, or shoulder, in ice water with immediate and continuous refrigeration is imperative. When blood is allowed to stand after removal from the circulation, the erythrocytes sediment at a rate that is characteristic for each subject. Before withdrawal of any aliquot for analysis, the whole blood sample must be thoroughly mixed by shaking or rotation to ensure identical composition of each. Transfer of the blood sample should also be done quickly to avoid such separation. In general, blood should be handled with care because erythrocytes are fragile and hemolysis produces complex changes that may be undesirable. If blood samples contain anesthetic gases, such as nitrous oxide, or volatile liquids, appreciable analytic errors can result because of their solubility in or reaction with absorbent solutions. Presence of such gases should be taken into account.

Blood pH is a function of temperature. The pH of human whole blood rises with falling temperature at a rate of 0.0147 pH unit/° C. The relationship of hemoglobin oxygenation to blood pH should not be ignored. If the pH of a highly saturated arterial blood sample is measured and its hemoglobin then completely reduced, holding P_{CO_2} constant, pH increases 0.06 to 0.07 unit. The P_{O_2} decreases as whole blood stands. This decrease is largely caused by the metabolism of the white blood cells. As whole blood stands, metabolic acidosis develops—fixed acids increase and pH falls. Initially, the pH decrease is about 0.001 pH unit/min. Subsequent changes are less predictable and also depend on whether fluoride has been added. Sodium fluoride should not be added to blood samples for pH determination because pH should be determined within minutes in any case and because the addition of sodium salts aggravates the glass electrode sodium error. Large P_{CO_2} gradients from blood sample to room air are always present and favor loss of CO_2, or respiratory alkalosis. *Dried* heparin minimizes dilution of the blood sample.

Several systems are commercially available, incorporating pH, P_{CO_2}, and P_{O_2} electrodes, for clinical service and research use. The *Astrup micromethod* for blood-gas and pH analysis is a widely used system in which P_{CO_2} is estimated from a nomogram rather than measured directly. This method involves the use of the *Siggaard-Andersen curve nomogram*, which is discussed in Chapter 11. A correction must be made when the oxyhemoglobin saturation of the blood sample is less than 100%; for each 1 gm/dL of unsaturated hemoglobin the pH−log P_{CO_2} line is moved 0.005 pH unit to the left. The Astrup micromethod gives values for CO_2 content that are about 2 mM/L lower than the results of standard methods. This problem is still unsolved and may be caused by metabolic acidosis, respiratory alkalosis, hemoglobin oxygenation, or the use of an assumed pK (6.11) that is too high. If *cutaneous* blood* must be used in place of the preferred *arterial* sample, the hand should be immersed in hot water for 3 to 5 minutes before puncture. Squeezing and consequent *dilution* of the cutaneous blood sample with tissue juice results in characteristic errors.

Blood O_2 capacity

Blood samples for determination of O_2 capacity must be obtained in relation to blood samples drawn for O_2 content not only at rest but also for each different physiologic state. For example, hemoglobin concentration and O_2 capacity may undergo considerable change during exercise or O_2 breathing. Arterial blood samples should be used for determination of blood O_2 capacity whenever possible. Samples of venous blood are less satisfactory for this purpose because of their lower and more variable initial O_2 content.

By exposure in a closed container to a volume of O_2 or by exposure to successive volumes of fresh air, the blood sample is brought toward equilibrium with the water vapor–saturated gas. The multiple air-equilibration method is preferable because (1) air has a sufficiently high P_{O_2} when ambient pressure is approximately that at sea level for almost complete saturation of the hemoglobin, (2) air is readily available, and (3) the composition of air is precisely known.

Note that this method of measuring blood O_2 capacity involves the near equilibration of whole blood with saturated air at *ambient* pressure and *room* temperature. Such blood samples are therefore different from blood samples drawn anaerobically from a subject. Dissolved O_2 content is larger at any given P_{O_2} than that in blood samples with the same P_{O_2} at body temperature.

---

*One should try to obtain the cutaneous blood sample from the *arterial* end of the capillaries.

Blood O_2 saturation

In calculation of oxyhemoglobin saturation, both total O_2 content and total O_2 capacity are corrected by subtraction of their respective values for dissolved O_2. The following three methods for obtaining dissolved O_2 are in general use:

1. Dissolved O_2 can be obtained by the estimation and assumption of standard values.

2. Calculation of approximate saturation can be made by dividing the uncorrected content by the uncorrected capacity. The resulting quotient is then used together with arterial pH to find P_{O_2} from the oxyhemoglobin dissociation curve (Fig. 10-4). This method can only be used when P_{O_2} is below 100 torr, where the slope of the oxyhemoglobin dissociation curve is appreciable.

3. After actual measurement of P_{O_2} with an O_2 electrode, dissolved O_2 can be calculated by multiplication with the factor for the appropriate temperature (Table 8).

O_2 method for detection of venous-to-arterial circulatory shunts

The brachial or radial arteries of either upper extremity may be used in this method, giving a choice of four possible sites. Although the femoral arteries are larger, they are less desirable if exercise is anticipated because exercise is awkward with the indwelling cannula in this location.

Venous-to-arterial circulatory shunts, also termed right-to-left shunts, can be detected by failure to achieve full arterial blood O_2 pressure and saturation after 15 minutes of O_2 breathing. Thebesian venous blood from the coronary circulation empties into the left ventricle, constituting a tiny physiologic right-to-left shunt. Pathoanatomic right-to-left shunts include intrapulmonary (arteriovenous fistula), intracardiac, and bronchial artery–to–pulmonary vein types. Pathoanatomic shunts may be quite large, diverting a sizable fraction of the cardiac output away from contact with alveolar gas. In chronic hepatic disease, shunts may occur that result in arterial O_2 saturation values of less than 90%. Anatomic localization of large venous-to-arterial shunts is possible in many cases with angiography; however, their existence and functional significance can be determined by the O_2 method.

The subject is given a high-O_2 breathing mixture for 15 minutes, with a deep breath each minute. The temptation to cut this period short must be resisted, or equivocal data will result in certain cases, and the question of venous-to-arterial shunt will remain unanswered. Concentrations of O_2 from 60% to 100% may be used for the test. Lower O_2 concentrations, such as 60%, are advantageous where only O_2 content, capacity, and saturation are measured and where a standard correction for dissolved O_2 is used. In this case the error introduced by assuming a value for dissolved O_2 is minimized because dissolved O_2 is a smaller value than that obtained if higher O_2 concentrations were breathed. Furthermore, if O_2 saturation is used, it is important to note that hemoglobin concentration and O_2 capacity decrease during O_2 breathing.

Actual measurement of P_{O_2} with an O_2 electrode is considerably more sensitive than measurement of O_2 content, capacity, and saturation. The correction for dissolved O_2 can then be calculated for each subject. Breathing 100% O_2 at sea level can be calculated to produce a maximum alveolar P_{O_2} of 673 torr. Water vapor tension and CO_2 pressure are subtracted from the barometric pressure : 760 − 47 − 40 = 673 torr. However, actual found values for arterial P_{O_2} in healthy subjects breathing 100% O_2 at sea level range from 610 to 660 torr. When pulmonary function is tested for clinical purposes, the highest arterial P_{O_2} achieved is used, and a value less than 550 torr is considered to indicate a venous-to-arterial shunt.

Formulas have been proposed for estimation of the magnitude of right-to-left shunts. These require arterial, mixed venous, and pulmonary end-capillary O_2 data. Such calculations ignore the effects of any ventilation/perfusion ($\dot{V}_A/\dot{Q}_c$) or diffusion abnormality that may be present, relying on the fact that their interference is minimized during high O_2 breathing. Determination of mixed venous blood O_2 involves catheterization of the right side of the heart and calculation of absolute values for shunt flow requires simultaneous measurement of cardiac output.

INTERPRETATION OF CARDIOPULMONARY LABORATORY DATA

Before cardiopulmonary laboratory data are interpreted, they should be examined for *internal consistency* and *credibility*. Data are internally consistent if there are no internal contradictions and credible if they are within bounds of the possible. Such examination sometimes leads to a question about a particular value in a set of data, so that certain tests can be repeated or calculations checked.

1. The respiratory exchange ratio (R_E), as calculated from measurement and analysis of expired gas, provides interesting and valuable information in fasting subjects. Because it is appreciably affected by both composition and quantity of food taken prior to study, interpretation is a complex matter in nonfasting subjects. The R_E, which equals the metabolic respiratory quotient (R) during steady state conditions, varies from about 0.70 to 0.86 in fasting subjects at rest. Factors that increase R_E are as follows:

   a. Hyperventilation, before attainment of a steady state of respiratory alkalosis or during recovery from hypoventilation.

   b. Exercise, where increase is the result of increased CO_2 exhalation, as metabolic acidosis develops, and later the result of preferential carbohydrate utilization by working muscles after achievement of a nearly steady state.

c. Postabsorptive metabolic conversion of nutrient substances, a process accelerated by exercise.

Factors that decrease R_E are as follows:

d. Hypoventilation, before attainment of a steady state of respiratory acidosis or during recovery from hyperventilation.

e. Exercise, before attainment of a steady state.

f. Loss of CO_2 when expired gas is permitted to stand in Douglas-type gas bags.

If an expired gas sample is simply mixed with atmospheric air, then calculated CO_2 output, O_2 uptake, and R_E all remain unchanged because $F_{E_{CO_2}}$ and $F_{E_{O_2}}$ are affected proportionately.

2. MVV in terms of percent predicted exceeds the MMEFR expressed in similar terms, except in cases where the process of inspiration is selectively affected or where the subject cannot or will not sustain the MVV effort.

3. Arterial blood O_2 saturation cannot exceed 100% under any conditions, including rest, hyperventilation, and breathing high O_2 mixtures. In cases where the calculated value does exceed 100%, this may be the result of incorrect values for (a) total whole blood O_2 content, (b) total whole blood O_2 capacity, (c) either of their respective corrections for dissolved O_2, or (d) any combination of these.

4. Hemoglobin concentration as calculated from O_2 capacity almost always decreases promptly when high O_2 mixtures are breathed and increases promptly during exercise.

5. If analyses are correct, the CO_2 content of simultaneously drawn mixed venous blood must exceed that of systemic arterial blood, which must in turn exceed that of a capacity blood sample prepared by the multiple air-equilibration method.

6. During exercise a metabolic acidosis characterized by decreased arterial blood pH and CO_2 content is almost always seen. This pattern may be complicated in certain cases by hyperventilation during exercise, producing concomitant respiratory alkalosis, or by superimposed respiratory acidosis in patients with severe ventilatory deficit.

To facilitate the interpretation of data obtained by study of their patients, the staff of each laboratory should make an effort to develop a concept of their own normal values for healthy subjects. Normal values vary from laboratory to laboratory because of differences in location, equipment, and personnel. The concept of normal values should include measures of central tendency (arithmetic means), reproducibility of the various test procedures (standard deviations), and comparative reproducibility of one test procedure with another (coefficients of variation, or dispersion relative to the mean).

DIFFERENTIAL DIAGNOSIS OF ARTERIAL HYPOXEMIA

Arterial hypoxemia is a clinically important manifestation, the differential diagnosis of which involves basic physiologic principles. The four causes of arterial hypoxemia are usually present in one or another combination but in certain instances may occur in almost pure form. They follow in order of their clinical frequency: (1) abnormality of $\dot{V}_A/\dot{Q}_c$ ratios, (2) alveolar hypoventilation, (3) loss of pulmonary diffusing capacity, and (4) pathoanatomic venous-to-arterial shunts.

It is possible to test for item 4 quite readily. Arterial blood samples are drawn for O_2 analysis both before and after the patient breathes

Table 11. Functional classification of cardiopulmonary insufficiency in bronchitis-emphysema syndrome (a chronic obstructive bronchopulmonary syndrome of multifactorial causation)

Functional stage	Pathologic physiology		Clinical manifestations	
	Pulmonary function evaluation	Comment	Bronchitis	Emphysema
IA	Reduced ventilatory capacity; Increased CV; Increased RV, TLC, and RV/TLC ratio	Low MMEFR may be the only spirometric evidence of reduced ventilatory capacity; Elevation of respiratory level seen in spirographically recorded MVV	May be asymptomatic	May be asymptomatic
IB	Impaired intrapulmonary mixing		Cough; Expectoration; Wheeze; Chronic or recurrent bronchitis	Exertional dyspnea
IIA	Arterial P_{O_2} falls during moderate exercise	Arterial hypoxemia during moderate exercise, but not at rest	TLC normal or slightly increased	TLC moderately or greatly increased
IIB	$\dot{V}_A/\dot{Q}_c$ abnormality; Arterial P_{O_2} and S_{O_2} low at rest; Arterial P_{CO_2} low or WNL*	Arterial hypoxemia at rest; Airway collapse may occur during forced expiration; Air-trapping may occur during forced expiration	Respiratory alkalosis with compensatory metabolic acidosis; Pulmonary arterial hypertension; Marked hypoxemia; Cyanosis	Respiratory alkalosis with compensatory metabolic acidosis; Weight loss; Pulmonary arterial hypertension; Slight hypoxemia; "Pink puffer"
IIIA	Arterial P_{CO_2} high; Arterial CO_2 content high	CO_2 retention, slight to moderate	Respiratory acidosis with compensatory metabolic alkalosis; Cor pulmonale; Cardiac insufficiency; Polycythemia; "Blue bloater"	
IIIB	Arterial pH WNL*; Arterial pH low	CO_2 retention, severe; Uncompensated respiratory acidosis	Susceptibility to O_2-induced CO_2 narcosis	

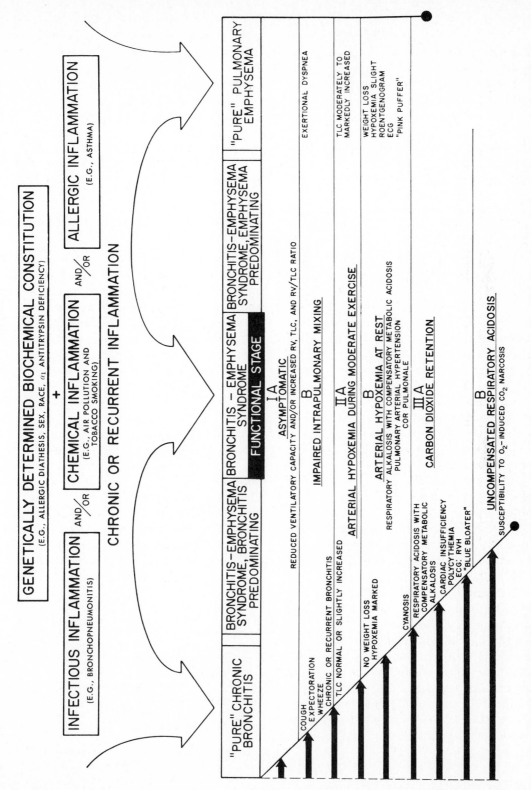

Fig. 17-9. Spectrum of the bronchitis-emphysema syndrome, a chronic obstructive bronchopulmonary syndrome of multifactorial causation.

60% to 100% O_2 for 15 minutes with a deep breath every minute. The resulting increased alveolar P_{O_2} is sufficient to overcome any bronchopulmonary factor, so that full arterial blood O_2 pressure and saturation result, unless pathoanatomic venous-to-arterial shunts are present.

If the subject's condition permits, he is next exercised by means of a bicycle ergometer or treadmill, erect or supine, at a steady work rate judged to be safe by the physician. The exercise period should be of at least 5 minutes duration and, if possible, should be standardized with respect to both work rate and duration. In follow-up studies it is highly desirable for purposes of comparison that any given subject repeat the same work stint done in the prior study. Treadmill work rate is determined by grade and speed. Bicycle ergometer work rate is determined by load setting and RPM. When venous-to-arterial shunts are present, exercise produces a further decrease of arterial P_{O_2} and saturation because the shunted mixed venous blood then contains even less O_2.

Two important clinical observations are relevant. First, arterial hypoxemia *always* precedes CO_2 retention in the course of chronic diffuse bronchopulmonary disease. Second, patients with sufficiently impaired pulmonary diffusing capacity demonstrate arterial hypoxemia, yet they have arterial P_{CO_2} values that are either low because of hyperventilation or are within normal limits. The explanation of these two observations involves the physiologic significance of $\dot{V}_A/\dot{Q}_c$ ratios, the slope of the two dissociation curves for O_2 and CO_2, and the fact that CO_2 is about 20 times as diffusible as O_2 across the alveolocapillary membrane.

In hypoxemia, rational clinical treatment includes efforts to increase alveolar ventilation, as with a mechanical respirator, and the use of increased concentrations of O_2 sufficient to restore arterial P_{O_2} to normal or near normal levels (70 to 100 torr). This can often be accomplished with O_2 administered at low flow rates, such as 1 to 3 L/min.

As already mentioned, the prevalence of chronic bronchopulmonary disease is increasing rapidly. The largest single clinical entity contributing to this increase is the *bronchitis-emphysema syndrome*,* a spectrum of chronic conditions of multifactorial causation. Because of its prevalence and the wide range of pathophysiologic problems it produces, we present Fig. 17-9 and Table 11, which give the basis for etiologic analysis and functional classification of patients.

MECHANICALLY ASSISTED AND CONTROLLED VENTILATION

If a healthy subject breathes gas at 20 to 30 torr above ambient pressure through a mask or mouthpiece, his lungs inflate rapidly to total lung capacity. *Continuous positive pressure breathing* (CPPB)† then involves periodic active, forced exhalations, which are followed automatically by passive inhalation from the pressurized source. However, such a system produces sustained intrathoracic pressure elevation, impeding the return of venous blood to the heart, thus limiting the pressure that can be used. Higher pressures seriously impede venous circulation unless the subject, at some time during the ventilatory cycle, inhales actively with sufficient force to reduce intrathoracic pressure, allowing venous blood to return to the chest. Hence, although CPPB increases the altitude ceiling for a pilot by increasing the total pressure in which the various constituent gases participate, it cannot be used above an altitude of 50,000 feet (15,250 M) because the high positive

---

Chronic bronchitis is characterized pathologically by hyperplasia and hypertrophy of the bronchial mucous glands, chronic inflammatory cell infiltration and edema of the bronchial mucosa, and squamous metaplasia of the respiratory epithelium. *Pulmonary emphysema* is characterized pathologically by widespread focal degeneration of elastic tissue, reticulum and collagen formation at the sites of elastic fiber damage, attenuation and disappearance of alveolar capillaries, and the fenestration and dissolution of alveolar septa.

†Also called *continuous positive airway pressure* (CPAP).

pressure required to maintain normal blood oxygenation pools blood excessively in dependent body regions, producing syncope.

Intermittent positive pressure breathing (IPPB) systems deliver positive pressure in bursts that inflate the lungs and chest but, in contrast with CPPB, passive exhalation occurs between bursts as pressure falls to ambient level in the mask or mouthpiece. IPPB machines can deliver pure O_2, room air, or a mixture of the two. High-O_2 breathing mixtures can be delivered directly from source to subject without change of composition, or they can be diluted with room air by routing them through an air-entraining venturi. The gas source is usually a cylinder of compressed medical gas or an air compressor.

A sensitivity control sets the inspiratory effort necessary to trigger the inspiratory phase over a range of subambient pressures. The inspiratory phase is triggered by the development of subambient pressure prior to each inspiration. Inspiratory flow rate is controlled by a variable orifice that impedes the constant-pressure gas stream beyond the regulator. Peak inspiratory pressure can be selected to stop the inspiratory phase at any desired cutoff pressure.

Expiratory flow can be retarded by a removable multiorificed cap placed over the exhaust port of the exhalation valve. Retardation of expiratory flow minimizes airway collapse and air-trapping and also favors aerosol retention. Moderately increased intrapulmonary pressure during expiration (PEEP) is of therapeutic value for patients who have pulmonary vascular congestion, pulmonary edema, or increased lung compliance. However, expiratory flow should be retarded carefully because, if too severe, increased intrathoracic pressure will impede venous return, decrease cardiac output, and produce syncope.

The respiratory therapist can thus adjust a mechanical respirator to compensate for such patient variables as thoracic compliance, R_{aw}, and TLC, thus assisting any breathing pattern.

Certain mechanical respirators can be adjusted to *control* ventilation automatically in the apneic patient. When it is necessary to override a patient's spontaneous breathing pattern (to *control* pulmonary ventilation), the respiratory therapist can independently control sensitivity, inspiratory flow rate, peak inspiratory pressure, and expiratory flow rate, creating almost any conceivable ventilatory pattern. Respirators can be connected directly to masks, to mouthpieces, or by adaptors, to endotracheal tubes, tracheotomy tubes, or spirometers. A respirator should have a safety valve that opens if a subject's inspiratory demand exceeds the rate of gas delivery from the respirator or if the gas supply should fail. An expiratory gas port allows expired gas to be collected for measurement and analysis.

In general, every effort should be made to minimize external (apparatus) dead space. However, IPPB often hyperventilates the lungs, causing hypocapnia and respiratory alkalosis. In such cases increased dead space is needed to prevent hyperventilation-induced hypocapnia. IPPB may also, especially in obtunded patients, distend the stomach. Hypovolemic patients are especially susceptible to the circulatory effects of IPPB and hence to syncope. The clinical indications for IPPB treatment include inordinate work of breathing, lung failure, pulmonary edema, atelectasis, prolonged apnea, and respiratory arrest. Contraindications include pulmonary hemorrhage, pneumothorax, and mediastinal or subcutaneous emphysema.

Medication in aerosol form is administered by inhalation in treatment of various bronchopulmonary diseases. Such aerosols are commonly administered by IPPB machines, which deposit minute droplets of medications such as bronchodilators, antimicrobials, or glucocorticosteroids in the airway. Sometimes larger volumes of aqueous liquids are administered to facilitate bronchial hygiene or to moisten the airway and its secretions. Synchronization of nebulization with the inspiratory phase of breathing conserves medication. Some nebulizers have a built-in port for connection to a liquid reservoir by means of tubing.

Positive end-expiratory pressure (PEEP) is a method of clinical importance. Used in conjunction with mechanical ventilation, it increases FRC, tends to prevent atelectasis, and tends to reduce alveolar-arterial (A-a) P_{O_2} difference. PEEP may also permit significant reduction of inspired O_2 concentration, while maintaining arterial blood P_{O_2} at acceptable levels. It is of particular value in patients who are hypoxemic as a result of venous-to-arterial shunting of blood in unventilated but perfused lung regions.

PEEP is essential in the treatment of adult respiratory distress syndrome (ARDS), a pulmonary complication of trauma, shock, aspiration, or fat embolization. In this syndrome, decreased lung compliance, microatelectasis, and intrapulmonary shunting produce respiratory alkalosis and hypoxemia that are unrelieved by pure O_2 administered by mask or even by IPPB. Death may occur within 48 to 72 hours unless effective treatment is given. From 5 to 15 cm H_2O of PEEP are usually applied. Blood oxygenation may improve in minutes or only after many hours. Full recovery is usual if the patient survives.

However, PEEP is not without risk. As with IPPB, it tends to decrease cardiac output in patients who are hypovolemic or who have lost sympathetic vascular tone as a result of anesthesia, morphine, or ganglionic blockade. Occasionally, diseased lung tissue ruptures, producing pneumothorax.

Proper sterilization of medical respirators and their accessories is extremely important. Failure to follow adequate aseptic procedure can cause serious bronchopulmonary infection. Any components exposed to high moisture levels, such as breathing tubes, nebulizer, exhalation valve, reservoirs of water or saline, and certain accessories, are potential culture media for pathogenic microorganisms. The segment of the system between the respirator and the patient who is under controlled ventilation must be replaced at regular intervals with a clean one. Transparent plastic construction permits inspection of internal parts for performance and cleanliness.

Some respirators fit snugly around the anterior chest. When the pressure is reduced within this shell, the chest is drawn forward, increasing lung volume. Such respirators can be set to operate at a variety of amplitude and frequency combinations, producing adequate ventilation if the airway is patent.

Drinker-type "iron lung" respirators enclose all the body below the neck. The subject's head protrudes and a rubber collar fits snugly around the neck. As pressure around the body decreases, the chest expands, causing air to flow down the airways into the lungs. This respirator can be operated at a variety of frequencies and amplitudes to produce adequate ventilation.

The phrenic nerve can be isolated as it passes down the anterior neck and may be stimulated at this point by a device that delivers an electric pulse of predetermined amplitude, duration, and frequency. When used properly, such an electrophrenic respirator produces unilateral diaphragmatic contraction of amplitude sufficient to simulate normal resting ventilation.

Barometric ventilation involves yet another device that encloses the body in one chamber and the head in a different but adjacent chamber. Pressures outside and within the chest change simultaneously. A small opening between the two chambers slows the pressure change in the chamber surrounding the body so that this change is in phase with gas flow into and out of the airways. This phase coincidence stops all chest and lung movement. During one phase of the ventilatory cycle the lungs contain many gas molecules; during the other the lungs contain far fewer. Gas flows up and down the airways, but the chest and lungs do not move. Subjects who have been in this respirator report experiencing more complete rest than ever before in their lives.

The variety of mechanical respirators now available affords a wide choice of mechanical characteristics. First, a decision must be made between a *pressure*-cycled versus a *volume*-cycled pressure breathing system. Because patients differ greatly with respect to respiratory resistance and compliance, no categoric statement can be made regarding the optimal settings of a mechanical respirator. In general, low breathing frequencies (8 to 12 breaths/min), large tidal volumes, slow flow rates, and an expiratory cycle longer than the inspiratory cycle are desirable. Some mechanical ventilators can be set to deliver an occasional deep breath (simulated sigh), decreasing the risk of atelectasis. Elevated P_{CO_2} in patients who have chronic respiratory acidosis should be reduced progressively but *gradually*. Rapid, large P_{CO_2} decreases (more than 20 torr/hr) can produce hazardous alkalosis. While alveolar ventilation is being artificially controlled, arterial blood gas and pH determinations are *indispensable* for adjustment of the mechanical respirator.

APPENDIX

Table A-1. Symbols and abbreviations for respiratory physiology (based on standardization of definitions and symbols in respiratory physiology, Fed. Proc. 9:602, 1950)

Symbol or abbreviation	Definition
Primary variables	
C	Concentration of gas in blood phase
D	Diffusing capacity in general; volume per unit time per unit pressure difference
F	Fractional concentration in dry gas phase
f	Breathing frequency; breaths per unit time
P	Gas pressure in general
$\bar{P}$	Mean gas pressure
Q	Volume of blood
$\dot{Q}$	Rate of blood flow
R	Respiratory exchange ratio in general—$\dot{V}_{CO_2}/\dot{V}_{O_2}$ (Use small uppercase subscript E when R is based on analysis of mixed expired gas.)
S	Saturation of hemoglobin with oxygen or carbon monoxide in percent
V	Gas volume in general (Pressure, temperature, and water vapor tension must also be given.)
$\dot{V}$	Gas volume per unit time; rate of gas flow
Secondary symbols for the gas phase*	
A	Alveolar gas
B	Barometric
D	Dead space gas
E	Expired gas
I	Inspired gas
L	Lung
T	Tidal gas
Secondary symbols for the blood phase	
a	Arterial blood (specify exact location)
b	Blood in general
c	Capillary blood (specify exact location)
v	Venous blood (specify exact location)
$\bar{v}$	Mixed venous blood

*All symbols are small uppercase letters.

240

Table A-1. Symbols and abbreviations for respiratory physiology—cont'd

Symbol or abbreviation	Definition
Other secondary symbols and abbreviations	
ATPD*	Ambient temperature, ambient pressure, dry
ATPS*	Ambient temperature, ambient pressure, saturated with water vapor
BTPD*	Body temperature, ambient pressure, dry
BTPS*	Body temperature, ambient pressure, saturated with water vapor
STPD*	Standard temperature, standard pressure, dry
$\underline{s}$	Subscript to denote the steady state
$\overline{X}$	Dash above any symbol used to indicate a mean value
$\dot{X}$	Dot above any symbol used to indicate a rate
Pulmonary function tests and measurements	
For lung volume and its subdivisions	
ERV	Expiratory reserve volume; maximal volume that can be expired from resting expiratory level
FRC	Functional residual capacity; volume of gas in lungs at resting expiratory level
IC	Inspiratory capacity; maximal volume that can be inspired from resting expiratory level
IRV	Inspiratory reserve volume; maximal volume that can be inspired from end-tidal inspiratory level
RV	Residual volume; volume of gas in lungs at end of maximal expiration
TLC	Total lung capacity; volume of gas in lungs at end of maximal inspiration
VC	Vital capacity; maximal volume that can be expired after maximal inspiration
For ventilatory capacity	
SINGLE BREATH TESTS†	
FEVC	Forced expiratory vital capacity; following maximal inspiration, entire vital capacity volume is expelled as rapidly as possible
FEV_T‡	Forced expiratory volume, timed; volume that has been expired at any time T during forced expiratory vital capacity
FEV_T%‡	Percent of vital capacity volume that has been expired at any time T during forced expiratory vital capacity
MEFR	Maximal expiratory flow rate; average rate of flow during expulsion of the liter from 200 to 1,200 ml during forced expiratory vital capacity
MET	Midexpiratory time; time required for expulsion of middle half of vital capacity during forced expiratory vital capacity
MMEFR	Maximal midexpiratory flow rate; average rate of flow during expulsion of middle half of vital capacity during forced expiratory vital capacity
PEFR	Peak expiratory flow rate

*Small uppercase letters.   *Continued.*
†To abbreviate corresponding *inspiratory* measurements, substitute I for E.
‡Subscript T is a small uppercase letter.

Table A-1. Symbols and abbreviations for respiratory physiology—cont'd

Symbol or Abbreviation	Definition
For ventilatory capacity—cont'd	
MULTIPLE BREATH TESTS	
MBC$_T$* or MVV$_T$*	Maximal breathing capacity or maximal voluntary ventilation calculated from an effort of T seconds' duration
MVV$_f$	Maximal voluntary ventilation at designated breathing frequency
MVV$_F$	Maximal voluntary ventilation at free breathing frequency

*Subscript T is a small uppercase letter.

Table A-2. Conversion table for units of measure

1 inch	2.54001 centimeters
1 centimeter	0.39370 inch
1 foot	0.30480 meter
1 meter	3.28083 feet; 39.3700 inches
1 pound	0.45359 kilogram
1 kilogram	2.20462 pounds
1 ounce	28.34953 grams
1 gram	0.03527 ounce
1 quart	0.94633 liter
1 liter	1.0561 quarts
1 micrometer (μm)	10^{-4} centimeter
1 angstrom unit (Å)	10^{-8} centimeter
1 watt (absolute)	10^7 ergs/sec
1 watt (absolute)	0.10197 kgm $\times$ m/sec

Table A-3. Mathematical constants

		Number	Square root
π	3.14159	2	1.41421
e	2.71828	3	1.73205
$\log_{10}$ e	0.43429	5	2.23607
$\ln_e$ 10	2.30259	6	2.44949
1 radian	57.29578° or 57° 17' 45"	7	2.64575
1 degree	0.01745 radian	8	2.82843
		10	3.16228

USEFUL DATA AND CONSTANTS

Absolute zero, $0°$ K $= -273.16°$ C
Water vapor tension, $P_{H_2O} = 47.067$ torr at $37.0°$ C
Avogadro's number $= 6.023 \times 10^{23}$ molecules/mole
Gas constant, R $= 8.31432 \times 10^7$ ergs/°K/mole
Gram-molecular volume of an "ideal" gas $= 22,414$ ml (STPD)
Gram-molecular volume of $CO_2 = 22,260$ ml (STPD); hence,

$$CO_2 \text{ content (mM/L)} = \frac{CO_2 \text{ content (vol\%)}}{2.226}$$

Air density (STPD) $= 1.2929$ gm/L
Mercury density at $0°$ C $= 13.5955$ gm/ml
Mercury density at $25°$ C $= 13.5340$ gm/ml
Water density, maximum at $3.98°$ C $= 1.0000$ gm/ml
Velocity of sound in air (STPD) $= 1,087.1$ feet/sec or $33,136$ cm/sec
Acceleration due to gravity, g, at sea level and $45°$ latitude $= 32.172$ feet $\times$ sec^{-2} or
    980.62 cm $\times$ sec^{-2}
1 atmosphere $= 760$ torr, 29.9 inches Hg; 1.03 kgm/cm^2; 14.7 pounds/square inch
1 gallon of water weighs approximately 8.3 pounds
1 cubic foot of water weighs approximately 62.4 pounds
Hydrostatic pressure increases with water depth by approximately 0.1 atm/M, the exact value
    depending on salinity, temperature, and latitude
Heat of fusion of water at $0°$ C $= 79.71$ cal/gm
Heat of vaporization of water at $100°$ C $= 539.55$ cal/gm
Whole blood: specific gravity $= 1.055$
Hemoglobin: 1 gm capable of combining with 1.36 ml (STPD) of O_2

VALUES PECULIAR TO EACH DIFFERENT LABORATORY

The value generally used to convert pressure from units of torr to CGS units of dynes/cm^2 is $1,330$ (mercury density $\times$ acceleration due to gravity). This value varies slightly with temperature (mercury density varies with temperature), altitude, and latitude (acceleration due to gravity, g, varies with *both* altitude and latitude).

Predicted values for certain pulmonary function tests vary somewhat from laboratory to laboratory, depending on technic and equipment. Altitude, in particular, affects certain tests.

RESPIRATORY CALCULATIONS

The ability to represent a relationship or problem in mathematical terms and the power to manipulate and solve it are invaluable. Mathematical manipulation of biologic data is a valuable exercise and sometimes leads to discovery of important facts and relationships. However, the results of such manipulation must always be finally interpreted in terms of what is biologically meaningful, what is biologically possible, and what is cause (independent variable) and what is effect (dependent variable).

    1. General gas law describing "ideal gas":

        A.   PV $=$ nRT

For calculating change of state, mass remaining constant:

B. $\dfrac{P_1 V_1}{T_1} = \dfrac{P_2 V_2}{T_2}$

The following formulas for conversion of gas volume are merely special cases of B:

C. $V_{STPD} = V_{ATPS} \times \dfrac{(P_B - P_{H_2O}) \times 0.35942}{(T°C + 273.16)}$

D. $V_{BTPS} = V_{ATPS} \times \dfrac{310.16}{273.16 + T°C} \times \dfrac{P_B - P_{H_2O}}{P_B - 47.067}$

E. $V_{BTPD} = V_{ATPS} \times \dfrac{310.16}{273.16 + T°C} \times \dfrac{P_B - 47.067}{P_B}$

F. $V_{STPD} = V_{BTPS} \times \dfrac{273}{310} \times \dfrac{(P_B - 47)}{760}$

2. For calculation of O_2 *uptake* (A) or CO_2 *output* (B) from measurement of volume and analysis of composition of mixed expired gas while breathing any mixture of O_2 and CO_2 in nitrogen or other inert gases (all gas volumes are STPD):

A. $\dot{V}_{O_2} = \dot{V}_E \times \dfrac{[F_{I_{O_2}} (1 - F_{E_{CO_2}}) - F_{E_{O_2}} (1 - F_{I_{CO_2}})]}{(1 - F_{I_{O_2}} - F_{I_{CO_2}})}$

B. $\dot{V}_{CO_2} = \dot{V}_E \times \dfrac{[F_{E_{CO_2}} (1 - F_{I_{O_2}}) - F_{I_{CO_2}} (1 - F_{E_{O_2}})]}{(1 - F_{I_{O_2}} - F_{I_{CO_2}})}$

Equation B divided by equation A gives the *respiratory exchange ratio* for expired gas:

C. $R_E = \dfrac{\dot{V}_{CO_2}}{\dot{V}_{O_2}} = \dfrac{[F_{E_{CO_2}} (1 - F_{I_{O_2}}) - F_{I_{CO_2}} (1 - F_{E_{O_2}})]}{[F_{I_{O_2}} (1 - F_{E_{CO_2}}) - F_{E_{O_2}} (1 - F_{I_{CO_2}})]}$

For the special case where CO_2 may be considered negligible in the inspired gas, equations A, B, and C reduce to simpler forms. If measurements are made in the steady state, then $R_E = R_s$ = metabolic respiratory quotient.

3. For calculation of *respiratory dead space* (all gas volumes are BTPS):

A. $V_D = \left(V_T - \dfrac{\dot{V}_A}{f}\right)$ or $\dot{V}_A = (V_T - V_D)f$

Bohr equation for *respiratory dead space to any gas, G:*

B. $V_{D_G} = \dfrac{(F_{E_G} - F_{A_G}) \times V_T}{(F_{I_G} - F_{A_G})}$

4. For calculation of *alveolar O_2 pressure* while breathing any mixture of O_2 with inert gas at any ambient pressure:

$P_{A_{O_2}} = F_{I_{O_2}} (P_B - P_{A_{H_2O}}) - P_{A_{CO_2}} \left[F_{I_{O_2}} + \dfrac{(1 - F_{I_{O_2}})}{R_A}\right]$

This equation is sometimes called the *alveolar gas equation*, although it applies equally well to any portion of expired gas that has undergone respiratory exchange. It is useful for determining equivalent altitudes and O_2 requirements for cabin or chamber atmospheres (Fig. A-1).

5. For calculation of *alveolar ventilation* from respiratory gas exchange:

$$\dot{V}_A = \frac{\dot{V}_{CO_2}}{F_{A_{CO_2}}} = \frac{R_A}{F_{A_{CO_2}}} \times \dot{V}_{O_2} = (P_B - P_{A_{H_2O}}) \times \frac{R_A}{P_{A_{CO_2}}} \times \dot{V}_{O_2}$$

6. For calculation of *pulmonary diffusing capacity* to O_2 by the Bohr method:

$$D_{L_{O_2}} = \frac{\dot{V}_{O_2}}{P_{A_{O_2}} - \overline{P}_{c_{O_2}}}$$

where $\overline{P}_{c_{O_2}}$ is the mean O_2 pressure in pulmonary capillary blood obtained by graphic integration of the oxyhemoglobin dissociation curve.

7. For calculation of *pulmonary blood flow* by the Fick principle:

$$\dot{Q}_b = \frac{\dot{V}_{O_2}}{(C_{a_{O_2}} - C_{\overline{v}_{O_2}})}$$

This equation assumes a steady state of the circulation and respiration and assumes that the two blood samples are simultaneously drawn midway during the mixed expired gas collection.

8. For calculation of the ratio of *alveolar ventilation* to *pulmonary blood flow*:

$$\frac{\dot{V}_A}{\dot{Q}_b} = R_s \,(P_B - P_{A_{H_2O}}) \times \frac{(C_{a_{O_2}} - C_{\overline{v}_{O_2}})}{P_{A_{CO_2}}}$$

This equation assumes a steady state of the circulation and respiration and assumes that the two blood samples are simultaneously drawn midway during the mixed expired gas collection.

9. *van der Waals' equation:*

$$P + \frac{a}{V^2} \times (V - b) = RT$$

where P and V are the pressure and volume at any constant temperature and a and b are constants; R is the gas constant and T is the absolute temperature. For values of R, a, and b, consult appropriate tables.

10. *Laplace's law* for bubbles (two surfaces):

A. $$P = \frac{4T}{r}$$

where P is pressure in dynes/cm^2 due to surface tension in a bubble of mean radius r cm for a liquid whose surface tension is T dynes/cm.
Laplace's law for drops (one surface):

B. $$P = \frac{2T}{r}$$

11. *Hydrostatic pressure:*

    P = hdg

    where d is the density of the liquid and h is the depth below the surface.
    Total force on an area A due to hydrostatic pressure:

    F = PA = Ahdg

    If h is in cm, d in gm/cc, and g in cm $\times$ sec^{-2}, then force will be in dynes and
    pressure in dynes/cm^2.

12. *Poiseuille's law* for laminar flow rate of fluids through a tube:

    $$\dot{V} = \frac{\pi \times \Delta P \times r^4}{8 \times L \times N}$$

    where L is the length of the tube, r is its radius, ΔP is the driving pressure, N is
    the coefficient of viscosity, and $\dot{V}$ is the volumetric flow rate per second. If L and
    r are in cm, ΔP in dynes/cm^2, and N in poises or dyne $\times$ sec $\times$ cm^{-2}, then
    volumetric flow rate is in cc/sec. Note that density does not appear in this equa-
    tion.

13. *Reynolds' number calculation:*

    $$N_R = \frac{v \times d \times 2r}{n}$$

    where N_R is Reynolds' number indicating the tendency to turbulence, v is *aver-
    age linear velocity* of gas in the airway, r is the radius of the airway, d is gas
    density, and n is absolute gas viscosity. If consistent units are used, the results
    are dimensionless.

14. *Bernoulli's law:* at any point in a tube through which a liquid is flowing, the sum
    of the pressure energy, potential energy, and kinetic energy is constant:

    P + hdg + ½ dv^2 = a constant

    where P is pressure, h is height above a reference plane, d is density of the
    liquid, and v is linear flow velocity.
    Diminution of pressure at the side of a moving stream:

    P = ½ dv^2

    for a fluid of density d, moving with a velocity v, the diminution of pressure P,
    neglecting viscosity, resulting from motion.

15. To prepare a gas mixture containing any intermediate concentration (F_3) of a gas
    (G) from two gas mixtures containing G in higher (F_1) and lower (F_2) concentra-
    tions, respectively.*†

---

*Resulting intermediate concentration will be only approximate, so that chemical analysis is required for ac-
curate determination of concentration.
†Gasometer dead space must be considered.

Case 1: $F_2 > 0$

A. $F_1V_1 + F_2V_2 = F_3V_3$

B. $V_1 + V_2 = V_3$

C. $\dfrac{V_1}{V_2} = \dfrac{F_3 - F_2}{F_1 - F_3}$

Case 2: $F_2 = 0$

A. $\dfrac{V_1}{V_2} = \dfrac{F_3}{F_1 - F_3}$

Table A-4. Altitude-pressure table*

Altitude (M)	Altitude (feet)	P_B† (torr)	$(P_B - 47)$‡ (torr)	$0.209\,(P_B - 47)$§ (torr)
0	0	760	713	149
610	2,000	707	660	138
1,220	4,000	656	609	127
1,830	6,000	609	562	118
2,440	8,000	564	517	108
3,050	10,000	523	476	100
3,660	12,000	483	436	91
4,270	14,000	446	399	83
4,880	16,000	412	365	76
5,490	18,000	379	332	69
6,100	20,000	349	302	63
6,710	22,000	321	274	57
7,320	24,000	294	247	52
7,930	26,000	270	223	47
8,540	28,000	247	200	42
9,150	30,000	226	179	37
9,760	32,000	206	159	33
10,370	34,000	187	140	29
10,980	36,000	170	123	26
11,590	38,000	155	108	23
12,200	40,000	141	94	20
12,810	42,000	128	81	17
13,420	44,000	116	69	14
14,030	46,000	106	59	12
14,640	48,000	96	49	10
15,250	50,000	187	40	8
19,215	63,000	47	0	0

*From Rahn, H., and Fenn, W. O.: A graphical analysis of the respiratory gas exchange, Washington, D.C., 1955, The American Physiological Society, p. 41. (Source of data: W. G. Brombacher, Nat. Adv. Com. Aer. Report 538, 1935.)

†P_B = barometric pressure.

‡$(P_B - 47)$ = (a) total pressure of the dry gases after the inspired gas has been saturated with water vapor at 37° C and (b) inspired O_2 pressure, P_{IO_2}, when pure oxygen is inspired.

§$0.209\,(P_B - 47)$ = inspired O_2 pressure, P_{IO_2}, when air is breathed.

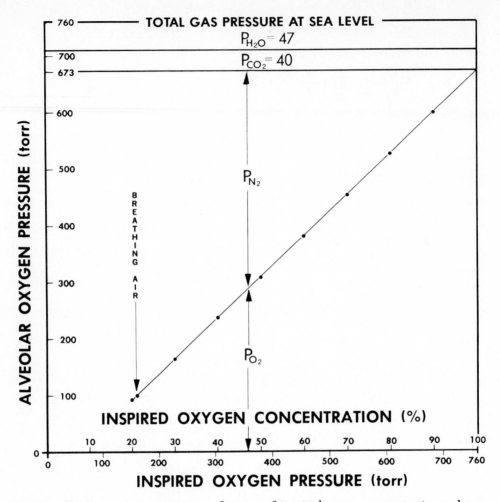

Fig. A-1. Alveolar oxygen pressure as a function of inspired oxygen concentration and pressure. This graph shows the alveolar O_2 pressure that results at sea level from breathing any given concentration or pressure of O_2 within the indicated range. Values for alveolar O_2 pressure were calculated using the alveolar gas equation, assuming barometric pressure to be 760 torr, alveolar water vapor tension to be 47 torr, alveolar CO_2 pressure to be 40 torr, and alveolar respiratory exchange ratio to be 0.85. Note that (1) total gas pressure is the simple arithmetic sum of the individual partial pressures (Dalton's law); (2) as inspired O_2 pressure increases to the maximum of 760 torr, alveolar O_2 pressure increases at the expense of alveolar nitrogen pressure to the maximum achievable (after denitrogenation) value of 673 torr; (3) the rightward displacement of the line from the undrawn line of identity represents the rate of O_2 uptake in the lungs; (4) the slope of the line (0.947) is less than 1 because lung gas is saturated with water vapor at 37° C and contains CO_2; and (5) despite the slope of less than 1, a slightly less than fivefold increase of inspired O_2 pressure results in a greater than sixfold increase of alveolar O_2 pressure. (Originator: N. Balfour Slonim.)

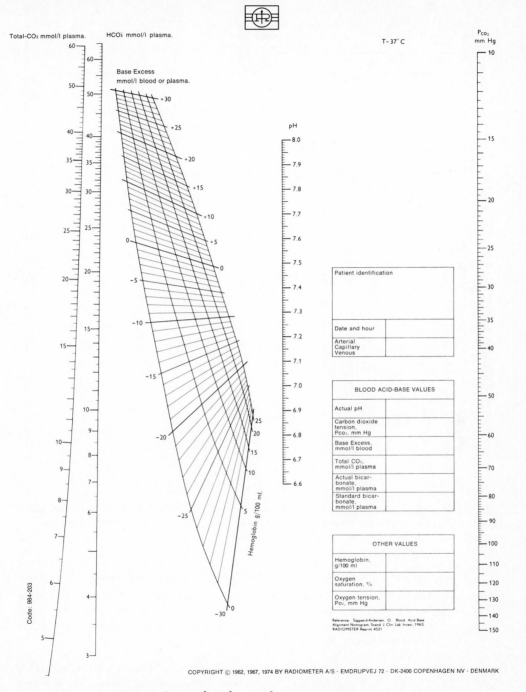

Fig. A-2. Siggaard-Andersen alignment nomogram.

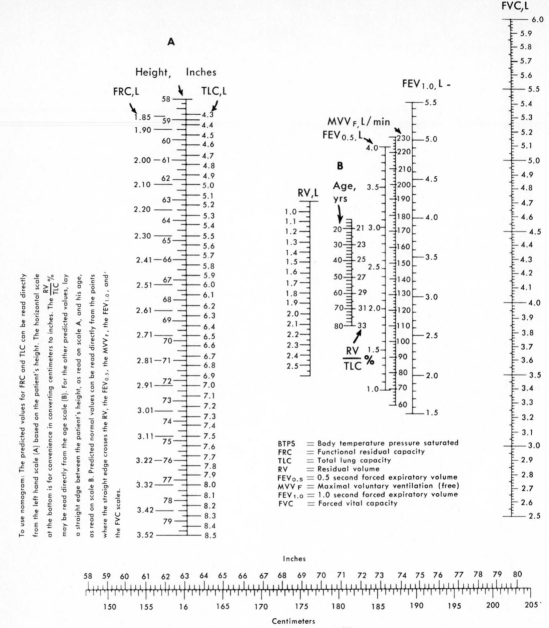

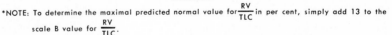

Fig. A-3. Pulmonary function prediction nomogram: healthy men. All gas volumes are BTPS. FRC, TLC, and RV are for semirecumbent position. $FEV_{0.5}$, MVV_F, $FEV_{1.0}$, and FVC are for standing position. (From Boren, H. G., Kory, R. C., and Syner, J. C.: Am. J. Med. **41**:96, 1966.)

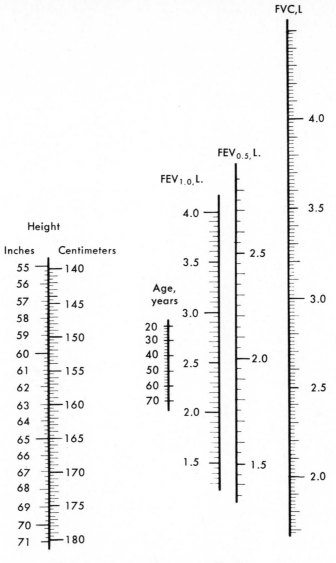

To use nomogram: Lay a straight edge between the patient's height as read on the height scale, and her age as it appears on the age scale. Predicted normal values for FEV$_{1.0}$ and FVC can be read directly from the points where the straight edge crosses the two right hand scales.

Fig. A-4. Pulmonary function prediction nomogram: spirometry in healthy women. This nomogram has been modified for use at 25° C (room temperature). Thus observed, volumes from a Vitalor spirometer record can be compared directly with these predicted values without temperature correction. FEV$_{0.5}$ is the forced expiratory volume in liters at one-half second, FEV$_{1.0}$ is the forced expiratory volume in liters at 1 second, and FVC is the forced expiratory vital capacity. (Unpublished work of Kory, R. A., and Callahan, R.)

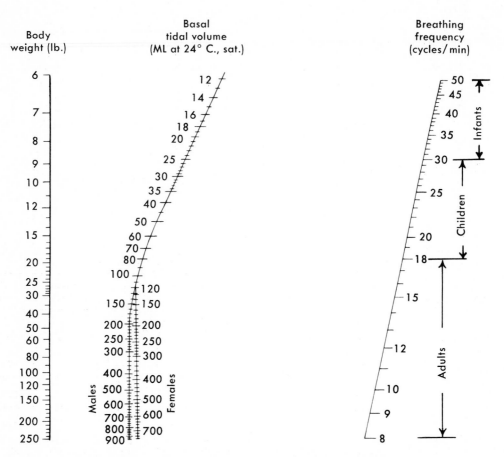

Fig. A-5. Radford prediction nomogram: body weight, tidal volume, and breathing frequency. Nomogram for predicting the basal tidal volume from breathing frequency, body weight, and sex. The following corrections may be needed: *daily activity,* add 10%; *fever,* add 5% for each degree above 99° F (rectal); *altitude,* add 5% for each 2,000 feet (610 M) above sea level; *metabolic acidosis during anesthesia,* add 20%; *tracheotomy and endotracheal intubation,* subtract a volume equal to 50% of the body weight; and *added dead space with anesthesia apparatus,* add volume of apparatus and mask dead space. Patients who have bronchopulmonary disease need larger tidal volumes. (From Radford, E. P., Jr., Ferris, B. Jr., and Kriete, B. C.: N. Engl. J. Med. **251:**877, 1954.)

Table A-5. Greek alphabet

Greek character		Greek name	Greek character		Greek name
A	α	alpha	N	ν	nu
B	β	beta	Ξ	ξ	xi
Γ	γ	gamma	O	o	omicron
Δ	δ	delta	Π	π	pi
E	ε	epsilon	P	ρ	rho
Z	ζ	zeta	Σ	σ	sigma
H	η	eta	T	τ	tau
Θ	θ	theta	Υ	υ	upsilon
I	ι	iota	Φ	φ	phi
K	κ	kappa	X	χ	chi
Λ	λ	lambda	Ψ	ψ	psi
M	μ	mu	Ω	ω	omega

Table A-6. Alphabetical table of the elements with international atomic weights

Element	Symbol	Atomic number	Atomic weight	Element	Symbol	Atomic number	Atomic weight
Actinium	Ac	89	227*	Cobalt	Co	27	58.9332
Aluminum	Al	13	26.98	Copper	Cu	29	63.54
Americium	Am	95	243*	Curium	Cm	96	247*
Antimony	Sb	51	121.75	Dysprosium	Dy	66	162.50
Argon	Ar	18	39.948	Einsteinium	Es	99	254*
Arsenic	As	33	74.9216	Erbium	Er	68	167.26
Astatine	At	85	210*	Europium	Eu	63	151.96
Barium	Ba	56	137.36	Fermium	Fm	100	253*
Berkelium	Bk	97	247*	Fluorine	F	9	18.9984
Beryllium	Be	4	9.0122	Francium	Fr	87	223
Bismuth	Bi	83	208.980	Gadolinium	Gd	64	157.25
Boron	B	5	10.811	Gallium	Ga	31	69.72
Bromine	Br	35	79.909	Germanium	Ge	32	72.59
Cadmium	Cd	48	112.40	Gold	Au	79	196.967
Calcium	Ca	20	40.08	Hafnium	Hf	72	178.49
Californium	Cf	98	249*	Helium	He	2	4.0026
Carbon	C	6	12.01115	Holmium	Ho	67	164.930
Cerium	Ce	58	140.12	Hydrogen	H	1	1.00797
Cesium	Cs	55	132.905	Indium	In	49	114.82
Chlorine	Cl	17	35.453	Iodine	I	53	126.9044
Chromium	Cr	24	51.996	Iridium	Ir	77	192.2

The atomic weights listed are those adopted in 1963 by the International Commission on Atomic Weights.
*Mass number of the isotope of longest known half-life or a better known one.

Table A-6. Alphabetical table of the elements with international atomic weights—cont'd

Element	Symbol	Atomic number	Atomic weight	Element	Symbol	Atomic number	Atomic weight
Iron	Fe	26	55.847	Radon	Rn	86	222*
Krypton	Kr	36	83.80	Rhenium	Re	75	186.2
Lanthanum	La	57	138.91	Rhodium	Rh	45	102.905
Lawrencium	Lr	103	257*	Rubidium	Rb	37	85.47
Lead	Pb	82	207.19	Ruthenium	Ru	44	101.07
Lithium	Li	3	6.939	Samarium	Sm	62	150.35
Lutetium	Lu	71	174.97	Scandium	Sc	21	44.956
Magnesium	Mg	12	24.312	Selenium	Se	34	78.96
Manganese	Mn	25	54.9380	Silicon	Si	14	28.086
Mendelevium	Md	101	256*	Silver	Ag	47	107.870
Mercury	Hg	80	200.59	Sodium	Na	11	22.9898
Molybdenum	Mo	42	95.94	Strontium	Sr	38	87.62
Neodymium	Nd	60	144.24	Sulfur	S	16	32.064†
Neon	Ne	10	20.183	Tantalum	Ta	73	180.948
Neptunium	Np	93	237*	Technetium	Tc	43	99*
Nickel	Ni	28	58.71	Tellurium	Te	52	127.60
Niobium	Nb	41	92.906	Terbium	Tb	65	158.924
Nitrogen	N	7	14.0067	Thallium	Tl	81	204.37
Nobelium	No	102	256*	Thorium	Th	90	232.038
Osmium	Os	76	190.2	Thulium	Tm	69	168.934
Oxygen	O	8	15.9994	Tin	Sn	50	118.69
Palladium	Pd	46	106.4	Titanium	Ti	22	47.90
Phosphorus	P	15	30.9738	Tungsten	W	74	183.85
Platinum	Pt	78	195.09	Uranium	U	92	238.03
Plutonium	Pu	94	242*	Vanadium	V	23	50.942
Polonium	Po	84	210*	Xenon	Xe	54	131.30
Potassium	K	19	39.102	Ytterbium	Yb	70	173.04
Praseodymium	Pr	59	140.907	Yttrium	Y	39	88.905
Promethium	Pm	61	147*	Zinc	Zn	30	65.37
Protactinium	Pa	91	231*	Zirconium	Zr	40	91.22
Radium	Ra	88	226*				

The atomic weights listed are those adopted in 1963 by the International Commission on Atomic Weights.
*Mass number of the isotope of longest known half-life or a better known one.
†Because of natural variations in the relative abundance of the isotopes of sulfur, the atomic weight of this element has a range of ±0.003.

GLOSSARY

acclimatization The physiologic process or the resulting state of adjustment of an individual that develops in response to repeated or prolonged exposure to an unaccustomed stressor or environment. Acclimatization usually results in increased tolerance to the given stressor. *Synonyms:* acclimation, adaptation.

acid A chemical substance that is a proton donor in aqueous solution.

acidemia Systemic arterial blood plasma pH less than the normal value of 7.41 ± 0.02 for healthy adult man at rest. The blood of human newborns, infants, and pregnant women may deviate from this value. *Antonym:* alkalemia.

acidosis A clinical term for the disturbance of acid-base balance in body fluids that results from an increase of acidic chemical substances (proton donors) and/or loss of basic chemical substances (proton acceptors). If the accumulating substance is CO_2 (an acid anhydride that reacts with water to form carbonic acid), the condition is *respiratory acidosis*. If the accumulating acidic substance is other than CO_2 (nonvolatile acids) or if basic substances are lost, the condition is *metabolic acidosis*. Homeostatic body mechanisms respond to acidemia initiating physiologic processes that tend to restore plasma pH to normal. In respiratory acidosis, the kidneys respond to acidemia by retaining HCO_3^- and thus increasing plasma HCO_3^- concentration; in metabolic acidosis, the lungs respond to acidemia by increasing alveolar ventilation rate and thus decreasing arterial blood P_{CO_2}. Such physiologic compensation may be complete (pH restored to normal) or incomplete (pH remains low). *Antonym:* alkalosis.

acidosis, metabolic Nonrespiratory acidosis.

acidosis, respiratory The acidotic condition of the body that results from hypercapnia. Acute hypercapnia produces acute respiratory acidosis, whereas during chronic hypercapnia homeostatic renal responses tend to correct the initial pH decrease by producing a secondary metabolic alkalosis. *Synonym:* CO_2 acidosis.

adaptation, genetic Genetic changes that increase the tolerance of a species to a stressor during generations of exposure. Adaptation favors survival in the presence of the given stressor.

air spaces All alveolar ducts, alveolar sacs, and alveoli. *Contrast:* airways.

airway conductance Instantaneous volumetric gas flow rate in the airway per unit of pressure difference between the airway opening (mouth, nares, or cannula opening) and the alveoli; the reciprocal of airway resistance. *Abbreviation:* G_{aw}. *Units:* liters $\times$ sec^{-1} $\times$ (cm H_2O)$^{-1}$.

airway resistance The ratio of pressure difference between the airway opening (mouth, nose, or cannula opening) and the alveoli to the simultaneously measured resulting instantaneous volumetric gas flow rate. *Abbreviation:* R_{aw}. *Units:* cm H_2O $\times$ liter^{-1} $\times$ sec^{-1}.

airways All conducting passageways of the respiratory tract from mouth or nares down to and including respiratory bronchioles. *Symbol:* aw. *Contrast:* air spaces.

alkalemia Systemic arterial blood plasma pH greater than the normal value of 7.41 ± 0.02 in healthy adult man at rest. The blood of human newborns, infants, and pregnant women may deviate from this value. *Antonym:* acidemia.

alkalosis A clinical term for the disturbance of acid-base balance in body fluids that results from an increase of basic chemical substances (proton acceptors) and/or loss of acidic chemical substances (proton donors). If the lost substance is CO_2 (an acid anhydride that reacts with water to form carbonic acid), the condition is *respiratory alkalosis*. If the lost acidic substance is other than CO_2 (nonvolatile acids) or if basic substances accumulate, the condition is *metabolic alkalosis*. Homeostatic body mechanisms respond to alkalemia initiating physiologic processes that tend to restore plasma pH to normal. In respiratory alkalosis, the kidneys respond to alkalemia by excreting HCO_3^- and thus decreasing plasma HCO_3^- concentration; in metabolic alkalosis, the lungs respond to alkalemia by decreasing alveolar ventilation rate and thus increasing arterial blood P_{CO_2}. Such physiologic compensation may be complete (pH restored to normal) or incomplete (pH remains high). *Antonym:* acidosis.

alkalosis, metabolic Nonrespiratory alkalosis.

alkalosis, respiratory The alkalotic condition of the body that results from hypocapnia. Acute hypocapnia produces acute respiratory alkalosis, whereas during chronic hypocapnia homeostatic renal responses tend to correct the initial pH increase by producing a secondary metabolic acidosis. The cause of hypocapnia and respiratory alkalosis is alveolar hyperventilation, which may be psychogenic, the result of fever or drugs such as salicylates, or a response to altitude. *Synonym:* CO_2 alkalosis.

alveolar Of or pertaining to pulmonary alveoli or the regions of the lungs in which respiratory gas exchange occurs.

alveolar-arterial end-capillary gas pressure difference The gas pressure difference that exists between alveolar gas and pulmonary capillary blood as the latter leaves the alveolus. *Units:* torr.

alveolar-arterial gas pressure difference The difference between the measured or calculated mean partial pressure of a gas such as O_2, CO_2, or N_2 in alveoli and the simultaneously measured partial pressure of that gas in systemic arterial blood. Such differences reflect, among other factors, ventilation-perfusion mismatching. By convention, a negative difference indicates that the partial pressure of the gas is higher in systemic arterial blood than it is in alveolar gas. *Units:* torr. *Symbol:* example for oxygen, $P_{A_{O_2}} - P_{a_{O_2}}$; also sometimes AaD_{O_2} or $(A-a)\Delta$.

alveolar gas In theory, the gas mixture present within gas-exchanging regions of the lungs, reflecting the combined effects of alveolar ventilation and respiratory gas exchange. In practice, expired gas that has come from the alveoli and gas-exchanging regions. Definition of alveolar gas composition is complicated by (1) the discontinuous nature of the process of pulmonary ventilation, (2) the regional variation of pulmonary capillary perfusion, (3) the regional variation of inspired gas distribution, (4) the imperfect matching of these two aspects of lung function, and (5) the technical problems of alveolar gas sampling. Alveolar gas is assumed to be saturated with water vapor at 37° C. *Contrast:* dead space gas.

alveolar gas volume The aggregate volume of gas in the lung regions within which respiratory gas exchange occurs. *Symbol:* V_A. *Contrast:* bronchopulmonary dead space.

alveolar ventilation If the bronchopulmonary system functioned perfectly, alveolar ventilation rate could be defined simply as the difference between tidal volume and anatomic dead space volume multiplied by the breathing frequency. However, physiologically alveolar ventilation rate can only be defined in terms of the arterial blood P_{CO_2}, which almost always reflects the total *effective* alveolar ventilation rate.

ambient Of or pertaining to an existing or prevailing environmental condition.

anaerobic Of or pertaining to the absence or exclusion of atmospheric air and, specifically, molecular O_2. For example, anaerobic microorganisms grow in the absence of O_2, and anaerobic metabolism proceeds in the absence of O_2.

anemia Generally, a quantitative lack or loss of blood. A quantitative blood deficiency of hemoglobin, red blood cells, or hematocrit. *Antonym:* polycythemia.

angiocardiography Visualization of selected segments of the cardiovascular system by roentgenography after rapid intravascular injection of a radiopaque contrast medium.

anlage An embryologic rudiment. The first discernible group of cells in a developing embryo that will ultimately form a given anatomic structure.

anoxia Absence or total lack of molecular oxygen.

apnea Cessation or absence of breathing movements, such as the transient cessation of breathing in anesthetized animals after hyperventilation.

apneusis A ventilatory pattern characterized by an intense sustained contraction of inspiratory muscles. Apneusis is observed in a vagotomized cat whose rostral pons has been transected, separating the pontine pneumotaxic center (NPBM) from the pontine apneustic center.

asphyxia A condition of restricted or even absent gas exchange characterized by increased CO_2 partial pressure above, and decreased O_2 pressure below, normal values. Hypoventilation causes asphyxia throughout the body; regional asphyxia results when the rate of blood flow through an organ is low relative to that organ's metabolic rate.

atelectasis *Absorption atelectasis* is the collapse of distal lung air spaces after obstruction of the proximal airway and consequent absorption of the trapped gas. The tendency for atelectasis increases if the lungs contain readily absorbable gas such as oxygen. *Primary atelectasis* is the failure of lung regions of the newborn infant to expand normally with air at birth.

ATPS conditions of a volume of gas The conditions of a volume of gas at ambient temperature, ambient pressure, and saturated with water vapor. These conditions exist in a water-sealed spirograph or gasometer when the water temperature equals ambient temperature. *Abbreviation:* volume (ATPS).

baroreceptor A specialized neural structure that senses changes of systemic arterial blood pressure and reflexly initiates compensatory changes of heart rate and systemic vascular resistance.

basal metabolic rate The rate of energy exchange of human beings measured with the subject at rest, in the postabsorptive state, and under conditions of thermal neutrality. The results are expressed as a percentage above or below a standard value established for healthy subjects of the same age and sex.

base A chemical substance that is a proton acceptor in aqueous solution.

base excess A measure of metabolic alkalosis or metabolic acidosis (negative values of base excess) expressed as the amount of strong acid or strong alkali required to titrate a sample of 1 L of blood to pH 7.40. While being titrated, the blood sample is kept at 37° C, fully oxygenated and, by equilibration, at a P_{CO_2} of 40 torr. *Abbreviation:* BE. *Units:* mEq/L.

blood buffer capacity The maximum amount of H^+ that can be made to combine with the solutes in 1 L of blood. Normal capacity is from 45 to 53 mEq/L. In practice, it is estimated as the sum of the bicarbonate ions, the anionic charges on hemoglobin and plasma proteins, and much smaller amounts of phosphate and other buffers. *Units:* mEq/L.

blood-gas tension The partial pressure of a gas in the blood. At equilibrium, the partial pressures of a given gas in a liquid and in the gas phase over the liquid are always equal regardless of solubility, buffer systems, partition coefficient, or dissociation curves. *Units:* torr.

Bohr effect The effect of CO_2 and H^+ on the affinity of hemoglobin for molecular O_2. In 1904 Bohr and associates described the effect of P_{CO_2} changes on oxyhemoglobin saturation. Now the usual practice is to relate the effect to changes of H^+ concentration or pH. Increasing P_{CO_2} and H^+ concentrations decrease oxyhemoglobin saturation, shifting the oxyhemoglobin dissociation curve to the right, whereas decreasing concentrations shift the curve to the left. In man, a decrease of pH from 7.4 to 7.3 at 40 torr P_{O_2} decreases oxyhemoglobin saturation by 6%, or about 1.2 ml (STPD) O_2/100 ml blood (oxygen capacity 20 ml [STPD] O_2/100 ml blood). The Bohr effect is very significant in the capillaries of working muscles, including myocardium, and in the maternal and fetal exchange vessels of the placenta. The Bohr effect is generally expressed as $\Delta \log P_{O_2}/\Delta pH$ at a given oxyhemoglobin saturation. For human blood between 10% to 90% oxyhemoglobin saturation the quotient at 37° C is 0.48 for a ΔpH of 0.1 unit. *Synonym:* Bohr shift.

Bohr integration A graphic integration procedure used to calculate the mean alveolocapillary O_2 diffusion gradient from mixed venous blood P_{O_2}, end-capillary blood P_{O_2}, alveolar gas P_{O_2}, and hemoglobin concentration.

breath-holding Voluntary apnea usually, but not necessarily, with a closed glottis. When maximally prolonged, voluntary apnea is terminated by an involuntary breaking point. While diving, certain seals and whales can hold their breath for more than 1 hour.

breathing Physiologically, the rhythmic process by which the ventilatory system draws a tidal volume of ambient gas or liquid into the lungs (inspiration) and then expels it (expiration).

breathing cycle A ventilatory cycle consisting of an inspiration followed by the expiration of a volume of gas, called the tidal volume. The duration of a breathing cycle is the breathing or ventilatory period; the reciprocal is the breathing frequency.

breathing frequency The number of breathing cycles per unit of time. *Symbol:* f. *Synonym:* respiratory rate.

breathing pattern A general term referring to the characteristics of the ventilatory activity, including tidal volume, breathing frequency, and shape of the spirographic (volume as a function of time) curve.

breathing, work of The energy required for breathing movements. The cumulative product of instantaneous pressure developed by the respiratory muscles and volume of air moved during a breathing cycle. Calculated as $\int PdV$ from volume-pressure diagrams of the passively driven respiratory system or from volume-transpulmonary pressure diagrams during spontaneous breathing, in which case the additional work done on the chest wall is computed from separate measurements made during voluntary relaxation. Rate of work (*Symbol:* $\dot{W}$) is calculated as the product of work per breathing cycle and breathing frequency. *Units:* kgm $\times$ M $\times$ min^{-1}. Work of inspiration (*Symbol:* W_{insp}) and work of expiration (*Symbol:* W_{exp}) can be stated separately. *Units:* kgm $\times$ M.

brisket disease A disease of cattle at high altitude initiated by hypoxic constriction of the pulmonary vasculature and often terminating in chronic cor pulmonale, right ventricular failure, and death. Named for edema of the brisket, a prominent sign of the disease.

bronchiole Any of several generations of the smallest ramifications of the branching tracheobronchial tree.

bronchiolitis Inflammation of the small airways, or bronchioles. Acute severe bronchiolitis can be serious, especially in children, causing fever, dyspnea, wheezing, cough, and cyanosis. The severe obstruction to pulmonary ventilation can cause hypoxemia, respiratory acidosis, and even death.

bronchomotor tone The state of contraction or relaxation of smooth muscle in the bronchial walls that regulates airway caliber. *Distinguish:* dynamic airway compression, dynamic airway expansion.

bronchospirometry Technic for study of the ventilation and gas exchange of each lung separately by introduction of a catheter into the left, or sometimes right, mainstem bronchus. A double-lumen tube, such as the Carlens catheter, permits simultaneous separate sampling of the gas from both lungs so that gas exchange, ventilation rates, and lung volumes can be measured and/or recorded.

BTPS conditions of a volume of gas The conditions of a volume of gas at body temperature, ambient pressure, and saturated with water vapor. These are the conditions that exist in the gas phase of the lungs. For man, normal respiratory tract temperature is taken as 37° C, the pressure as ambient pressure, and the partial pressure of water vapor at 37° C as 47 torr. *Abbreviation:* volume (BTPS).

carbaminohemoglobin Hemoglobin carbamate. Compounds formed by the reaction of some of the free amino groups of hemoglobin with CO_2 to form carbamino compounds and hydrogen ions:

$$Hb\text{-}NH_2 + CO_2 \rightleftharpoons Hb\text{-}NHCOO^- + H^+$$

carbon monoxide uptake: kinetic constant The rate at which erythrocytes take up CO. This rate is affected by the simultaneously present O_2 tension. *Units:* ml (STPD) CO $\times$ min^{-1} $\times$ torr^{-1} $\times$ (ml of blood)$^{-1}$. *Abbreviation:* θ.

carbonic anhydrase A zinc-containing enzyme present in many cell types, including erythrocytes, that catalyzes the reaction: $CO_2 + OH^- + H^+ \rightleftharpoons H^+ + HCO_3^-$. This enzyme facilitates CO_2 transport first from the metabolizing cells, where it forms to the systemic capillary blood, and then from pulmonary capillary blood to alveolar gas. Carbonic anhydrase accelerates the reaction 2,090 times in erythrocytes and 13,000 times in aqueous solution.

carboxyhemoglobin Hemoglobin in which the iron atoms are associated with CO. *Symbol:* HbCO. The affinity of hemoglobin for carbon monoxide is 200 to 300 times greater than that for O_2. Carboxyhemoglobin formation shifts the oxyhemoglobin dissociation curve to the left.

carcinogen A chemical substance or physical agent capable of inducing cancer.

chemoreceptor A chemosensitive structure in a sense organ that detects chemical changes. For example, the receptors within the carotid and aortic bodies detect chemical changes in the bloodstream, especially reduced O_2 content, and reflexly increase both pulmonary ventilation and systemic arterial blood pressure. Also a receptor adapted for excitation by chemical substances, for example, gustatory and olfactory receptors.

Cheyne-Stokes breathing A pattern of breathing in which tidal volume first progressively increases and then progressively decreases, followed by a period of apnea at relaxation volume (midposition) after which the breathing sequence is repeated.

chloride shift As blood flowing through systemic capillaries takes up CO_2, increasing erythrocyte HCO_3^- concentration produces a HCO_3^- concentration gradient that favors diffusion of HCO_3^- from red blood cells into plasma. In exchange, Cl^- diffuse from plasma into red blood cells, maintaining electroneutrality. This movement is called the chloride shift. Because the concentration of intracellular solute increases as CO_2 enters the erythrocyte and forms HCO_3^-, and because this concentration is not further changed by the HCO_3^--Cl^- exchange, water also diffuses into the cell, swelling it very slightly. As CO_2 leaves the blood in the pulmonary capillaries, all these processes reverse. *Synonym:* Hamburger effect.

choanal atresia A congenital obstruction by either membranous or bony structures of the posterior nares (choanae narium), which normally open into the nasopharynx.

closed-circuit breathing system Any breathing system used in cardiopulmonary technology in which the contained gas mixture is rebreathed, either directly or after recirculation through a water- or CO_2-absorbing unit, for example, the spirograph. *Compare:* open-circuit breathing system.

CO_2 concentration The amount of CO_2 that can be extracted from a given volume of liquid by acidification and evacuation. In the case of blood, this includes physically dissolved CO_2, carbonic acid, bicarbonate, carbonate, and CO_2 bound to hemoglobin as carbamate. *Units:* ml (STPD) CO_2/100 ml sample or mmole CO_2/liter. *Symbol:* C_{CO_2}. Although appropriate for HCO_3^-, mEq is not an appropriate expression for an amount of CO_2.

CO_2, endogenous Carbon dioxide produced within the body by metabolic processes.

CO_2 narcosis The impaired state of consciousness, ranging to unconsciousness and produced by hypercapnia.

CO_2 output The amount of CO_2 eliminated by the lungs in the expiratory gas stream. CO_2 output is determined by measurement and analysis of mixed expired gas, with correction for any inspired CO_2. It is usually expressed as a rate in volume units per unit time. *Units:* ml (STPD)/min. *Symbol:* $\dot{V}_{CO_2}$. *Distinguish:* CO_2 production, which is the amount of CO_2 produced by the metabolizing cells. During a steady state of the respiration and circulation, CO_2 output rate equals CO_2 production rate and body CO_2 stores remain constant.

CO_2 pressure The tension, or partial pressure, of CO_2 within a defined region, system, or space. A measure of CO_2 fugacity, or escaping tendency. *Abbreviation:* P_{CO_2}.

CO_2 retention Increased partial pressure and body stores of CO_2 as a result of impaired pulmonary CO_2 elimination in conditions such as alveolar hypoventilation, strangulation, apnea, and bronchopulmonary conditions associated with ventilation-perfusion abnormality. *Hypercapnia* means any increased CO_2 tension in lung gas, blood, and body fluids and may result from CO_2 retention, inhalation of CO_2-containing gas mixtures, rebreathing, or asphyxia. *Respiratory acidosis* is the general pathophysiologic state, including pH, electrolyte, and other biochemical changes, which results from acute or chronic hypercapnia of any cause.

CO_2 stores The amount of CO_2 stored throughout the body as CO_2, carbonic acid, carbonate, bicarbonate, and carbaminohemoglobin. CO_2 stores amount to several liters (STPD) in an adult human subject. During a steady state of the respiration and circulation, CO_2 output rate equals CO_2 production rate and the quantity of body CO_2 stores remains constant.

CO_2 titration curve A curve or line on any graph of the Henderson-Hasselbalch equation describing the blood (or separated or true plasma) pH and total CO_2 concentration changes that result from addition (increasing P_{CO_2}) or removal (decreasing P_{CO_2}) of CO_2. Hence, a curve describing the titration of blood with carbonic acid. *Synonyms:* CO_2 dissociation curve, blood buffer curve, CO_2-blood (or -plasma) equilibrium curve. *Abbreviations:*

CBEC, CPEC. In vitro curves are plotted by equilibration of shed whole blood or separated plasma samples with gas mixtures containing various partial pressures of CO_2. The relationship for fully oxygenated hemoglobin is obtained by equilibrating the blood with a P_{O_2} of at least 200 torr. In vivo (whole body) curves are obtained by inhaling gas mixtures that contain various concentrations of CO_2 for an appropriate equilibration time and then measuring the resulting CO_2 concentration and pressure in blood or true plasma samples. In vitro CO_2 titration curves for shed whole blood differ from in vivo CO_2 titration curves; because extravascular compartments equilibrate in vivo, HCO_3^- concentration is less than that measured in vitro at CO_2 pressures greater than 40 torr. The slope of a CO_2 titration curve is a measure of blood buffer capacity.

collateral ventilation Ventilation of pulmonary air spaces through indirect pathways, for example, through pores in alveolar septa or anastomosing respiratory bronchioles.

compliance A measure of distensibility. The lung volume change produced by a unit pressure change. Absolute values of compliance vary with lung size. *Symbol:* C. The reciprocal of elastance. *Static compliance* is the slope of a static volume-pressure curve at any given point, or the slope of a linear approximation to a nearly straight portion of such a curve in the tidal volume range. *Units: L (BTPS)/cm H_2O. Symbol:* C_{st}. Because the static volume-pressure characteristics of lungs are nonlinear (static compliance decreases as lung volume increases) and vary depending on the immediately preceding volume history (static compliance at a given volume increases after full inflation and decreases after deflation), one must specify the relevant conditions of measurement. *Dynamic compliance* is the ratio of the tidal volume to the intrapleural pressure difference between the points of zero gas flow at the two extremes of tidal volume. *Units:* L (BTPS)/cm H_2O. *Symbol:* C_{dyn}. Because volume acceleration is usually not 0 at the points of zero gas flow at the extremes of tidal volume and because, particularly in abnormal states, gas may still be flowing within lungs between regions that are exchanging volume, dynamic compliance may differ from static compliance, the latter pertaining to conditions of zero volume acceleration and zero gas flow throughout the lungs. In healthy lungs at ordinary volumes and breathing frequencies, static and dynamic compliance are equal.

conceptional age Total gestational age of an infant at birth, the duration of pregnancy calculated from 2 weeks after the first day of the last menstrual period.

conductance Volumetric flow rate produced per unit of pressure difference; the reciprocal of resistance. *Symbol:* G. *Units:* L $\times$ sec^{-1} $\times$ (cm $H_2O)^{-1}$.

coryza Acute rhinitis; a common cold.

countercurrent gas exchange Gas exchange between two media flowing in opposite directions. Exchange of this type occurs in many aquatic animals. Examples include exchange (1) between blood flowing in the lamellae of the gill filaments and water flowing along the lamellae from the buccal cavity to the opercular cavity, and (2) in the rete mirabile of the gas gland of certain fish. Such an anatomic arrangement facilitates gas transfer.

cyanosis A bluish purple discoloration of the skin, mucous membranes, and nail beds resulting from O_2 deficiency in the blood producing an abnormally high concentration of deoxyhemoglobin. It has been empirically determined that cyanosis first becomes apparent when arterial blood O_2 saturation decreases to about 83% in a subject with normal hemoglobin concentration. In other terms, cyanosis first becomes apparent when the concentration of deoxyhemoglobin in the capillary blood of the skin, mucous membranes, or nail beds exceeds about 5 gm/100 ml blood. The brownish discoloration of methemoglobinemia and the grayish discoloration of argyria are sometimes mistaken for cyanosis.

dead space, anatomic The total volume of all non–gas-exchanging or conducting airways in the lung. This space normally consists of the upper airway and the bronchial tree down to, but not including, the respiratory bronchioles where, during air breathing, respiratory gas exchange begins to occur at the entrance of the alveolar ducts. *Symbol:* $V_{D_{anat}}$. *Synonym:* inert gas dead space.

dead space, phsyiologic A calculated or virtual, not an actual topographic, volume that accounts for the difference between the pressures of CO_2 in mixed expired and alveolar gas (or arterial blood). Physiologic dead space differs from anatomic, or inert gas, dead space in that it expresses the degree of nonuniformity of $\dot{V}_A/\dot{Q}_c$ ratios in the lung; it is the sum of anatomic dead space and alveolar dead space, the volume of the latter increasing with increasing nonuniformity of ventilation/perfusion ratios in the lung. For a particular gas, physiologic dead space is the number that must be used for V_D in the Bohr equation to compute the correct arterial blood gas tension from inspired and mixed expired gas concentrations. *Symbol:* $V_{D_{phys}}$. *Synonym:* functional dead space.

decompression sickness A group of syndromes characterized by formation of gas bubbles in blood and other body fluids. When ambient pressure decreases at sufficient rate and to sufficient extent, physically dissolved gases emerge from solution, forming bubbles. The most common symptom is limb pain occurring soon after emergence from a hyperbaric environment. Decompression sickness may also result from abrupt exposure to very low pressures, for example, at high altitude, in which case symptoms other than limb pain may occur. The best treatment is immediate recompression. Some treatment schedules also use high inspired O_2 concentrations. Decompression sickness should be distinguished from other conditions associated with decreased ambient pressure, such as traumatic air embolism resulting from overdistention of the lungs. Decompression sickness can be avoided by gradual decompression. For example, 9 days are required to decompress safely from 50 ATA pressure. *Synonyms:* compressed air illness, bends, caisson disease.

denitrogenation The process of elimination of lung and body nitrogen during a period of pure O_2 breathing.

diffusing capacity The rate of gas transfer through a unit area of a permeable membrane per unit of gas pressure difference across it. Although a simple physical concept, diffusing capacity is usually a complex biologic measurement because it is difficult to determine accurately the effective pressure difference. O_2 or CO are usually used to measure *total pulmonary diffusing capacity. Units:* ml (STPD) of gas (O_2, CO, or CO_2) diffusing between alveolar gas and pulmonary capillary blood $\times$ (mean gas pressure difference in torr)$^{-1} \times$ min^{-1}. *Synonyms:* diffusion factor, transfer factor. *Symbols:* D_L, D_{LO_2}, D_{LCO_2}, D_{LCO}, T_L.

diffusion coefficient, membrane A component of total pulmonary diffusing capacity. The sum of all factors affecting CO transfer other than pulmonary capillary blood volume (V_c) and the kinetic constant (θ). It includes qualitative and quantitative characteristics of the alveolar surface, as well as other additive factors. *Symbol:* D_M.

2,3-diphosphoglyceric acid A biochemical compound in the anaerobic glycolytic cycle of carbohydrate metabolism. Within the erythrocyte this intermediate compound affects the affinity of hemoglobin for molecular O_2 and is thus an important link in the biochemical feedback control system that regulates the release of O_2 to the tissues. *Abbreviation:* 2,3-DPG.

dissolved gas Gas in simple physical solution, as distinguished from gas that has reacted chemically with the solvent or other solutes and is chemically combined.

distribution The concept or mathematical description of the manner in which the volume of inspired gas and the volume of pulmonary blood flow are distributed to the large number of functional units throughout the lungs. The matching of these two distributions is a subject of great physiologic importance. *Inert gas distribution* is the distribution of a nonexchanging gas among alveoli, theoretically perfect (ideal) only when each alveolus receives the same volume of inspired gas from the tidal volume in relation to its original volume as every other alveolus receives.

ductus arteriosus The fetal vascular shunt between pulmonary artery and descending aorta that allows blood to bypass the nonfunctioning lungs. Normal during intrauterine life, this structure closes spontaneously soon after birth to form the ligamentum arteriosum.

dynamic A condition of changing volume; hence, flow is not 0.

dyne Unit of force. The force required to accelerate a free mass of 1 gm 1 cm per second per second. One dyne equals 10^{-5} newton.

dysbarism Any morbid condition, syndrome, or disease resulting from exposure to a change of ambient pressure; usually a sudden or great change.

dysplasia Abnormal development; alteration of size, shape, and organization of adult cells.

dyspnea Difficult or labored breathing. The uncomfortable awareness of the need for increased breathing. Subjective by definition, dyspnea is not a sign but a symptom usually related to decreased ventilatory capacity and increased work of breathing. The sensation of dyspnea felt by patients is probably not experienced by healthy highly trained individuals.

effluent A liquid, solid, or gaseous emission. The discharge or waste outflow from a machine or industrial process.

elastance The reciprocal of compliance. *Units:* cm H_2O/liter or cm H_2O/ml. *Symbol:* E.

elastic recoil The difference between intrapleural pressure and alveolar pressure at a given lung volume under static conditions. *Abbreviation:* P_{st}.

endoderm The innermost of the three primary germ layers of the developing embryo. It gives rise to the bronchopulmonary system as well as the digestive epithelium, bladder, vagina, and urethra. *Synonyms:* entoderm, hypoblast.

environment The totality of all elements—matter, energy, and force fields—that interact directly or indirectly with an organism at any level of physiologic organization.

environment of a living organism An arbitrarily limited region of space containing the matter, energy, and force fields that interact with the organism directly or indirectly at any level of organization—physicochemical, biologic, or psychologic.

environmental physiology The branch of the science of physiology concerned with the physiologic responses of presently existing forms of life to environmental change and environmental stressors.

environmental stressor An environmental change sufficient to evoke a regulatory counterresponse in an organism.

enzyme A highly specific biologic catalyst of protein nature produced by living cells and necessary for in vivo catalysis of biochemical reactions under ordinary conditions of life.

equivalent lung volume A virtual volume of dilution. A hypothetic volume of pulmonary gas used to calculate changes of alveolar partial pressures of CO_2 and O_2 when these gases are added to or removed from the gas phase within the lung. Equivalent lung volume is the sum of the actual intrapulmonary gas volume plus a hypothetic volume that reflects the fixation of CO_2 or O_2 in lung tissue and pulmonary blood. For CO_2, equivalent lung volume is about 15% greater than actual lung volume; for O_2, it is only slightly more than actual lung volume. The physiologic phenomenon referred to by the term equivalent lung volume decreases the amplitude of the P_{CO_2} and P_{O_2} fluctuations that normally occur during the breathing cycle. *Abbreviation:* ELV.

erythrocyte Red blood cell. Human erythrocytes are circular, biconcave hemoglobin-containing discs about 1 μm thick and about 7.7 μm in diameter. There are normally about 5 million in each cubic millimeter of blood. The average life span is about 120 days. Erythrocytes are important in both O_2 and CO_2 transport. Circulating erythrocytes of mammals have no nuclei.

erythropoietin An α_2-globulin glycoprotein hormone normally produced by the kidney that stimulates bone marrow erythropoiesis. Erythropoietin release is enhanced by hypoxia and decreased by hyperoxia.

eupnea Normal comfortable breathing at rest.

exposure, acute A brief or transient exposure. Often a brief exposure to a high concentration or intense level of some agent. *Chronic exposure* is a continuous or frequently recurring long-term exposure. Often a long-term exposure to low concentrations or levels of some agent.

fibrin An insoluble filamentous protein formed in blood by the action of thrombin on fibrinogen. The resulting deposit of fine interlacing protein filaments is the matrix of the blood clot, or thrombus.

fibrinolysis The dissolving of clots. An example is the action of the proteolytic enzyme plasmin, formed in blood from its precursor, plasminogen.

fibrosis Excessive formation of fibrous tissue within an organ such as the lungs or heart. Usually, this is a response to some identifiable insult, such as hypoxia or inflammation that injures or destroys cells. Because of its stiffness, relative impermeability, and tendency to shrink, fibrous tissue, although an important element of the healing process, may impair heart or lung function. Pulmonary interstitial fibrosis sometimes results from interstitial pneumonitis. Although the term *fibrosis* is often used loosely to describe certain chest roentgenographic patterns or diminished lung volume, it is properly a histopathologic diagnosis requiring tissue examination by a pathologist.

flow rate of a fluid, linear Linear flow velocity. The velocity of a particle within a moving stream. *Units:* cm/sec.

flow rate of a fluid, volumetric The rate at which a volume of fluid flows past a designated point. *Units:* L or ml/sec.

flow-volume curve Graph of the instantaneous volumetric flow rates achieved during a forced expiratory vital capacity maneuver plotted as a function of the lung volume. When recorded for the full range of vital capacity, the curve includes maximum expiratory flow rates at all possible lung volumes and is called a *maximum expira-tory flow-volume curve* (*abbreviation:* MEFV). A partial expiratory flow-volume curve is one that describes maximum expiratory flow rate within only a selected range of the vital capacity (*abbreviation:* PEFV).

foramen ovale The opening in the interatrial septum of the fetal heart through which blood shunts past the lungs from right to left atrium. The foramen ovale normally closes soon after birth, separating the two upper cardiac chambers.

forced expiratory flow The average volumetric flow rate during any stated volume interval while a forced expired vital capacity is performed. *Abbreviation:* FEF. The volume interval is usually expressed as a percent of vital capacity. *Example:* FEF_{25-75}.

forced expired vital capacity A pulmonary function test. The maximal volume of gas that can be forcefully and rapidly exhaled starting from the position of full inspiration. *Abbreviation:* FEVC. *Units:* L or ml (BTPS). *Synonym:* timed vital capacity.

forced expired volume The volume of gas exhaled during a specified time interval while a forced expired vital capacity is performed. *Abbreviation:* FEV. *Units:* L or ml (BTPS). Commonly used time intervals are 0.5, 0.75, or 1 second. The elapsed time in seconds during which the forced expired volume has been measured is indicated by appropriate subscripts as follows: $FEV_{0.5}$, $FEV_{0.75}$, $FEV_{1.0}$. It is also useful to express forced expired volume as a percent of the total forced expired vital capacity. *Example:* $FEV_{1.0}/FEVC \times 100$.

functional residual capacity The volume of gas that remains in the lungs and airways at the end of a quiet spontaneous expiration; end-expiratory lung volume. *Abbreviation:* FRC. *Units:* L or ml (BTPS).

gas pocket A gas-filled cavity created artificially by injecting gas into subcutaneous tissue. The composition of gas in the pocket reflects the partial pressures of gases in the surrounding tissue. Pneumoperitoneum, pneumothorax, obstructed middle ear, and subcutaneous emphysema are analogous to artificial subcutaneous gas pockets.

gas solubility coefficient The volume of gas physically dissolved in 1 ml of fluid at 1-atm test gas pressure and at a given temperature. *Units:* ml (STPD) of gas/ml of fluid/atm or vol%/torr. *Symbol:* α. Example for O_2, α_{O_2}. For O_2 in water at 37° C, α = 0.0239. For O_2 in blood (15 gm Hb) at 37° C, α = 0.0223.

gasp A ventilatory movement consisting of a sudden, brief, inspiratory effort.

gestational age Total age of the infant at birth, the duration of pregnancy calculated from the first day of the last menstrual period.

glutathione A biochemical compound containing three amino acids: glutamic acid, cysteine, and glycine. This ubiquitous tripeptide is the most abundant sulfhydryl compound in cells and is important in maintaining enzymes in their active state by means of a sequence of reduction-oxidation reactions. Glutathione is functionally associated with glucose-6-phosphate dehydrogenase and reduced triphosphopyridine nucleotide in the maintenance of red blood cell integrity. Glutathione deficiency predisposes erythrocytes to the oxidant and hemolytic effects of certain drugs, such as the antimalarial agents.

gradient The rate of increase or decrease of any variable, or the curve that represents it; usually with reference to pressure. Also, the rate of change of pressure or concentration with respect to distance in a medium, across a membrane, or between two points. The term gradient is often mistakenly used to refer to a simple arithmetic pressure difference between two points.

Haldane effect Increasing oxyhemoglobin saturation decreases blood CO_2 binding capacity. Fully deoxygenated human blood at 40 torr CO_2 pressure and 37° C binds about 6 ml (STPD) CO_2/100 ml blood more than fully oxygenated blood (O_2 capacity 20 ml [STPD] O_2/100 ml blood). The Haldane effect results from decreasing affinity between protons and oxygenating hemoglobin. As O_2 uptake in the lungs of a healthy resting subject at sea level increases oxyhemoglobin saturation from 75% to 98%, the Haldane effect releases 1.4 ml (STPD) CO_2/100 ml blood. *Synonym:* Christiansen-Douglas-Haldane effect.

hematoma A collection of blood in tissues as a result of extravasation or hemorrhage. Hematomas may occur spontaneously or as a result of trauma.

hemoglobin Any of a class of hemoproteins that occur naturally in the blood of most vertebrates. The protein moiety, or globin, which differs for each different hemoglobin, consists of four polypeptide chains, each attached to a heme group. Each of the four heme groups consists of a cyclic protoporphyrin structure containing four pyrrole rings linked by methene bridges and an atom of divalent ferrous iron (Fe^{++}) that combines reversibly with molecular O_2. *Symbol:* Hb.

hemoglobin-O_2 affinity The affinity under stated conditions between a given hemoglobin and molecular O_2. Affinity is usually expressed as the degree of O_2 saturation of a blood sample or of a hemoglobin solution at a specified P_{O_2}, pH, and temperature which, for most homeotherms, are 7.4 and body temperature, respectively. The affinity between a given hemoglobin and O_2 is characterized completely by an oxygen-hemoglobin equilibrium curve. A simpler but much less complete characterization of affinity is the P_{50}, or O_2 pressure that produces one-half (50%) saturation of a blood sample or of a hemoglobin solution.

hemolysis Rupture of erythrocyte membranes with resulting release of their contents into the blood plasma.

Henderson-Hasselbalch buffer equation This equation defines the equilibrium relationship of the different forms of CO_2 in an aqueous solution to the acidity:

$$pH = pK_1' + \log \frac{[total\ CO_2] - S \times P_{CO_2}}{S \times P_{CO_2}} = pK_1' + \log \frac{[HCO_3^-]}{S \times P_{CO_2}}$$

where pK_1' is the negative logarithm of the apparent first ionization constant of carbonic acid corrected for the ratio of CO_2 to H_2CO_3 and S is a factor relating the partial pressure of CO_2 to the sum of the millimolar concentrations of carbonic acid and dissolved CO_2 in plasma (0.0301). The Henderson-Hasselbalch buffer equation is used in various forms to calculate any one of the three variables, pH, P_{CO_2}, and $[HCO_3^-]$, from the other two. The equation is valid only for single-phase aqueous systems such as plasma or serum; hence, it does not apply to whole blood.

Hering-Breuer reflexes Reflexes originating in the lungs that tend to limit breathing excursion. The reflexes originate in slowly adapting pulmonary mechanoreceptors located in bronchi and bronchioles, and impulses proceed through vagal afferent fibers, the brainstem respiratory centers, the medullospinal pathway, and finally motoneurons to the respiratory muscles. Increased intratracheal pressure, airway distention, and pulmonary inflation stimulate pulmonary stretch receptors. There are three types of Hering-Breuer reflexes: (1) an inflation reflex in which lung inflation tends to inhibit inspiration and stimulate expiration, (2) a deflation reflex in which lung deflation tends to inhibit expiration and stimulate inspiration, and (3) a paradoxic reflex in which sudden inflation may stimulate the inspiratory muscles. In the type (1) reflex, impulses from the mechanoreceptors affect medullary respiratory center activity, inhibiting inspiration to an extend that depends on the existing degree of lung inflation; the afferent link informs the respiratory centers of the lung volume state or of the rate of change of volume. Whether Hering-Breuer receptors influence the medullary respiratory centers directly or act indirectly modifying the tonic effect of pontine centers on the medulla remains unknown.

homeostatic system The coordinated and integratively functioning hierarchy of systems and subsystems of regulatory processes that maintains a steady physiologic state in the healthy living organism. Many of the subsystems function as negative feedback control mechanisms, such as those that regulate P_{O_2}, P_{CO_2}, and pH.

homeotherm A warm-blooded animal, such as a mammal or bird; an animal whose relatively constant normal body temperature is well maintained by its thermoregulatory homeostatic system despite environmental temperature fluctuations.

hydrogen ion concentration An important physicochemical variable of aqueous solutions. The acidity of an aqueous solution is a manifestation of hydrogen ion concentration (activity). *Symbol:* $[H^+]$. *Units:* nanomoles of hydrogen ion per liter (nM/L). The negative logarithm of the hydrogen ion concentration is pH.

hyperbaric Of or pertaining to pressure in excess of atmospheric pressure. *Antonym:* hypobaric.

hyperbaric oxygenation The administration of O_2 in a pressure chamber at partial pressures greater than that of pure O_2 at sea level (760 torr). Hyperbaric oxygenation is used to treat CO intoxication and gangrene associated with anaerobic bacterial infection.

hyperbarism Any morbid condition, syndrome, or disease resulting from exposure to increased ambient pressure. Usually it results from sudden exposure or significant increase of pressure.

hypercapnia Abnormally high CO_2 pressure within a biologic system; excess of CO_2 in the blood. Any state in which the systemic arterial blood P_{CO_2} is significantly greater than 40 torr. Hypercapnia occurs when the alveolar ventilation rate is low for a given metabolic rate (hypoventilation), during CO_2 inhalation, and in patients who have diffuse bronchopulmonary disease (CO_2 retention). *Synonym:* hypercarbia. *Antonyms:* hypocapnia, hypocarbia.

hyperoxia Increased or abnormally high O_2 concentration or pressure. Inspired O_2 pressure greater than the pressure of O_2 in air at sea level (159 torr) but not greater than 1 ATA (760 torr). *Antonym:* hypoxia. *Compare:* normoxia.

hyperpnea Increased breathing frequency and/or tidal volume. *Example:* hyperpnea of exercise. *Distinguish:* hyperventilation. *Antonym:* hypopnea.

hyperresonance The exaggerated hollow, tympanic quality of the sound elicited by percussion of an overinflated or emphysematous chest or other overdistended gas-filled body cavity.

hyperventilation Generally, a pulmonary ventilation rate that exceeds the metabolically required rate for respiratory gas exchange. It may result from increased breathing frequency, increased tidal volume, or any combination of these two. Hyperventilation is most meaningfully expressed in terms of *alveolar* ventilation rate. There are three ways of considering hyperventilation: (1) an alveolar ventilation rate that decreases alveolar CO_2 pressure to a value less than the normal 40 torr; this definition has the virtue of relating alveolar ventilation rate to P_{CO_2}, which is normally the controlled variable; (2) in terms of ventilation equivalent, the ratio of pulmonary ventilation rate to oxygen uptake rate; (3) by comparison with predicted normal values for healthy subjects of the same age, size, sex, race, and in the same geographic location. Hyperventilation *increases* alveolar and arterial blood O_2 tension and *decreases* alveolar and arterial blood CO_2 tension. The resulting hypocapnia produces dizziness, numbness, tingling, arterial hypotension, respiratory alkalosis, and, if continued, significant psychomotor impairment. *Synonym:* overventilation. *Antonym:* hypoventilation.

hypobaric Of or pertaining to ambient pressure less than atmospheric pressure. *Antonym:* hyperbaric.

hypobarism Any syndrome, morbid condition, or disease resulting from exposure to decreased ambient pressure. Hypobarism is usually the result of sudden exposure or significant decrease of pressure.

hypobarogenous aerobullosis A neologism; generalized emergence and growth of gas bubbles from solution in fluids and tissues throughout the body as a result of decompression. *Distinguish:* aeroembolism has been used in this sense but, as the term suggests, it should mean the *intravascular* emergence, growth, and *transport* of gas bubbles as a result of decompression.

hypocapnia Abnormally low CO_2 pressure within an organism. Deficiency of CO_2 in the blood. Systemic arterial blood P_{CO_2} significantly less than 40 torr. Usually caused by alveolar hyperventilation. *Synonym:* hypocarbia. *Antonyms:* hypercapnia, hypercarbia.

hypokalemia Abnormally low blood potassium ion concentration. Blood serum potassium ion concentration below the normal range of 3.5 to 5.5 mEq/L.

hyponatremia Abnormally low blood sodium ion concentration. Blood serum sodium ion concentration below the normal range of 135 to 147 mEq/L.

hypoplasia Arrested or defective anatomic development of a structure or organ, which as a result remains less than normal size or in an immature state.

hypopnea Decreased breathing frequency and/or tidal volume compared to breathing at rest. Less precise than and not to be confused with hypoventilation. *Synonym:* oligopnea. *Antonym:* hyperpnea.

hypoventilation Generally, a pulmonary ventilation rate less than the rate metabolically required for respiratory gas exchange. Decreased pulmonary ventilation rate allowing alveolar P_{CO_2} to rise above the normal value of 40 torr. Hypoventilation is most meaningfully expressed in terms of *alveolar* ventilation rate. It may result from decreased breathing frequency, decreased tidal volume, or any combination of the two. It decreases alveolar and arterial blood O_2 tension and increases alveolar and arterial blood CO_2 tension. Hypoventilation produces hypoxemia, hypercapnia and, if continued, CO_2 retention and respiratory acidosis. *Synonym:* underventilation. *Antonym:* hyperventilation. *Chronic alveolar hypoventilation* is an important clinical syndrome; the combination of hypoxemia and respiratory acidosis constricts the pulmonary vascular bed producing pulmonary arterial hypertension, cor pulmonale, and right heart failure.

hypoxemia Deficient blood oxygenation. Low blood O_2 tension and low oxyhemoglobin saturation. Oxygen pressure and/or O_2 concentration in arterial and/or venous blood is lower than the normal values at sea level. Normal O_2 pressures at sea level are 85 to 100 torr in arterial blood and 37 to 44 torr in mixed venous blood. In adult human subjects the normal O_2 concentration is 17 to 23 ml (STPD) O_2/100 ml arterial blood; in mixed venous blood at rest it is 13 to 18 ml (STPD) O_2/100 ml blood. *Colorimetric hypoxemia* is hypoxemia as determined by oximetry and thus abnormally low oxyhemoglobin saturation.

hypoxia Generally, low or reduced O_2 concentration or pressure. Deficiency of O_2 in the inspired air or gas mixture or low O_2 content or pressure at any specified point in the O_2 transport system, including lung, blood, and metabolizing tissues, compared with that of healthy resting man breathing air at sea level. Low ambient P_{O_2}, whether caused by decreased barometric pressure or by decreased O_2 concentration, is termed *environmental hypoxia*. Blood hypoxia is termed *hypoxemia*. Insufficient O_2 pressure or concentration of free O_2 molecules to meet the requirements of aerobic cell or tissue metabolism is *histohypoxia*. Even without arterial hypoxemia, tissues can be hypoxic as in stagnant hypoxia when local circulation is insufficient to meet local metabolic requirements. *Hypoxidation* is a state of reduced aerobic metabolism associated with the reduced energy requirements of hypothermia, hibernation, hypothyroidism, or with the effect of certain drugs. *Hypoxidosis* is a condition of impaired aerobic metabolism in hypoxia, enzyme deficiency or dysfunction, substrate lack, or excessive accumulation of metabolites. Paradoxically, hyperbaric oxygenation may produce hypoxidosis.

hypoxia threshold The O_2 pressure at or below which O_2 deficiency in inspired gas or arterial blood stimulates breathing.

hysteresis The influence of the previous condition or treatment of a body on its subsequent response to a given force. The physical effect on a body lags behind a force applied to it. Hysteresis is an elastic property of the lung. For example, at any given lung volume the elastic recoil pressure within the airways during expiration is less than that which exists at the same lung volume during the process of inflation.

infant, immature An infant whose birth weight is less than 1,000 gm, regardless of gestational age.

infant, low birth weight An infant who weighs less than 2,500 gm at birth.

infant, premature An infant whose gestational age is less than 37 weeks, regardless of birth weight.

infant, small-for-date An infant whose gestational age is

greater than 37 weeks, but who weighs less than 2,500 gm at birth.

inspiratory capacity The maximum volume of gas that can be inhaled, starting from the resting end-expiratory position. *Abbreviation:* IC.

inspiratory reserve volume The maximal volume of gas that can be inhaled, starting from the end of a spontaneous inspiration. This volume equals the inspiratory capacity minus the tidal volume. *Abbreviation:* IRV.

isobar A line connecting points of equal pressure or tension on a graph. *Example:* the lines connecting points of equal CO_2 tension on the pH-bicarbonate diagram.

isocapnia Having equal CO_2 pressure.

isohydric shift The shift of buffer capacity (proton affinity) of hemoglobin as it oxygenates and deoxygenates. As a result, most of the H^+ generated as CO_2 hydrates are taken up by deoxygenating hemoglobin without change of H^+ concentration. Conversely, as H^+ are removed in the dehydration of carbonic acid, they are replaced by oxygenating hemoglobin. The isohydric shift thus facilitates CO_2 loading in systemic capillaries and CO_2 unloading in pulmonary capillaries.

isovolume pressure-flow curve A curve describing the relationship of driving pressure to the resulting volumetric flow rate in the airways at any given lung inflation. The infinite set of such curves for the entire range of lung volume comprises the volume-pressure-flow surface. *Abbreviation:* IVPF curves.

kyphoscoliosis An abnormal condition characterized by combined backward and lateral curvature of the spinal column. This condition interferes with both respiratory and circulatory function, predisposing afflicted patients to eventual cardiopulmonary failure.

kyphosis Abnormal backward or posterior convexity or curvature of the thoracic spinal column. If severe, this condition interferes with breathing, predisposing to chronic alveolar hypoventilation and its consequences.

ligamentum arteriosum The structure formed by closure of the normal fetal ductus arteriosus. Hence, a fibrous cord that extends from the left pulmonary artery to the aortic arch.

lung capacities Lung volumes that consist of two or more of the four primary nonoverlapping volumes. Functional residual capacity is the sum of residual volume and expiratory reserve volume. Inspiratory capacity is the sum of tidal volume and inspiratory reserve volume. Total lung capacity, the lung volume at the end of maximal inspiration, is the sum of two capacities: functional residual capacity and inspiratory capacity. Total lung capacity is thus also the sum of inspiratory reserve volume, tidal volume, expiratory reserve volume, and residual volume.

maximal midexpiratory flow rate A pulmonary function test. The average volumetric rate of gas flow during the middle half (in terms of volume) of a forced expired vital capacity maneuver. More sensitive than the $FEV_{1.0}$, this test is used to detect and evaluate chronic diffuse obstructive bronchopulmonary diseases, such as bronchitis, emphysema, and asthma. *Abbreviation:* MMEFR. *Units:* L (BTPS)/sec. *Synonym:* Forced expiratory flow, 25% to 75% (FEF_{25-75}).

maximal voluntary ventilation A pulmonary function test. The maximal volume of gas that a subject can ventilate by voluntary effort per unit time breathing as quickly and as deeply as possible. Although the actual performance time for this tiring test is usually limited to 12 to 20 seconds, the results are expressed in volume units per minute. *Abbreviation:* MVV. *Units:* L (BTPS)/min. *Synonym:* Maximal breathing capacity (MBC).

mesenchyme The meshwork of primitive embryonic tissue in the mesoderm, which eventually forms all the connective tissues of the body and also the lymphatic vessels, the blood vessels, the heart, and the blood. *Synonym:* mesenchyma.

metabolism The sum of all genetically determined chemical processes and associated energy transformations that occur within a living biologic system. The regulated and integratively functioning web of chemical reaction sequences or pathways that comprise the biochemical subsystem of a living organism. Metabolic transformations are (1) synthetic (anabolic) and usually endergonic, (2) degradative (catabolic) and usually exergonic, or (3) in many cases not readily classifiable as either. Metabolism supplies the substance and energy for all intrinsic functions, including growth, repair, reproduction, and all kinds of biologic work.

methemoglobin The compound produced from hemoglobin by oxidation of the iron atoms from the ferrous to the ferric state. Erythrocytes normally contain a biochemical redox system that maintains heme iron in the reduced state. Methemoglobin occurs in certain hereditary disorders and is also produced by various drugs. Methemoglobin does not combine with O_2 or CO and thus transports neither. Certain methods for hemoglobin measurement involve methemoglobin formation (chlormethemoglobin, cyanmethemoglobin). *Synonyms:* ferrihemoglobin, hemiglobin.

midposition The end-expiratory or end-tidal level or position of the lung-chest system under any given conditions, defining the functional residual capacity. Sometimes called *respiratory level.* Do not confuse with midcapacity.

milieu Environment; surroundings.

minute volume of breathing Pulmonary ventilation rate per minute. The volume of gas inspired or expired per minute under any given conditions. Usually, *expiratory minute volume* expressed as expired gas volume in L (BTPS)/min. Note that *expired* gas almost always differs from *inspired* gas with regard to temperature and the content of water vapor, CO_2, and O_2.

mixed venous blood Blood composed of a mixture of the venous blood from the heart and all systemic tissues in proportion to their venous returns. In the absence of abnormalities of the heart and great vessels, mixed venous blood is present in the main pulmonary artery. Blood samples drawn from right atrium or even right ventricle may be incompletely mixed. *Symbol:* $\bar{v}$.

mountain sickness Pathophysiologic state induced by high altitude. During their first few days at high altitude, unacclimatized subjects often experience headache, dyspnea, disturbances of sensory and intellectual functions, insomnia, nausea, and even vomiting. This symptom complex is called acute mountain sickness, or soroche. Symptoms rarely last more than a few days and are usually relieved by breathing an O_2-enriched mixture. Permanent residents at high altitude may develop chronic mountain sickness (Monge's disease) with diminished alveolar ventilation and signs and symptoms referable to the cardiovascular and central nervous systems. Relative hypoventilation aggravates the hypoxemia, and right heart failure develops. Extreme polycythemia with hematocrit ratios as high as 75% may be seen. The syndrome is relieved by a return to sea level.

Müller's maneuver Inspiratory effort against a closed airway or glottis. The effort decreases intrapulmonary and intrathoracic pressures and expands pulmonary gas.

myoglobin A heme protein occurring naturally in muscle cells. It consists of a single polypeptide chain to which a heme group is attached. The heme group is a protoporphyrin, consisting of four pyrrole rings joined by methene bridges, within which a divalent (ferrous) iron atom combines reversibly with molecular O_2. The great affinity of myoglobin for O_2 facilitates O_2 transfer from blood to cells. *Symbol:* Mb. *Synonym:* myohemoglobin.

neonate A newborn infant; an infant during the first 4 weeks of life.

nitrogen narcosis Depression of central nervous system function by high partial pressure of nitrogen. For example, during a deep dive, breathing air at 7 ATA may cause N_2 narcosis. In such a situation, dangerously high P_{N_2} may be avoided to a certain extent by replacing N_2 with O_2 in the breathing mixture. However, above a certain O_2 pressure there is danger of O_2 toxicity and N_2 is often replaced by helium.

nitrogen washout curve The curve obtained by plotting the concentration of N_2 in expired alveolar gas during O_2 breathing as a function of time. A subject, who has been breathing ambient air, begins to inhale pure O_2. The curve shows a progressive decrease of N_2 concentration that can be analyzed into two or more exponential phases. After 4 minutes of breathing pure O_2, healthy subjects have a N_2 concentration in expired alveolar gas of less than 2%.

normoventilation The alveolar ventilation rate that produces an alveolar CO_2 pressure of about 40 torr at any metabolic rate. *Synonym:* eupnea.

normoxia An ambient O_2 pressure of about 150 ± 10 torr; namely, the partial pressure of O_2 in atmospheric air at sea level.

O_2 capacity of blood The maximum amount of O_2 that can be made to combine chemically with the hemoglobin in a unit volume of blood. Oxygen capacity does not include physically dissolved oxygen. Mammalian blood requires a P_{O_2} of at least 150 torr for 100% saturation of hemoglobin with oxygen. The mean hemoglobin content of human male blood is about 15.3 gm/100 ml blood, which corresponds to an O_2 capacity of about 21 ml (STPD) O_2/100 ml blood. Although theoretically 1 gm of hemoglobin can bind a maximum of 1.391 ml (STPD) O_2, this value is never actually achieved in vivo because of several variable factors that operate to prevent it. These include the formation of carboxyhemoglobin and inactive hemoglobins, such as methemoglobin, which tends to increase in concentration as P_{O_2} increases. Thus, *calculation* of blood O_2 content and capacity using a figure such as 1.34, 1.36, or 1.39 is likely to be less precise than actual laboratory measurement. *Units:* ml (STPD) O_2/100 ml blood or mmole O_2/liter blood.

O_2-CO_2 concentration diagram A plot of CO_2 concentration versus O_2 concentration used almost exclusively for blood. O_2 and CO_2 concentrations of arterial and venous blood can be represented simultaneously for various organs. The slope of a line through an arterial point and a venous point for an organ in a steady state indicates the respiratory quotient of that organ.

O_2-CO_2 pressure diagram Plot of the CO_2 partial pressure versus the O_2 partial pressure in biologic media, such as alveolar gas, arterial and venous blood, inspired gas or water, and expired gas or water. Points representing all the O_2 and CO_2 pressures throughout the body can be represented simultaneously on this diagram. Because for a given fluid O_2 and CO_2 concentrations are completely defined by the O_2 and CO_2 pressures, a family of O_2 and CO_2 isoconcentration lines can be drawn on the O_2-CO_2 pressure diagram, demonstrating quantitatively and simultaneously the Haldane and Bohr effects. Respiratory gas exchange ratio lines for both gas and blood can also be plotted on the diagram. *Synonyms:* O_2-CO_2 diagram, Fenn-Rahn-Otis diagram.

O_2 concentration in blood The concentration of O_2 in a blood sample, including both O_2 combined with hemoglobin and O_2 that is physically dissolved. *Units:* ml (STPD) O_2/100 ml blood, or mmole O_2/L. *Symbol:* For arterial blood, C_{aO_2}. *Synonym:* O_2 content of blood.

O_2 consumption The quantity of O_2 utilized by a cell, tissue, or organism. When expressed as a quantity of O_2 per unit time, it is an O_2 consumption *rate.* For whole organisms O_2 consumption is usually expressed per unit

surface area or as a power of the body weight. *Symbols:* $\dot{V}_{O_2}$ or $\dot{Q}_{O_2}$. *Units:* $\dot{V}_{O_2}$ = L or ml (STPD) $O_2 \times$ kgm^{-1} $\times$ min^{-1} or L or ml (STPD) $O_2 \times$ kgm$^{-1} \times$ hr^{-1}. For tissue samples or isolated cells $\dot{Q}_{O_2}$ = μL (STPD) $O_2 \times$ (mgm dry weight)$^{-1} \times$ hr^{-1}. *Distinguish:* O_2 uptake.

O_2 cost of breathing The rate at which the respiratory muscles consume O_2 as they ventilate the lungs. *Units:* ml (STPD) O_2/L (BTPS) of pulmonary ventilation.

O_2 debt The quantity of O_2 taken up by the lungs during recovery from a period of exercise or apnea that is in excess of the quantity needed for resting metabolism during the preexercise period. Hence, O_2 debt represents repayment of O_2 and energy stores that were depleted during the time that O_2 uptake from the environment was inadequate for aerobic metabolism.

O_2 half-saturation pressure of hemoglobin The O_2 pressure necessary for 50% saturation of hemoglobin at body temperature and at pH 7.4 or 40 torr CO_2 pressure. This value is widely used as a measure of the affinity between O_2 and hemoglobin. *Symbol:* P_{50}.

O_2 intoxication All deleterious biologic effects of hyperoxia. Any functional and/or structural impairment of an organism resulting from exposure to O_2 at high partial pressures. Hyperoxia disturbs the oxidation-reduction potential within cells, oxidizing a variety of biochemical compounds, including proteins such as sulfhydryl-dependent dehydrogenase enzymes. Short-term hyperoxia causes pulmonary edema, hemorrhage, congestive atelectasis, hyaline membranes, and retrolental fibroplasia in premature infants. Chronic hyperoxia causes increased erythrocyte fragility, depression of erythropoiesis, anemia, and eventually death. It also causes infertility in experimental animals. Hyperbaric oxygen causes convulsions. *Synonym:* O_2 poisoning. Although O_2 therapy depresses the pulmonary ventilation of patients who have lung failure and may thus occasionally precipitate CO_2 narcosis, this effect should not be called O_2 intoxication.

O_2 stores The total quantity of O_2 stored at any given time in the various body compartments—lungs, arterial and venous blood, and tissues. In a 70-kgm man, blood contains about 800 ml (STPD) O_2 as oxyhemoglobin, muscles contain about 150 ml (STPD) as oxymyoglobin, alveolar gas contains a few hundred ml (STPD) of O_2, and about 50 ml (STPD) are dissolved in the tissues.

O_2 tolerance Increased capacity to withstand the toxic effects of hyperoxia as a result of any adaptive change occurring within an organism.

O_2 uptake Generally, the amount of O_2 that an organism *removes* from its environment; the amount of O_2 that the lungs remove from the ambient atmosphere, that the blood removes from the alveolar gas in the lungs, or the rate at which an organ or tissue removes O_2 from the blood perfusing it. When the amount of O_2 is expressed in volume units per unit of time, it is an O_2 uptake *rate.*

Symbol: $\dot{V}_{O_2}$. *Synonym:* O_2 intake. *Distinguish:* O_2 consumption, the amount of O_2 *used* by the metabolizing tissues. When a steady state of the respiration and circulation exists, O_2 *uptake* rate equals O_2 *consumption* rate and body O_2 stores remain constant. Oxygen consumption rate may also be thought of as the sum of the individual O_2 uptake rates of all the metabolizing tissues of the body. *Compare:* CO_2 output, as opposed to CO_2 *production.*

ontogeny Ontogenesis; a history of the process of growth and development in the early life of an organism.

open-circuit breathing system A type of breathing system used in cardiopulmonary technology in which rebreathing does not occur. Gas is inspired through a breathing branch or limb that is connected to a gas source or open to the ambient atmosphere and then expired through a directional valve into a collecting reservoir or vented back into the ambient atmosphere. *Contrast:* closed-circuit breathing system and rebreathing.

organism A living plant or animal; a living biologic system.

orthopnea Dyspnea in the recumbent, especially supine, position that is relieved by sitting or standing up. More characteristic of cardiac than pulmonary conditions. *Synonym:* dyspnea decubitus.

oxyhemoglobin dissociation curve A graphic representation of the amount of O_2 chemically bound at equilibrium to the hemoglobin in blood as a function of P_{O_2}. The curve is thus an expression of the affinity between O_2 and the hemoglobin. To define a curve completely, the pH, P_{CO_2}, and temperature must also be stated. The amount of O_2 plotted on the vertical axis is given in ml (STPD) O_2/100 ml blood, or in mmole O_2/L blood, or as a percent of the O_2 capacity (percent saturation). The total amount of O_2 in the blood, that combined with hemoglobin and that free in solution, can also be plotted. *Abbreviation:* OHDC. *Synonyms:* oxygen-hemoglobin equilibrium curve, oxygen dissociation curve of hemoglobin.

oxyhemoglobin saturation The amount of O_2 actually combined with hemoglobin, expressed as a percentage of the O_2 capacity of that hemoglobin. *Symbol:* S_{O_2}; *Example:* for arterial blood, S_{aO_2}.

panting Rapid, shallow breathing. A ventilatory pattern characterized by high breathing frequency and small tidal volume. Certain animals, for example the cow and the dog, pant when exposed to heat; thus the terms thermal panting and thermal tachypnea. Panting moves gas back and forth in the dead space of the upper airways at a high flow rate, which evaporates water, removes heat with little or no increase of alveolar ventilation rate, and avoids hypocapnia.

partial pressure of a gas The pressure or tension exerted by any one component gas in a gas mixture. A significant measurement with respect to the physicochemical behavior of a gas and the physiologic responses to it. As described by Dalton's law, the total pressure of a gas mixture is the arithmetic sum of all the individual partial pressures of the constituent gases. *Synonyms:* gas pressure, gas tension. *Example:* P_{CO_2} is the partial pressure, tension, or pressure of CO_2. An intensive property of a system, pressure alone does not define a system and may not tell one all one would like to know. For example, at any given O_2 pressure, the presence of an inert gas strongly affects the tendency to absorption atelectasis in the lung and the process of combustion in a sealed atmosphere. To define a system, the extensive property *content* is also needed and within any given system is predictably related to pressure.

particulates Minute discrete particles or fragments of a substance or material.

partition coefficient of a gas The ratio at equilibrium of the concentrations of a given gas in two or more solvents.

perinatal Near the time of birth. Occurring shortly before or soon after birth. The period beginning at about 28 weeks of gestation and ending at about 1 to 4 weeks after birth, hence including antenatal and neonatal periods.

periodic breathing Any of several abnormal patterns of breathing in which groups of ventilatory cycles are separated by pauses. *Examples:* Cheyne-Stokes breathing, Biot's breathing, apneustic breathing, coupled breathing.

pH A measure of the acidity or alkalinity of an aqueous solution on a scale of 0 to 14 on which 7 (neutrality) is the value for pure water at 25° C. Values less than 7 represent increasing H^+ concentration and increasing acidity, whereas values greater than 7 represent decreasing H^+ concentration and increasing alkalinity. The negative common logarithm of the effective H^+ concentration (H^+ activity) in gram-equivalents per liter or, identically, the common logarithm of the reciprocal of the H^+ concentration. pH is usually determined using a glass electrode, using a hydrogen electrode, or colorimetrically with indicators. The pH notation was introduced in 1909 by Sorensen to avoid the use of extremely small fractions. Although convenient, it has the disadvantage of being a logarithmic function of the actual acidity. Thus, some scientists prefer to express acidity in terms of H^+ concentration.

Pickwickian syndrome Obesity-hypoventilation syndrome; chronic alveolar hypoventilation occurring in obese subjects. It involves both extreme obesity and relative insensitivity to hypoxia and hypercapnia. A clinical syndrome named for the novel *Pickwick Papers* by Charles Dickens in which he accurately describes a fat boy with this syndrome.

plasma, separated Plasma separated from blood cells. Because the plasma is no longer in contact with erythrocytes, the results of equilibrating it with various gas pressures differ from those of plasma that has been separated from blood after equilibration (true plasma). Separated plasma is sometimes used in studies of acid-base balance, for example, equilibration with various CO_2 pressures and measurement of CO_2 concentration. Its composition under new conditions of equilibration does not include any influence of exchanges with erythrocytes because they have been removed.

plasma, true Plasma separated anaerobically from whole blood. Analysis of true plasma reveals the composition it had while still in contact with the blood cells. True plasma samples are often used in studies of acid-base balance.

plethysmograph Generally, an instrument consisting of a rigid chamber placed around a living structure to measure and record volume and volume changes of a body part, such as those resulting from circulatory variations. In respiratory measurements, a *body plethysmograph* ("body box") encloses the entire body of the subject and measures gas volume changes in the system produced by (1) solution and volatilization (for example, uptake of foreign gases by the blood), (2) changes of temperature or pressure (for example, gas compression in the lungs or expansion of gas on passing into the moist warm lungs), or (3) breathing through a tube to the outside. Three types of body plethysmograph are used: (1) pressure, (2) volume, and (3) pressure-volume. In type (1) the body chamber has fixed volumes, and volume changes are measured in terms of pressure changes secondary to gas compression (within the chamber, outside the body). In type (2) the body chamber serves as a conduit between body surface and instruments (spirometers or integrating flowmeters) that measure gas displacements. Type (3) combines types (1) and (2) by appropriate summing of chamber volume and pressure displacements. The body plethysmograph measures thoracic gas volume and its compartments, as well as airway resistance.

pneumatocele A hernial protrusion of the lung.

pneumoconstriction The dimple of collapsed tissue that results from mechanical stimulation of the exposed lung. It is produced by local reflex muscular closure of alveolar ducts and alveoli.

pneumograph An apparatus that records the movements of breathing, for example, by means of an inflated coil around the chest. A pneumograph measures the duration of the ventilatory cycle exactly but does not usually record the amplitude of breathing movements accurately. The record produced is a *pneumogram.*

pneumonitis, interstitial Pneumonias that affect primarily the interstitial tissue of the lung, sometimes resulting in interstitial fibrosis. Pulmonary function tests of patients with interstitial pneumonitis show a restrictive spirographic pattern of ventilatory impairment, normal or low P_{CO_2}, and hypoxemia with increased A-a P_{O_2} difference. Some cases resolve spontaneously; some are therapeuti-

cally reversible; whereas others do not respond to treatment. *Synonyms:* interstitial fibrosis, fibrosing alveolitis, Hamman-Rich syndrome.

pneumoperitoneum The presence of air or gas within the peritoneal cavity of the abdomen. It may be *spontaneous*, as from rupture of a hollow gas-containing organ, or *induced* for diagnostic or therapeutic purposes.

pneumotachograph An instrument for measuring instantaneous gas flow rates during breathing by recording the pressure decrease across a device of fixed flow resistance that has known pressure-flow characteristics. The device is commonly connected to the airway by means of a mouthpiece, face mask, or cannula. The flow-resistive device usually consists of either fine-mesh screen (Silverman-Lilly type) or parallel capillary tubes (Fleisch type). *Synonym:* pneumotachometer.

pneumotaxic center Bilateral anatomic structures located in the rostral pons that play a role in the rhythmic respiratory activity of certain mammals. In vagotomized cats transection of the brainstem caudal to these structures arrests breathing activity. *Synonym:* nucleus parabrachealis medialis (NPBM).

pneumothorax The presence of air or gas outside the lungs and within either or both pleural cavities, resulting in a corresponding degree of lung collapse. Air enters the pleural space through a chest wound, lung perforation, ruptured superficial lung bulla or cavity, or through burrowing abscesses. Symptoms of pneumothorax are the sudden onset of sharp, severe chest pain and rapidly increasing dyspnea. Unexpected lung rupture without known cause is *spontaneous* pneumothorax. Chest injuries that puncture the lung cause *traumatic* pneumothorax. If a lung is torn in such a way that a tissue flap forms a directional valve favoring passage of air from airways to pleural space, an emergency termed *tension* pneumothorax results. When gas or air is deliberately injected into the pleural space for diagnostic or therapeutic purposes, the condition is termed *induced* or *artificial* pneumothorax.

poikilotherm An animal whose body temperature fluctuates with the ambient temperature. Such animals are usually capable of enduring extremes of heat and cold.

poise A unit of liquid or gas (fluid) viscosity expressed in gm/cm/sec. The centipoise, or one-hundredth of a poise, is more commonly used.

polarograph An instrument that records the current-voltage curve produced in electroanalysis by means of a dropping mercury cathode. The record is a polarogram.

pollutant A foreign or extraneous substance, material, or agent that impairs the quality or diminishes the life-supporting capacity of an environment. In its most general sense, a pollutant is an undesired substance, not naturally present, that is added to an environment; it may be present in air, water, or soil.

polycythemia Excess of blood, especially its formed elements. The degree of polycythemia is usually expressed in terms of hemoglobin concentration, hematocrit, or erythrocyte count. *Polycythemia vera*, or *erythremia*, is a disease characterized by excessive blood formation, increased blood volume, and increases of all formed elements in the blood. Other polycythemias include those secondary to hypoxemia in the following conditions: (1) normal fetal condition, (2) high altitude exposure, (3) chronic diffuse bronchopulmonary disease, (4) chronic alveolar hypoventilation, and (5) venous-to-arterial circulatory shunt. Hypoxemia increases production of the bone marrow–stimulating hormone, erythropoietin. *Erythrocytosis* refers simply to increased red blood cell count. *Contrast:* anemia.

polypnea Rapid or panting breathing. *Synonym:* panting.

pressure Force per unit area. Pressure at any given point relative to ambient (unless otherwise specified) pressure. *Units:* cm H_2O, torr.

pressure, alveolar Total gas pressure in alveoli usually expressed relative to ambient pressure. *Symbols:* P_A, P_{alv}. *Units:* cm H_2O. *Synonyms:* intrapulmonary pressure, intrapulmonic pressure.

pressure breathing apparatus A respirator; any mechanical device to *assist* spontaneous respiration, for O_2 therapy, for delivery of aerosol medication to the respiratory tract, or to *control* pulmonary ventilation. Pressure breathing systems are either *pressure-cycled* or *volume-cycled* and may provide *continuous* or *intermittent, positive* or *"negative"* (subatmospheric) pressure. Systems vary with respect to their dynamic flow-pressure characteristics. Proper selection and effective application of a pressure breathing system in a given clinical case challenges the knowledge and skill of the respiratory therapist.

pressure, intrapleural The normally subambient pressure that exists within the potential or actual space between visceral and parietal pleura (between lungs and chest wall). Intrapleural pressure results from elastic lung recoil and is approximately equal to intraesophageal pressure. Average local lung surface pressures can be measured directly by means of small induced pneumothoraces or indirectly by means of esophageal balloon catheters. Pressures in the pleural liquid normally present within the intrapleural space reflect an equilibrium between the colloid osmotic pressures and hydrostatic pressures of both capillary blood and pleural liquid. Pleural liquid pressures may be less than average local surface pressures because the lung surface is exposed not only to pleural liquid but also to contact with the solid parietal pleura that exerts the equivalent of positive pressure on the lung surface, compensating for differences between liquid and average surface pressures. Intrapleural pressure is used to estimate transpulmonary pressure, which is the pressure difference between the airway opening and the pleural surface of the lung. *Symbol:* P_{pl}. *Units:* cm H_2O. *Synonyms:* pleural pressure, intrathoracic pressure.

pressure, intrapleural, maximal static negative The difference between intrapleural and alveolar pressure at full inspiration.

pressure, intrapulmonary Alveolar pressure. *Synonym:* intrapulmonic pressure.

pressure, intrathoracic Intrapleural pressure; pleural pressure.

pressure, pulmonary artery wedge The pressure recorded through an opening in the tip of a catheter wedged in a small branch of the right or left pulmonary artery. Pulmonary artery wedge pressure reflects changes of left atrial pressure.

pressure, transpulmonary The difference between alveolar and intrapleural pressure. Hence, the pressure acting across the lung from the intrapleural space to the alveoli. Also, the pressure difference between airway opening (mouth, nares, or cannula opening) and the visceral pleural surface; thus used, the term transpulmonary includes extrapulmonary structures such at the trachea and extrathoracic airways. Transpulmonary is used for lack of an anatomic term that includes the lungs and all airways. *Symbol:* P_l. *Units:* cm H_2O.

pressure, transthoracic The pressure difference between body surface and parietal pleural surface. Transthoracic in this sense means across the chest wall. This misnomer came into use for lack of an adjectival term meaning chest wall. *Symbol:* P_w.

prolapsed cord Premature expulsion of the umbilical cord during the process of labor.

pulmonary capillary blood volume The volume of blood in the lung that is in contact with alveolar gas at any instant. *Abbreviation:* V_c.

pulmonary edema A fluid transudate within the alveolar spaces of the lung. It may result from increased pulmonary capillary pressure or from increased pulmonary capillary permeability. Edema fluid interferes with respiratory gas exchange and may cause hypoxemia, metabolic acidosis, and respiratory acidosis. *Pulmonary interstitial edema*, an accumulation of transudate fluid within the interstitial tissues of the lung, precedes frank pulmonary edema.

pulmonary perfusion Pulmonary capillary blood flow, supplying terminal airways and alveoli.

radiolucent Relatively permeable to, and thus permitting the passage of, radiant energy; usually said of body structures or materials in relation to roentgen rays (x-rays).

rebreathing Breathing into a closed system. Exhaled gas mixes with the gas in the closed system, and some of this mixture is then reinhaled. Unless the O_2 removed from and the CO_2 added to the breathing mixture are respectively replaced and removed, O_2 concentration decreases progressively and CO_2 concentration increases progressively within the closed sytem and correspondingly in the subject's alveolar gas. Although rebreathing is uncommon under ordinary conditions of life, partial rebreathing occurs in poorly ventilated spaces and during the use of diving equipment, such as scuba and snorkels. Rebreathing has been used to equalize alveolar gas and mixed venous blood CO_2 pressures in an attempt to estimate the latter; at rest, the values given by this method are usually within 6 torr of the true value.

residual volume The volume of gas that remains in the lungs and airways after a maximal voluntary expiratory effort; hence, total lung capacity minus vital capacity. *Units:* L or ml (BTPS). *Abbreviation:* RV.

resistance to flow The pressure differential required to produce a unit flow change; the ratio of the flow-resistive components of a pressure drop across an element or system to the simultaneous flow produced by that pressure drop. Flow-resistive components of pressure are calculated by subtracting any elastic or inertial components, proportional respectively to volume and volume acceleration. Most flow resistances in the respiratory system are nonlinear functions of magnitude and direction of flow, lung volume, lung volume history, and possibly volume acceleration. Hence, it is necessary to specify fully the conditions of measurement. The concept of flow resistance is applicable not only to gas flow but is also used to describe tissue flow resistance. *Symbol:* R. *Units:* cm $H_2O \times liter^{-1} \times sec^{-1}$.

respirator A mechanical device used to produce or to assist pulmonary ventilation. Respirator systems are generally of two types—volume-cycled and pressure-cycled.

respiratory centers Bilateral brainstem structures whose periodic activity produces the rhythmic alternation of inspiratory and expiratory outputs.

respiratory distress syndrome A pulmonary syndrome that may occur even in previously healthy subjects after a variety of insults to the lungs, including severe trauma, circulatory shock, overwhelming infection, pneumonia, massive fat embolism, and narcotic overdose. It is characterized pathophysiologically by loss of lung compliance and clinically by dyspnea, tachypnea, intercostal retraction, expiratory grunting, refractory cyanosis, and bilateral diffuse alveolar infiltrates on the chest roentgenogram. Although potentially fatal, if alveolar ventilation and blood oxygenation are maintained and if the underlying disease process is effectively treated, clinical recovery is possible. *Abbreviation:* RDS. *Synonyms:* shock lung, traumatic wet lung, stiff lung, postperfusion lung, acute pulmonary injury syndrome, adult hyaline membrane disease. A similar syndrome develops in about 10% to 15% of premature newborn infants weighing less than 2,500 gm at birth; the incidence increases with decreasing gestational age (increasing prematurity). In in-

fants the syndrome is characterized pathophysiologically by pulmonary surfactant deficiency, decreased lung compliance, increased work of breathing, alveolar instability, and transudation of fluid into the alveoli. Clinical manifestations include chest retraction, tachypnea, expiratory grunting, and decreased alveolar ventilation. Postmortem examination often reveals a hyaline membrane lining the pulmonary alveoli. *Abbreviation:* RDS of the newborn.

respiratory muscles Muscles whose actions produce the volume changes of the thorax during breathing. The inspiratory muscles include the hemidiaphragms, external intercostals, and the following accessory muscles: scaleni, sternomastoids, trapezius, pectoralis major, pectoralis minor, subclavius, latissimus dorsi, serratus anterior, and all muscles that extend the back. The expiratory muscles include the internal intercostals, the abdominals, and all muscles that flex the back.

respiratory quotient The ratio of the volume of CO_2 produced to the volume of O_2 consumed by an organism, organ, or tissue during a given period of time. Respiratory quotients are calculated by comparing the composition of the incoming with that of the outgoing medium, for example, inspired and expired gas, inspired gas and alveolar gas, or arterial and mixed venous blood. *Symbol:* RQ. Metabolic respiratory quotient (*Symbol:* R) means the ratio of CO_2 production rate to O_2 consumption rate by metabolizing tissues, whereas *respiratory exchange ratio* (*Symbol:* R_E) is the ratio of CO_2 output rate to O_2 uptake rate in the lungs. Hence, respiratory quotient and respiratory exchange ratio are equal during a steady state, a condition that also implies constancy of body O_2 and CO_2 stores. Respiratory quotient is calculated as follows: $RQ = \dot{V}_{CO_2}/\dot{V}_{O_2}$.

reticulogranular A term used to describe the characteristic roentgenographic appearance of the lungs of infants who have respiratory distress syndrome; a cloudy "ground glass" appearance of the lungs.

retrolental fibroplasia A condition characterized by the presence of opaque tissue behind the lens of the eye, leading to retinal detachment, arrest of eye growth, and sometimes blindness. It is generally attributed to the use of excessive O_2 concentrations in the care of premature infants. *Synonym:* retinopathy of prematurity.

Rohrer's constants Constants in an empiric equation for airway resistance: $R = K_1 + K_2\dot{V}$, where R is resistance, $\dot{V}$ is the instantaneous volumetric flow rate, K_1 is a constant representing gas viscosity and airway geometry (laminar flow, or flow-independent, component of the resistance), and K_2 is a different constant representing gas density and airway geometry (turbulent flow, or flow-dependent, component of the resistance). Although the theoretic basis of Rohrer's original equation has been disproved, the expression nevertheless fits observed flow-resistive pressure-flow relationships reasonably well, if applied over a narrow range of flows and if expiratory plateaus are excluded. *Symbols:* K_1 and K_2.

Root effect A property of many fish hemoglobins. Increasing H^+ concentration displaces the oxyhemoglobin dissociation curve down and to the right. This effect differs from the Bohr effect in that even at high O_2 pressures (sometimes as much as several hundred ATA) complete saturation of hemoglobin with O_2 is never achieved.

sensitivity The quantitative extent of a given reaction or response evoked by an acute unit change of concentration, pressure, or intensity of a given stimulus or agent. *Distinguish:* threshold.

shock organ The organ or organ system that manifests the greatest reaction to a stressor or toxicant.

shunt A vascular communication that bypasses alternate circulatory channels; a passage or connection between two natural channels. Shunts are (1) physiologic and intermittently open, (2) the result of abnormal fetal development, (3) the result of failure of normal fetal communications to undergo postnatal closure, or (4) the result of trauma. Some shunts divert venous blood into vessels that normally contain only arterial blood (right-to-left shunt, venous-to-arterial shunt, venous admixture), whereas other shunts do the reverse (left-to-right shunt). Congenital right-to-left shunts within the heart, lungs, and between large vessels are important in respiratory physiology. Left-to-right shunt flow is marked with a minus sign ($-$).

somatotype The body build of a human subject as determined by certain physical characteristics or anthropometric measurements. Examples: ectomorphic, endomorphic, and mesomorphic somatotypes.

spirograph A mechanical device, including bellows or other sealed moving parts, that provides a graphic record of gas volume changes and can also be used to collect and store gases.

spirometer An apparatus similar to a spirograph but without recording facility.

standard bicarbonate The bicarbonate ion concentration of plasma separated anaerobically from whole blood that has been saturated with O_2 and equilibrated at $P_{CO_2} = 40$ torr at $38°$ C. Standard bicarbonate is a measure of the metabolic disturbance of acid-base balance in a sample of blood after any respiratory disturbance present has been corrected. The normal range is 21 to 26 mEq/L.

static Stationary, not moving. In pulmonary mechanics, static denotes a condition of zero flow and thus unchanging (constant) volume. *Antonym:* dynamic.

stethomeiotic A neologism; any condition causing or associated with a reduction of chest volume below its normal value. Such conditions may be congenital, acquired, temporary, or permanent.

STPD conditions of a volume of gas Standard temperature, standard pressure, and dry. The conditions of a volume of gas at 0° C, at 760 torr, and containing no water vapor. A volume (STPD) of any gas contains a calculable number of moles of that gas. *Abbreviation:* volume (STPD).

surface tension A property of liquids. The tension upon the surface of a liquid in contact with another fluid with which it does not mix. The force resulting from intermolecular attraction (cohesion) and from the specific orientation of molecules at the surface, boundary, or interface between a liquid and another substance, such as a gas, solid, or another liquid that is immiscible with the first. This force is exerted in the plane of the interface and acts to preserve the integrity of the surface of separation and to resist rupture of the surface film. It tends to pull the surface molecules of the exposed liquid together and, if the surface is convex, tends to contract the volume of liquid to the smallest possible surface area, forming spheroidal drops (one surface) or bubbles (two surfaces). Laplace's law relates surface tension and radius to pressure. *Units:* dynes/cm or ergs/cm^2.

surfactant A generic term for compounds that orient themselves at the phase boundary between two fluids, for example, the boundary between alveolar gas and the liquid alveolar lining layer. Pulmonary surfactants in the alveolar lining layer concentrate at the gas hypophase boundary, altering the surface tension of the liquid in which they reside.

surfactant, pulmonary The protein-phospholipid (mainly dipalmitoyl lecithin) complex that lines the terminal air spaces (alveoli and possibly small airways). It reduces surface tension and makes air-space patency possible at low transpulmonary pressures.

synergism The total biologic effect of two or more chemical substances or physical agents acting together is greater than the simple algebraic sum of the separate effects of each; the action of one substance or agent enhances the action of another. *Compare:* potentiation.

system, closed, equilibrium state According to thermodynamic principles, a dynamic physicochemical balance of the matter and energy within a system that exchanges neither matter nor energy with its surroundings. *Compare:* steady state of an open system.

system, open, steady state According to kinetic principles, the state of dynamic physicochemical balance within a system that takes in matter and energy from its surroundings, subjects them to physicochemical transformations, and expels matter and energy as waste. A living organism is an open system in a steady state. Physiologists often say steady state when they really mean *nearly* steady state, especially in speaking of physical exercise. *Compare:* equilibrium state of a closed system.

system, open, transient state An unsteady state; a transitory condition of dynamic imbalance produced by displacement of a steady state within an open system. Hence, a condition intermediate between successive steady states. *Contrast:* steady state of an open system.

tachypnea Rapid breathing; increased breathing frequency at rest.

tetany A condition characterized by increased neuromuscular excitability and muscular spasm. It is usually associated with alkalosis and deficiency of calcium ions in extracellular body fluids.

threshold The critical level of concentration, pressure, or intensity at which acute exposure to a given stimulus or substance begins to exert an effect or evoke a response in an organism. Threshold may be altered in the process of acclimatization or adaptation. *Distinguish:* sensitivity.

tidal volume Volume of gas that is either inspired or expired during one ventilatory cycle. *Units:* L or ml (BTPS). *Symbol:* V_T.

time constant In pulmonary mechanics, the product of compliance and airway resistance.

tolerance The inherited or acquired capacity of an organism to endure the effects of chemical substances, physical agents, or environmental stressors with minimal displacement of its physiologic steady-state processes.

tonometry A method for measuring the gas pressure in a fluid. A small gas bubble is equilibrated at known pressure and temperature with a relatively large volume of fluid, after which the bubble is analyzed. Unfortunately, sometimes used to mean any equilibration of gas and liquid phases, including situations in which the volume of gas is relatively large and the volume of liquid is relatively small, so that the gas phase determines the gas pressure in the liquid rather than vice-versa.

torr A unit of pressure equal to 1,333.22 dynes/cm^2, or 1.33322 millibars. One torr is the pressure required to support a column of mercury 1 mm high when the mercury is of standard density and subjected to standard acceleration. These standard conditions are 0° C and 45° latitude, where the acceleration of gravity is 980.6 cm/sec^2. In reading a mercury barometer at other temperatures and latitudes, corrections commonly exceeding 2 torr must be made for these factors and for the thermal expansion of the measuring scale used. For physiologic purposes, the torr is interchangeable with the pressure unit mm Hg.

total lung capacity The volume of gas contained in the lungs at the end of a full inspiration. *Abbreviation:* TLC. *Units:* L or ml (BTPS).

trimester The first, second, or third 3-month period of a human pregnancy.

"true oxygen" The calculated concentration as either percent or fraction which, when multiplied by the expiratory minute volume at STPD, gives O$_2$ uptake.

Valsalva maneuver Expiratory effort against a closed glottis or airway. This maneuver increases intrathoracic pressure and decreases venous return and cardiac output. *Examples:* straining at stool or straining during childbirth. *Contrast:* Müller maneuver.

ventilation, alveolar Gas flow through the gas-exchanging regions of the lung, usually expressed as a rate. *Symbol:* $\dot{V}_A$. Alveolar ventilation rate is always less than total pulmonary ventilation rate. As a tidal volume of gas is exhaled, the last portion, consisting of alveolar gas, remains within the dead space to be reinhaled at the start of the next inspiration. Hence, tidal volume minus dead space volume equals the volume of alveolar gas. Alveolar ventilation rate is calculated as the product of alveolar volume and breathing frequency.

ventilation/perfusion ratio The ratio of pulmonary alveolar ventilation to pulmonary capillary perfusion, both measured quantities being expressed in the same units. Ventilation/perfusion ratios describe the degree of matching or mismatching of *gas* distribution (ventilation) with *blood* distribution (perfusion) in the lung. Ventilation/perfusion ratios are a fundamental determinant of gas exchange and more precisely of the O$_2$ and CO$_2$ pressures of alveolar gas and end-capillary blood in the lung. Although an overall average ventilation/perfusion ratio for both lungs can be calculated, ratios normally vary from one lung region or unit to another. This mismatching, which can be extreme in certain bronchopulmonary diseases, is termed variously unevenness, inequality, or nonuniformity. Mismatching causes variation of both the composition of alveolar gas and the composition of end-capillary blood and is the most common cause of alveolo-arterial P_{O_2} difference and thus clinical arterial hypoxemia. To distinguish this hypoxemia from the true venous admixture caused by pathoanatomic venous-to-arterial shunts, the terms venous admixture–like or shuntlike effect are used. *Symbol:* $\dot{V}_A/\dot{Q}_c$.

ventilation, pulmonary Physiologically, the rhythmic movement of gas in and out of the lungs, usually expressed as a rate. Total pulmonary ventilation, the product of tidal volume and breathing frequency, is an aspect of the supply and distribution of inspired air to the gas-exchanging regions of the lung. *Distinguish:* alveolar ventilation. *Synonyms:* minute volume of breathing, ventilatory minute volume. Because the composition of inspired gas almost always differs from that of expired gas, the terms expiratory minute volume (*Symbol:* $\dot{V}_E$) and inspiratory minute volume (*Symbol:* $\dot{V}_I$) are used for precise work and in calculations. *Units:* L(BTPS)/min.

ventilatory equivalent Ratio of the total pulmonary ventilation rate (BTPS) to the O$_2$ uptake rate (STPD) under any given conditions. This ratio indicates how many volumes BTPS of air are being breathed to obtain one volume STPD of O$_2$ and is hence an expression of relative breathing drive. A typical figure for healthy man is 28 L (BTPS) of air breathed for 1 L (STPD) of O$_2$ taken up.

The reciprocal of the ventilatory equivalent ratio is a measure of ventilatory efficiency for O_2.

vital capacity, expiratory The maximum volume of gas that can be voluntarily exhaled after a full inspiration, with no time limit for duration of the expiratory effort. *Abbreviation:* EVC. Forced expired vital capacity is the maximum volume of gas that can be expired as rapidly as possible from a position of full inspiration. *Abbreviation:* FEVC.

vital capacity, inspiratory The maximum volume of gas that can be voluntarily inhaled after a complete expiration, with no time limit for duration of the inspiratory effort. *Abbreviation:* IVC. Forced inspired vital capacity is the maximum volume of gas that can be expired as rapidly as possible from a position of complete expiration. *Abbreviation:* FIVC.

volume The space occupied by an element or system of elements. *Units:* liters or milliliters.

SUGGESTIONS FOR FURTHER READING

GENERAL

Berger, A. J., Mitchell, R. A., and Severinghaus, J. W.: Regulation of respiration, N. Engl. J. Med. **297:** 92-97, 138-143, 194-201, 1977.

Bouhuys, A.: Breathing: physiology, environment, and lung disease, New York, 1974, Grune & Stratton.

de Reuck, A. V. S., and Porter, R., editors: Development of the lung, a CIBA Foundation symposium, Boston, 1967, Little, Brown & Co.

Fenn, W. O., and Rahn, H., editors: Handbook of Physiology, section 3, Respiration, vols. 1 and 2, Bethesda, Md., 1964-65, American Physiological Society.

Forster, R. E., and Crandall, E. D.: Pulmonary gas exchange, Annu. Rev. Physiol. **38:**69-93, 1976.

Fraser, R. G., and Paré, J. A. P.: Structure and function of the lung: with emphasis on roentgenology, ed. 2, Philadelphia, 1977, W. B. Saunders Co.

Murray, J. F.: The normal lung: the basis for diagnosis and treatment of pulmonary disease, Philadelphia, 1976, W. B. Saunders Co.

Nunn, J. F.: Applied respiratory physiology, ed. 2, London, 1977, Butterworth & Co.

Phillipson, E. A.: Respiratory adaptations in sleep, Annu. Rev. Physiol. **40:**133-156, 1978.

Wagner, P. D.: Ventilation-perfusion relationships, Annu. Rev. Physiol. **42:**235-247, 1980

West, J. B.: Ventilation/blood flow and gas exchange, ed. 2, Oxford, 1970, Blackwell Scientific Publications.

West, J. B.: Respiratory physiology—the essentials, Baltimore, 1974, The Williams & Wilkins Co.

West, J. B.: Pulmonary pathophysiology—the essentials, Baltimore, 1977, The Williams & Wilkins Co.

Wyman, R. J.: Neural generation of the breathing rhythm, Annu. Rev. Physiol. **39:**417-448, 1977.

MECHANICS OF BREATHING

Agostoni, E., Mognoni, P. Torri, G., and Saracino, F.: Relation between changes of rib cage circumference and lung volume, J. Appl. Physiol. **20:**1179-1186, 1965.

Bohn, D. J. Miyasaka, K., Marchak, B. E., Thompson, W. K., Froese, A. B., and Bryan, A. C.: Ventilation by high-frequency oscillation, J. Appl. Physiol.: Respir. Environ. Exercise Physiol. **48:**710-716, 1980.

Briscoe, W. A., Forster, R. E., and Comroe, J. H., Jr.: Alveolar ventilation at very low tidal volumes, J. Appl. Physiol. **7:**27-30, 1954.

DuBois, A. B., Botelho, S. Y., Bedell, G. N., Marshall, R., and Comroe, J. H., Jr.: A rapid plethysmographic method for measuring thoracic gas volume: a comparison with a nitrogen washout method for measuring functional residual capacity in normal subjects, J. Clin. Invest. **35:**322-326, 1956.

Hart, M. C., Orzalesi, M. M., and Cook, C. D.: Relation between anatomic respiratory dead space and body size and lung volume, J. Appl. Physiol. **18:**519-522, 1963.

Ingram, R. H., Jr., and McFadden, E. R., Jr.: Localization and mechanisms of airway responses, N. Engl. J. Med. **297:**596-600, 1977.

Macklem, P. T.: Relationship between lung mechanics and ventilation distribution, Physiologist **16:**580-588, 1973.

Mazzone, R. W., Modell, H. I., and Farhi, L. E.: Interaction of convection and diffusion in pulmonary gas transport, Respir. Physiol. **28:**217-225, 1976.

Morris, J. F., Koski, A., and Johnson, L. C.: Spirometric standards for healthy nonsmoking adults, Am. Rev. Respir. Dis. **103:**57-67, 1971.

Reichel, G., and Islam, M. S.: Measurement of static lung and thorax compliance in health and pulmonary diseases, Respiration **29:**507-515, 1972.

PHYSICS AND CHEMISTRY OF GAS AND BLOOD

Davenport, H. W.: The ABC of acid-base chemistry, ed. 4, Chicago, 1958, University of Chicago Press.

Garby, L., and Meldon, J.: The respiratory functions of blood, New York, 1977, Plenum Medical Book Co.

Rahn, H., and Fenn, W. O.: A graphical analysis of the respiratory gas exchange; the O_2-CO_2 diagram, Washington, D.C., 1955, American Physiological Society.

Siggaard-Andersen, O.: The acid-base status of the blood, ed. 4, Baltimore, 1974, The Williams & Wilkins Co.

Slonim, N. B.: Blood-gas and pH abnormalities. In Friedman, H. H., and Papper, S., editors: Problem-oriented medical diagnosis, Boston, 1975, Little, Brown & Co., pp. 278-289.

NEURAL AND CHEMICAL CONTROL OF BREATHING

Cherniack, N. S., and Fishman, A. P.: Abnormal breathing patterns, DM; Disease-a-month, July 1975.

Cohen, M. I., and Feldman, J. L.: Models of respiratory phase-switching, Fed. Proc. **36**:2367-2374, 1977.

Cohen, M. I., Piercey, M. F., Gootman, P. M., and Wolotsky, D.: Respiratory rhythmicity in the cat, Fed. Proc. **35**:1967-1974, 1976.

Leusen, I.: Regulation of cerebrospinal fluid composition with reference to breathing, Physiol. Rev. **52**:1-56, 1972.

St. John, W. M., Glasser, R. L., and King, R. A.: Rhythmic respiration in awake vagotomized cats with chronic pneumotaxic area lesions, Respir. Physiol. **15**:233-244, 1972.

Sorensen, S. C.: The chemical control of ventilation, Acta Physiol. Scand. [Suppl.] **361**:1-72, 1971.

Wyman, R. J.: Neurophysiology of the motor output pattern generator for breathing, Fed. Proc. **35**:2013-2023, 1976.

NEONATAL RESPIRATORY PHYSIOLOGY

Chiswick, M. L., and Milner, R. D. G.: Crying vital capacity: measurement of neonatal lung function, Arch. Dis. Child. **51**:22-27, 1976.

James, L. S., and Adamsons, K., Jr.: Respiratory physiology of the fetus and newborn infant, N. Engl. J. Med. **271**:1352-1409, 1964.

Longo, L. D., and Ching, K. S.: Placental diffusing capacity for carbon monoxide and oxygen in unanesthetized sheep, J. Appl. Physiol.:Respir. Environ. Exercise Physiol. **43**:885-893, 1977.

Milner, A. D., Hull, D., Hatch, D. J., and Cogswell, J. J.: A new method for measuring static compliance in infants and young children, Clin. Sci. **43**:689-694, 1972.

Rigatto, H.: Respiratory control and apnea in the newborn infant, Crit. Care Med. **5**:2-9, 1977.

Slonim, N. B., Schneider, S. N., Weng, T. R., and Fields, L. J.: Pediatric respiratory therapy: an introductory text, Monsey, N.Y., 1974, Year Book Medical Publishers.

Thurlbeck, W. M.: Postnatal growth and development of the lung, Am. Rev. Respir. Dis. **111**:803-844, 1975.

VENTILATION-PERFUSION RELATIONSHIPS

Wagner, P. D., Laravuso, R. B., Uhl, R. R., and West, J. B.: Continuous distributions of ventilation-perfusion ratios in normal subjects breathing air and 100% O_2, J. Clin. Invest. **54**:54-68, 1974.

West, J. B.: Ventilation-perfusion relationships, Am. Rev. Respir. Dis. **116**:919-943, 1977.

West, J. B.: Regional differences in the lung, Chest **74**:426-437, 1978.

CLINICAL AND PATHOLOGIC PULMONARY PHYSIOLOGY

Altose, M. D.: The physiological basis of pulmonary function testing, Clinical Symposia, vol. 31, no. 2, Summit, N. J., 1979, Ciba Pharmaceutical Co.

Fairshter, R. D., and Wilson, A. F.: Relative sensitivities and specificities of tests for small airways obstruction, Respiration **37**:301-308, 1979.

Gelb, A. F., and MacAnally, B. J.: Early detection of obstructive lung disease by analysis of maximal expiratory flow-volume curves, Chest **64**:749-753, 1973.

Peslin, R., Bohadana, A., Hannhart, B., and Jardin, P.: Comparison of various methods for reading maximal expiratory flow-volume curves, Am. Rev. Respir. Dis. **119**:271-277, 1979.

Tockman, M., Menkes, H., Cohen, B., Permutt, S., Benjamin, J., Ball, W. C., Jr., and Tonascia, J.: A comparison of pulmonary function in male smokers and nonsmokers, Am. Rev. Respir. Dis. **114**:711-722, 1976.

MISCELLANEOUS

Askanazi, J., Silverberg, P., Hyman, A., Foster, R., Yaremchuk, M., and Kinney, J. M.: Effects of the mask and mouthpiece plus noseclip on spontaneous breathing pattern, Crit. Care Med. **6**:143-146, 1978.

Ebert, R. V.: Small airways of the lung, Ann. Intern. Med. **88**:98-103, 1978.

Fenn, W. O., and Dejours, P.: Composition of alveolar air during breath holding with and without prior inhalation of oxygen and carbon dioxide, J. Appl. Physiol. **7**:313-319, 1954.

MacKlem, P. T.: Physiology of cough, Ann. Otol. Rhinol. Laryngol. **83**:761-768, 1974.

Melville, G. N., and Iravari, J.: Factors affecting ciliary beat frequency in the intrapulmonary airways of rats, Can. J. Physiol. Pharmacol. **53**:1122-1128, 1975.

Meyer, B. J., Meyer, A., and Guyton, A. C.: Interstitial fluid pressure. V. Negative pressure in the lungs, Circ. Res. **22**:263-271, 1968.

Nunn, J. F.: Measurement of pulmonary shunt, Acta Anaesthesiol. Scand. [Suppl.] **70**:144-153, 1978.

Polgar, G., and Weng, T. R.: The functional development of the respiratory system: from the period of gestation to adulthood, Am. Rev. Respir. Dis. **120**:625-695, 1979.

Weibel, E. R., and Bachofen, H.: Structural design of the alveolar septum and fluid exchange. In Fishman, A. P., and Renkin, E. M., editors: Pulmonary edema, Bethesda, Md., 1979, American Physiological Society, pp. 1-20.

INDEX